Barcode in Back

MW01121278

Current Issues in Developmental Disorders

Cognitive development in children is a highly complex process which, while remarkably resilient, can be disrupted in a variety of ways. This volume focuses on two types of neurodevelopmental disorder: syndromic conditions such as fragile X syndrome, Down syndrome, Williams syndrome and velocardiofacial syndrome; and non-syndromic conditions including dyslexia, specific language impairment, autism spectrum disorder and attention deficit hyperactivity disorder.

The book provides a state-of-the-art review of current research and covers key topics across the full range of developmental disorders. Topics include:

- diagnosis and comorbidity
- genetics
- longitudinal studies
- computational models
- distinguishing disorder from disadvantage
- language and culture
- the modern beginnings of research into developmental disorders.

The book also looks at how the study of developmental disorders has contributed to our understanding of typical development, and themes emerge that are common across chapters, including intervention and education, and the neurobiological bases of developmental disorders. The result is a fascinating and thought-provoking volume that will be indispensable to advanced students, researchers and practitioners in the fields of developmental psychology, neuropsychology, speech and language therapy, and other developmental disorders.

Chloë R. Marshall, PhD, is Senior Lecturer in Psychology and Human Development at the Institute of Education, University of London, and a former Montessori nursery teacher and teacher-trainer.

Current Issues in Developmental Psychology
Series Editor: Margaret Harris
Head of Psychology, Oxford Brookes University, UK

Current Issues in Developmental Psychology is a series of edited books that reflect the state-of-the-art areas of current and emerging interest in the psychological study of human development. Each volume is tightly focused on a particular topic and consists of seven to ten chapters contributed by international experts. The editors of individual volumes are leading figures in their areas and provide an introductory overview. Example topics include: developmental disorders, implicit knowledge, gender development, word learning and categorisation.

Published titles in the series

Current Issues in Developmental Disorders
Edited by Chloë R. Marshall

Current Issues in Developmental Disorders

Edited by Chloë R. Marshall

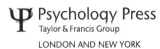

Psychology Press
Taylor & Francis Group
LONDON AND NEW YORK

First edition published 2013
27 Church Road, Hove, East Sussex, BN3 2FA

Simultaneously published in the USA and Canada
by Psychology Press
711 Third Avenue, New York, NY 10017

Psychology Press is an imprint of the Taylor & Francis Group, an informa business

British Library Cataloguing in Publication Data
A catalogue record for this book is available from the British Library

Library of Congress Cataloging-in-Publication Data
    Current issues in developmental disorders /
    edited by Chloe Marshall.—1st ed.
    p. cm.—(Current issues in developmental psychology)
    1. Developmental disabilities–Etiology.
    2. Pediatric neuropsychology.
    3. Cognitive neuroscience.
    4. Developmental neurobiology. I. Marshall, Chloe.
    RJ506.D47C87 2012
    618.928—dc23
    2012007633

ISBN13: 978–1–84872–084–8 (hbk)
ISBN13: 978–0–20310–028–8 (ebk)

Typeset in Times New Roman
By Swales & Willis Ltd, Exeter, Devon

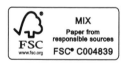

Printed and bound in Great Britain by the MPG Books Group

Contents

PART II
Reflections on the study of developmental disorders 171

Figures

Contributors

Dr Caspar J. M. Addyman, Centre for Brain and Cognitive Development, Department of Psychological Sciences, Birkbeck, University of London, Malet Street, London WC1E 7HX, UK (c.addyman@bbk.ac.uk).

Dr Frank D. Baughman, School of Psychology, Curtin University, Bentley, Perth, Australia (frank.baughman@curtin.edu.au).

Professor Brian Byrne, Department of Behavioral Sciences, Linköping University, Linköping, Sweden; and School of Behavioural, Cognitive and Social Sciences, University of New England, Armidale NSW 2351, Australia (bbyrne@une.edu.au).

Professor Shula Chiat, Department of Language and Communication Science, City University London, 10 Northampton Square, London EC1V 0HB, UK (shula.chiat.1@city.ac.uk).

Professor Kevin K. H. Chung, Department of Special Education and Counselling, The Hong Kong Institute of Education, 10 Lo Ping Road, Tai Po, New Territories, Hong Kong, China (kevin@ied.edu.hk).

Dr Roberto Filippi, Developmental Neurocognition Lab, Centre for Brain and Cognitive Development, Department of Psychological Sciences, Birkbeck, University of London, Malet Street, London WC1E 7HX, UK; and Department of Psychology, Anglia Ruskin University, East Road, Cambridge CB1 1PT, UK (roberto.filippi@anglia.ac.uk).

Dr Paula Hellal, Applied Linguistics and Communication, School of Social Sciences, History and Philosophy, Birkbeck, University of London, 30 Russell Square, London WC1B 5DT, UK (paulahellal@googlemail.com).

Dr Themis Karaminis, Developmental Neurocognition Lab, Centre for Brain and Cognitive Development, Department of Psychological Sciences, Birkbeck, University of London, Malet Street, London WC1E 7HX, UK (themkar@googlemail.com).

Professor Annette Karmiloff-Smith, Centre for Brain and Cognitive Development, Department of Psychological Sciences, Birkbeck, University of

London, 32 Torrington Square, London WC1E 7JL, UK (a.karmiloff-smith@bbk.ac.uk).

Dr Sophie E. Lind, Psychology Department, Durham University, Science Laboratories, South Road, Durham DH1 3LE, UK (sophie.lind@durham.ac.uk).

Professor Marjorie P. Lorch, Applied Linguistics and Communication, School of Social Sciences, History and Philosophy, Birkbeck, University of London, 30 Russell Square, London WC1B 5DT, UK (m.lorch@bbk.ac.uk).

Dr Chloë R. Marshall, Department of Psychology and Human Development, Institute of Education, University of London, 25 Woburn Square, London WC1H 0AA, UK (c.marshall@ioe.ac.uk).

Dr Dianne Newbury, Wellcome Trust Centre for Human Genetics, University of Oxford, Roosevelt Drive, Oxford OX3 7BN, UK (dianne@well.ox.ac.uk).

Professor Richard K. Olson, Department of Behavioral Sciences, Linköping University, Linköping, Sweden; and Department of Psychology, University of Colorado, Boulder, CO 80309-0345, USA (rolson@psych.colorado.edu).

Professor Penny Roy, Department of Language and Communication Science, City University London, 10 Northampton Square, London EC1V 0HB, UK (p.j.roy@city.ac.uk).

Professor Stefan Samuelsson, Department of Behavioral Sciences, Linköping University, Linköping, Sweden (stefan.samuelsson@liu.se).

Professor Michael S. C. Thomas, Developmental Neurocognition Lab, Centre for Brain and Cognitive Development, Department of Psychological Sciences, Birkbeck, University of London, Malet Street, London WC1E 7HX, UK (m.thomas@bbk.ac.uk).

Dr David M. Williams, Psychology Department, Durham University, Science Laboratories, South Road, Durham DH1 3LE, UK (david.williams@durham.ac.uk).

Dr Simpson W. L. Wong, Department of Psychological Studies, The Hong Kong Institute of Education, 10 Lo Ping Road, Tai Po, New Territories, Hong Kong, China (swlwong@ied.edu.hk).

Dr Moon X. Y. Xiao, Department of Special Education and Counselling, The Hong Kong Institute of Education, 10 Lo Ping Road, Tai Po, New Territories, Hong Kong, China (xyxiao@ied.edu.hk).

Acknowledgements

Editing this book has been a pleasure, not least because I've learnt a huge amount in the process, and for that I thank all the authors and reviewers. I'm grateful to Margaret Harris, the series editor, for her guidance throughout. The team at Psychology Press have been terrific. Finally, I would like to acknowledge an Early Career Fellowship from the Leverhulme Trust, which supported (among many things) my time on this book.

Chloë R. Marshall

Introduction

Chloë R. Marshall

The subject of this book, the first in the series "Current Issues in Developmental Psychology", is neurodevelopmental disorders. Two types of condition fall under its remit: (1) syndromic conditions of known genetic aetiology, such as Fragile X Syndrome, Down Syndrome, Williams Syndrome and Velocardiofacial Syndrome; and (2) non-syndromic conditions whose aetiology is likely to be multifactorial and therefore complex, including Dyslexia, Specific Language Impairment, Autism Spectrum Disorder, and Attention Deficit Hyperactivity Disorder. Crucially, the book is not divided into individual chapters devoted to each of these disorders (as is the case, for instance, for those under (2) in the book by Hulme & Snowling, 2009). Rather, each of the first six chapters considers a current issue or "hot topic", which authors have been encouraged to address from the broader perspective of more than just one disorder. The book concludes with two reflective chapters, whose authors again consider their subject across several disorders. The aim therefore is to give a review of key areas in the field that are common across disorders. A glossary is included for readers who might not be familiar with all the disorders that are discussed.

The planning of this book started with the selection of the "current issues" to be featured, from, inevitably, a considerably larger number of candidates. These issues are: diagnosis and comorbidity, genetics, longitudinal studies, computational models, distinguishing disorder from disadvantage, and language and culture. The final two chapters reflect on the modern beginnings of research into developmental language disorders, and on how the study of developmental disorders contributes to our understanding of typical development. There are, of course, other current issues that could have been allocated dedicated chapters, but every book has a page limit, and tough decisions had to be made. Other very relevant issues, such as neurobiology, cognitive theories, intervention and education, are discussed throughout the book.

The authors have done a superb job of contributing chapters that are characterised by breadth and original insight, and that make a valuable contribution to the study of atypical development. The chapters vividly illustrate the vibrancy of current research in this field. In the remainder of this introduction I discuss each chapter in turn, picking out the authors' main points, and adding my own views to the mix.

Part 1: Current issues in the study of developmental disorders

The first chapter, by **David Williams and Sophie Lind,** tackles what is probably the thorniest issue, and the one that forms the most obvious starting point because so much else rests on it: diagnosis. The use of terms such as "Specific Language Impairment" (SLI), "developmental dyslexia" and "Autism Spectrum Disorder" (ASD) assumes both that such a classification exists and that children will fall neatly into these different categories. It also assumes that these categories reflect the underlying nature of those disorders, that they are "natural kinds" (to use the terminology of Tomblin, 2011). But, as Williams and Lind discuss, this is only the case for disorders that have a straightforward and known genetic aetiology, which are the ones under (1) in the opening paragraph of this introduction, i.e., Fragile X Syndrome (FXS), Down Syndrome (DS) and Williams Syndrome (WS) etc. For these disorders, not only is a clear set of clinical characteristics associated with the syndrome, but a genetic test exists for confirmation of the diagnosis.

In contrast, behaviourally-defined disorders, i.e., those that come under (2), are identified by a battery of standardised cognitive assessment tests. Given that scores on these tests are unimodal in distribution, "impairment" lies on one side of an arbitrary cut-off. There is little certainty in diagnosis of such disorders, and children may change diagnostic category as they get older (e.g., for ASD: Eaves & Ho, 2004; for SLI and literacy difficulties: Stothard, Snowling, Bishop, Chipchase, & Kaplan, 1998). To further complicate matters, diagnostic criteria evolve over time, which can have a considerable effect not only on how particular disorders are conceptualised, but also on their prevalence rates. This is perhaps most dramatically exemplified by autism, where prevalence rates have increased from 4.5 cases per 10,000 children in the 1960s (Lotter, 1966), to anything between 20 and 40 cases per 10,000 in the past decade, and up to around 60–110 per 10,000 when the broader autism spectrum is considered (see Charman et al., 2009, for a short review). Much of this increase is due to the broadening of the diagnostic category during that time. (Although, such a broadening arguably does not fully account for the increase; Charman et al., 2009.)

On the other hand, there have also been moves to define certain disorders more narrowly. For example, there is considerable heterogeneity in the children classed as having SLI and dyslexia, and there have been attempts to subcategorise both of these disorders (e.g., surface and phonological dyslexia, Castles & Coltheart, 1993; syntactic-SLI, lexical-SLI and pragmatic-SLI, Friedmann & Novogrodsky, 2011; grammatical-SLI, van der Lely, Rosen, & McClelland, 1998), although such attempts have been widely criticised (as Byrne, Olson, & Samuelsson discuss for dyslexia in this volume). Yet such subtyping might have value in the search for the neural correlates of impaired language and literacy processing. The hundreds of brain imaging studies of dyslexia to date have identified many different regions of the brain with atypical structure, but differences between dyslexic and control groups are weak and inconsistent across studies, arguably because groups are small and average over different subtypes of dyslexia (Price, 2011).

A related issue is the tension between diagnoses that are used in research, and those that are required for clinical and educational purposes. The former are critical if we are to understand the underlying causes of these disorders, whereas the latter help us to work out how best to support affected individuals and their families. The two are not necessarily identical. For example, there is a long-running debate over whether non-verbal IQ should play a role in the diagnosis of SLI and dyslexia. Research studies tend to select participants whose non-verbal IQs are in the normal range, and who therefore have a discrepancy between language, or reading, and non-verbal IQ, but it is not clear whether such a distinction is important for remediation. Williams and Lind argue that it might be for SLI, citing research that finds that language-impaired children with non-verbal IQ in the normal range tend to have better outcomes than those with low IQ, perhaps because they have more compensatory skills available to them. This makes intuitive sense, but is not inevitably the case. For example, Bishop and Edmundson (1987) found that children with both poor language and poor non-verbal IQ indeed have a poor prognosis with respect to language, but that prognosis is also poor for many children with good non-verbal scores. This book is being written as the new *Diagnostic and Statistical Manual of Mental Disorders* (*DSM-5*; American Psychiatric Association, due May 2013) is being planned. There will be substantial revisions to many diagnostic categories and, as Byrne et al. discuss in this volume, the *DSM-5* is relaxing its discrepancy criterion for dyslexia; they support this relaxation because the nature of reading impairments, and how well they respond to intervention, does not appear to differ much according to non-verbal IQ. Hence, while including normal non-verbal IQ as a criterion for SLI and dyslexia might be important for research studies (allowing researchers to argue that, for such children, their language and reading impairments are not caused by low non-verbal IQ (e.g., van der Lely et al., 1998), this may not be as important a consideration for teachers and speech and language therapists.

There are further tensions between definitions of special educational needs that might be politically expedient versus the diagnostic categories that are more useful for research and practice. For example, Lindsay (2011) discusses the use of the term "speech, language and communication needs" (SLCN), a term that is currently in widespread use in the UK. In a recent review of children and young people with speech, language and communication difficulties (Bercow, 2008), the term SLCN was used in a very broad sense to cover three groups of children, (1) those whose SLCN is primary, for example those with SLI, (2) those whose SLCN is secondary, as is the case for those with ASD or a hearing impairment, and (3), those who have had limited experience, for example as a result of socioeconomic disadvantage. This broad definition is motivated by a desire for inclusivity of the full range of children and young people with speech, language and communication needs, and is an important, and entirely appropriate, political decision. However, it conflicts with the narrower definition that English state school teachers are required to use when categorising the special educational needs of pupils, which includes just those with primary speech and language difficulties. Furthermore, in the medical and speech and language therapy literature, the term SLI is preferred, which might in turn reflect the preference of speech and language therapists for a diagnosis-based approach and of teachers for a needs-based approach (Lindsay, Dockrell, Mackie, & Letchford, 2005).

Issues of terminology aside, diagnosis of developmental disorders can ulti-mately only be as accurate as the instruments devised for assessment. As Wil-liams and Lind discuss, the largely subjective measurements used to assess ASD are not without their problems, including low specificity (i.e., over-identification) and disagreement over which children are identified. However, at least for ASD there *are* two "gold-standard" assessments: the Autism Diagnostic Observation Schedule-Generic (ADOS-G; Lord et al., 2000) and the Autism Diagnostic Inter-view-Revised (ADI-R; LeCouteur, Lord, & Rutter, 2003). Such a "gold-standard" is lacking for the assessment of language impairments in children with SLI. A vast array of standardised language assessments exists, but there is no unanimity as to which ones should be used and where the cut-off for impairment lies. Fur-thermore, such "static" tests only give a snapshot in time of children's language abilities, and do not reveal *why* children perform poorly. Children might fail a test for different reasons, and these differences could potentially be important for remediation. Educationalists and clinicians are therefore increasingly embracing "dynamic" assessment. Dynamic assessment is an interactive approach to con-ducting assessments that focuses on the ability of the learner to respond to inter-vention, i.e., the learner's capacity for change or "modifiability" (Hasson & Joffe, 2007; Peña, Reséndiz, & Gillam, 2007). Unlike traditional psychometric testing, dynamic assessment employs a test, teach, retest procedure to assess the child's learning processes. This approach is able to distinguish between children whose language is delayed, but who have unimpaired capacity to learn language, ver-sus those with a language disorder. It is able to identify children with SLI with high degrees of specificity and sensitivity that compare extremely favourably with static assessments, while at the same time giving practitioners additional informa-tion about what might help each particular child to learn.

The issue of diagnosis is complicated yet further when we consider, as Williams and Lind do, the issue of comorbidity between disorders. Complex developmental disorders occur in the same individuals at substantially higher levels than would be expected by chance, suggesting some common aetiology. As an illustration, dyslexia shows significant comorbidity with ADHD, SLI, speech sound disorder, central auditory processing disorder, dyscalculia, and developmental coordina-tion disorder (see Messaoud-Galusi & Marshall, 2010, and references therein). Comorbidity challenges our categorisation of developmental disorders, and our understanding of their underlying causes. For example, progress in exploring the neurobiology of SLI has been hampered by the inclusion of individuals with comorbid disorders in study samples (Hulme & Snowling, 2009). As Williams and Lind convincingly argue, when searching for explanations of comorbidity we need to be clear at what level – genetic, neurobiological, cognitive – our explana-tions are based, and we need to aim for a complete understanding of the causal chain between genes and behaviour, via neurobiology and cognition.

In our efforts to explain comorbidity, the search for "endophenotypes" is gaining pace. Endophenotpyes are cognitive markers that are associated with a particular disorder, are present at all stages of the disorder (even when superficial behav-ioural difficulties have resolved), are heritable (which makes them particularly useful in genetic studies), and are present in non-affected family members at greater-than-chance levels. Williams and Lind discuss a proposed endophenotype for SLI, namely non-word repetition, a task where participants hear and immediately repeat made-up words. However, non-word repetition is impaired not only in SLI, but also in dyslexia (Marshall & van der Lely, 2009), ASD (Whitehouse, Barry, & Bishop, 2008), and DS (Cairns & Jarrold, 2005). Does this mean that the neuro-cognitive underpinnings of impaired non-word repetition are the same in each disorder? Not necessarily.

As Williams and Lind argue, one has to look more closely at the relative patterns of performance on non-word repetition tasks, including error patterns. For example, children with dyslexia, but not those with SLI, are disadvantaged by consonant clusters at the onset of unstressed syllables compared to clusters at the onset of stressed syllables (Marshall & van der Lely, 2009), and whereas both groups are particularly disadvantaged compared to typically developing controls for onset clusters in the middle of a word, as opposed to onset clusters that occur word-initially, children with ASD do not show this disadvantage (Williams, Payne, & Marshall, 2012). Furthermore, although children with SLI show a dramatic reduction in repetition accuracy as non-words get longer (Gathercole & Baddeley, 1990), this is not the case for children with ASD (Whitehouse et al., 2008). It is difficult to argue that these different patterns of performance can be captured by the same underlying cause. (Filippi and Karmiloff-Smith make a similar argument for visual selective attention in FXS and WS in this volume.)

As has long been discussed, non-word repetition taps various cognitive skills, including phonological short-term memory, speech perception, articulation, the ability to create an accurate phonological representation, and lexical knowledge (for a review, see Coady & Evans, 2008), and potentially one or all of these could be the source of non-word repetition difficulties. Marshall and van der Lely (2009) argue that the poor performance of children with SLI is caused by an impairment at the level of complex phonological representations, while others argue for a phonological short-term memory deficit (Gathercole & Baddeley, 1990). In DS the non-word repetition deficit is argued to rest on impaired phonological short-term memory (Cairns & Jarrold, 2005). As for ASD, the finding that non-word repetition performance does not differ on any measure to that of typically developing children matched for verbal mental age raises the question as to whether we should be talking about a non-word repetition impairment in that population at all (Williams et al., 2012). Finally, although children with WS do not appear to be impaired in non-word repetition, they have been argued to rely less on the support of lexical knowledge than do typically developing children when completing the task (see Brock, 2007, for a review and counter-arguments).

There are no easy answers to the issues surrounding diagnosis and comorbidity, and they are therefore likely to remain "current" for many years to come.

Although Williams and Lind touch on genetics in the context of diagnosis and comorbidity, the aim of **Dianne Newbury**'s chapter is to provide a much more thorough account of the genetic basis of developmental disorders. The genetics of syndromic conditions are relatively well understood, even though there is still work to be done relating specific phenotypic characteristics to, for example, the deletion of specific genes in Velocardiofacial Syndrome, and to specific genes on the third copy of chromosome 21 in individuals with DS. Much of the current research in the genetics of developmental disorders concerns non-syndromic disorders, and this is also Newbury's focus. She stresses that such disorders are genetically complex, and the search to identify genes involved is far from straightforward. It is very unlikely that a single genetic mutation will map on to a specific disorder or behaviour, but rather that many genes will be associated with multiple traits across related disorders. Newbury argues that this is what we should expect, given our current understanding of how gene products – i.e., proteins – function. The search for relevant genes is not helped by the fact that studies choose participants on the basis of different criteria, a point that harks back to Williams and Lind's chapter.

There was considerable excitement in the scientific and popular press with the discovery a decade ago of the gene *FOXP2*, a mutation of which is associated with a rare form of verbal dyspraxia (Lai, Fisher, Hurst, Vargha-Khadem, & Monaco, 2001). As Fisher and his colleagues have taken pains to stress, *FOXP2* is not a "gene for language", however attractive that sobriquet might be to headline writers. It has, nevertheless, provided an extraordinary window on to the molecular biology, neurobiology and evolution of the biological networks involved in speech and language, as Newbury discusses. She also discusses an aspect of genetics that might be less familiar to the reader, namely the submicroscopic genomic duplications or deletions, termed copy number variants, that are found in autism. These can occur *de novo*, and therefore affect individuals who have no family history of autism.

One possible explanation for the rise in the incidence of autism – beyond the widening of diagnostic boundaries discussed earlier – is the rising age of parenthood. For example, an Israeli study found evidence that high paternal age is associated with an increased rate of autism in offspring (Reichenberg et al., 2006). It is possible that age increases the rate of the *de novo* mutations that are being found in individuals with autism. This certainly seems a more likely explanation for the increased prevalence of autism than the MMR (measles, mumps, rubella) vaccine, which continues to receive coverage in the popular press, despite a failure to replicate the initial study on which these fears are based (see discussion in Rutter, 2009). It is also consistent with previous work showing that increased *maternal* age is associated with an increased rate in DS (Penrose, 1967), and with both mild and severe mental retardation of unknown cause (Croen, Grether, & Selvin, 2001).

Genetic research advances extremely rapidly, and there was much that could not be included in this chapter. Newbury helpfully provides list of review papers on genetics of individual disorders, for readers who wish to explore this vast literature further.

In chapter 3, **Brian Byrne, Richard Olson, and Stefan Samuelsson** argue persuasively for the merits of longitudinal studies, using dyslexia as an example, but also touching upon ADHD, autism, dyscalculia, and poor reading comprehension. Not least, of course, tracking the same children over time eliminates between-subject variation. As evidence in favour of longitudinal studies, Byrne et al. illustrate how the relationship between difficulties in word recognition/decoding and difficulties in reading comprehension changes during development, and how the subtypes of dyslexia differ in stability over time; both of these points have implications for how we define dyslexia, and therefore for how we approach diagnosis and remediation. Byrne et al. also discuss how the relative influences of genetics and the environment on dyslexia can be studied longitudinally, and how longitudinal studies of comorbidity show that children with both dyslexia and the inattention component of ADHD fare particularly poorly with respect to long-term educational and social outcomes. Hence much in this chapter relates back to the material in chapters 1 (diagnosis and comorbidity) and 2 (genetics).

Longitudinal studies can reveal precursors to developmental disorders, e.g., early language and phonological weaknesses in children at family risk of developing dyslexia. This is particularly valuable in the case of reading difficulties, which can only be diagnosed once the child is old enough to have to failed to make the expected progress in reading after several years of literacy instruction. These findings are important not only for early diagnosis and intervention, but also for understanding the underlying causes of the disorder (the logic being that if phonological deficits precede reading deficits, they are likely to be causal).

Particularly exciting is evidence that atypical speech-processing in the right hemisphere of Finnish newborn infants at risk of dyslexia, as revealed by event-related potentials (ERPs), predicts receptive language and phonological memory skills at 2.5 and 5 years of age, and pre-reading skills at 6.5 years (which in Finland is before the onset of formal education; Guttorm, Leppänen, Hämäläinen, Eklund, & Lyytinen, 2010). Similar results have been reported by Benasich and her colleagues for American-English children at risk of language-learning impairments: ERP responses to non-speech sounds (tones) in 6-month-olds predict language and cognitive scores at 24 months (Benasich et al., 2006). Both sets of authors predict that ERP techniques might allow the very early identification of literacy and language impairments in infants. As yet, however, ERPs are not reliable enough at the level of the individual participant to play a useful role in diagnosis.

Finally, longitudinal studies are important with respect to intervention because they inform us about whether any gains are maintained for longer than just the treatment period. Interestingly, Byrne et al. discuss a project that incorporated a measure of rate of learning of phoneme identity, which turned out to be a reasonable indicator of future decoding and spelling ability (Byrne, Shankweiler, & Hine, 2008), and which is consistent with dynamic assessment approaches to testing.

Michael Thomas, Frank Baughman, Themis Karaminis, and Caspar Addyman, in chapter 4, discuss how computational modelling can allow researchers to investigate mechanisms of developmental change in both typical and atypical development. Because modelling generates testable predictions (e.g., whether proposed deficits can indeed account for observed behaviours), it is a particularly valuable method of testing cognitive theories of disorders. Thomas and his colleagues critically discuss the contribution of modelling to our understanding of a range of developmental disorders, including SLI, dyslexia, autism, and WS, and in so doing cover a range of modelling methods, including associative artificial neural networks, reinforcement learning, dynamical systems modelling, and population modelling. Together, such models hold great promise in helping us to understand issues that are raised elsewhere in this volume, such as: why intervention and remediation might or might not be successful, how specific the cognitive effects of developmental disorders really are, and how different levels of explanation, including the cognitive, neurobiological, and genetic, can be integrated.

The next two chapters consider issues that rarely make their way into a discussion of developmental disorders, but that are arguably critical to understanding them: how we separate disorder from disadvantage, and how language and culture affect the manifestation of developmental disorders.

Many chronic childhood disorders and developmental disorders increase in prevalence with decreasing levels of socioeconomic status (SES; Durkin, Schupf, Stein, & Susser, 2007). In chapter 5, **Penny Roy and Shula Chiat** examine the effect of SES on children's development, with a specific focus on the disproportionate number of children from low-SES backgrounds who have moderate to severe language problems. As well as reviewing the often contradictory literature in this area, the authors present results from their recent study of speech and language abilities in young children from a borough of London with high levels of socioeconomic disadvantage. Studies of this type are important because the diagnosis of complex disorders such as SLI, as we have seen, is far from straightforward. We need to be able to tease apart children with SLI, who have language-learning difficulties despite adequate input, from those children have adequate learning potential but poor input, all the while recognising that some children will fall into both categories. We need to make this distinction not only so that we can better understand the causes and developmental trajectories of atypical language development, but also so that we can provide effective intervention.

Roy and Chiat's chapter goes beyond previous analyses of language in children with low SES by considering not only the different factors that contribute to SES and how they differ in their effects on early language experience, but also the varied components of language that standardised language tests measure and how differing experiences of language might affect performance on them. Not surprisingly, they conclude that a consideration of SES factors is fundamental for understanding the heterogeneity of early language problems, and is very relevant to the early detection and intervention for language delay and language impairment. Interestingly, Thomas and his coauthors discuss in chapter 4 how computational models are beginning to model the effects of SES on language development, and have the potential to elucidate causal relations.

Although Roy and Chiat's chapter focuses on language development, the effects of SES go beyond language. Carroll, Maughan, Goodman, and Meltzer (2005), in a large UK study of 9- to 15-year-olds, found striking variation in children's reading ability according to SES. They found that children in the lowest social class were ten times more likely to have specific literacy problems than children from the highest social class. It is likely to take more than good schooling to close this gap: during the long summer holidays, children who are economically disadvantaged experience declines in reading achievement, while middle and high income children improve, presumably because the latter have more reading opportunities at home. Although summer literacy camps, with instruction targeted to phonemic awareness, phonics, vocabulary, fluency, and reading comprehension skills, can be effective in helping such children make progress relative to a control group who do not attend, maintaining progress over the longer term is a challenge (Schacter & Jo, 2005).

In stark contrast to the lower levels of language and reading achievement among children of lower SES, the pattern appears to be the opposite for ASD: ASD has a higher prevalence amongst children from higher SES backgrounds (Durkin et al., 2010). This may partly be a result of ascertainment bias rather than a direct link between SES and ASD: conceivably as parental education and wealth increase, children have better access to diagnostic services and are more likely to receive an accurate diagnosis. However, Durkin et al. (2010) raise the intriguing possibility that factors associated with socioeconomic advantage (such as increased parental age) might be causally associated with the risk for developing autism. Again, this underscores the importance of considering SES factors in research on developmental disorders.

In chapter 6, **Simpson Wong, Moon Xiao, and Kevin Chung** address issues of culture and language relevant to developmental disorders through the prism of dyslexia in Chinese-speaking children.

Developmental disorders occur across cultures; they are not culture-bound. For example, Leung et al. (1996) studied the prevalence of ADHD in Hong Kong children, and in so doing established that ADHD is not specific to Western, "permissive", culture, but is actually a universal disorder with a strong biological basis. This does not mean, of course, that cultural differences, including differences in schooling, language, orthography, and expectations of behaviour, have *no* impact on the manifestation of developmental disorders. On the contrary, cross-linguistic work has been invaluable in helping us to understand language and literacy disorders, and in particular, for testing cognitive models of the disorder. There is a large body of work comparing SLI across languages (Leonard, 1998), and comparing dyslexia across languages and orthographies (Ziegler et al., 2010). This work has helped elucidate the cognitive causes of these disorders. For example, the recent identification of SLI in deaf children who are acquiring British Sign Language (BSL; Mason et al., 2010) strongly suggests that even if deficits in processing the rapid auditory transitions of speech can cause SLI (Benasich et al., 2006), they cannot be the *sole* cause (because BSL is processed visually). A focus on non-word repetition across languages has revealed that although non-word repetition deficits are characteristic of SLI in many languages, this is *not* the case for two very diverse languages: Cantonese (Stokes, Wong, Fletcher, & Leonard, 2006) and BSL (Mason et al., 2010). Cantonese has very simple phonological structure, while that of BSL is arguably complex and less predictable than that of spoken languages (Marshall,

Mann, & Morgan, 2011). In the former language, children with SLI repeat novel phonological forms with ease, while in BSL even non-impaired signers find the repetition of nonsense signs a difficult task. Both sets of findings illustrate the role of phonological structure in short-term memory, and give clues to the possible locus of the breakdown in SLI.

Wong et al.'s chapter considers the specific case of dyslexia in Chinese. Whereas English has an alphabetic script, Chinese orthography is best described as morpho-syllabic, with each basic graphic unit being a character that links a morpheme (i.e., meaning unit) to an entire syllable. Learning to read in Chinese places a heavy load on the rote memorisation of such associations. Wong et al. argue that whereas weaknesses in phonological awareness are the hallmark of dyslexia in English, dyslexia in Chinese is characterised additionally by weaknesses in visual-orthographic knowledge, morphological awareness, rapid naming, and verbal memory. However, the complete picture is complicated by Chinese having a variety of spoken forms and orthographies as a result of its cultural history; furthermore, different teaching methods are used in different Chinese-speaking countries. Putonghua (also known as Modern Standard Chinese and Mandarin) is the language of mainland China, Taiwan, and Singapore, whereas Cantonese is spoken in southern mainland China and Hong Kong. In mainland China and Singapore, children are taught a system of phonetic symbols, Hanyu Pinyin, that represent the sounds of Putonghua. Pinyin is learnt first, and later, when characters are introduced, they are presented with their Pinyin symbols. A similar phonological coding system, Zhuyin fuhao, is used in Taiwan. No such phonological coding system is used to teach the Chinese characters in Hong Kong, however, and teaching there relies heavily on the "look-and-say" method. Furthermore, while the traditional characters are taught in Hong Kong and Taiwan, a simplified script is used in mainland China and Singapore. As a result of these regional variations, the manifestation of dyslexia appears to differ in different parts of the Chinese-speaking world (Luan, 2005).

Wong et al. focus on dyslexia, but the issues they raise are also relevant to other developmental disorders. In a very general way of course, the human impact of developmental disorders depends to a large extent on the skills that a culture values most. In cultures where spoken and written language skills are highly prized and are essential for well-paid employment, there is a growing recognition that dyslexia and SLI have a long-lasting effect on individuals' academic and vocational success. This contrasts quite strikingly with a developmental condition called congenital amusia, which is characterised by a life-long failure to recognise familiar tunes or tell one tune from another (Stewart, 2011), but which presumably does not have quite as severe an impact on the lives of affected individuals. However, as Stewart discusses, the case of amusic individuals learning a tonal language (e.g., Chinese) would make a fascinating topic for investigation: does amusia make the acquisition of tonal languages more challenging, or alternatively does learning a tonal language have a protective effect and reduce an individual's amusia?

Part 2: Reflections on the study of developmental disorders

The book finishes with two reflective chapters. In chapter 7, **Paula Hellal and Marjorie Lorch** present a fascinating review of the modern beginnings of research into developmental language disorders. In so doing they illustrate why studying the history of the study developmental disorders – a topic that, at first glance, might strike the reader as an unusual choice for inclusion in a book on "current" issues – is indeed relevant to researchers today.

Developmental disorders existed long before they formed the subject of scientific study. Although the first official appearance of "autism" was in the 1940s (Kanner, 1943), autism spectrum disorders have always existed – either misdiagnosed (e.g., as mental retardation or schizophrenia), or "culturally accommodated" (as in the examples of the "blessed fools" of Russia and Brother Juniper in 12th century Italy; Frith, 2003). Similarly, it is probable that the elves of European folklore were based on the facial and social features and short stature of individuals with WS (Lenhoff, 1999). WS, however, did not gain medical attention, as idiopathic hypercalcaemia, until the late 1950s (Bongiovanni, Eberlein, & Jones, 1957). Nevertheless, developmental language disorders, which are the focus of Hellal and Lorch's chapter, were actually being studied and treated by doctors as long ago as the second half of the 19th century. Language disorders arguably benefitted from the interest at that time in acquired language disorders (e.g., Broca's pioneering work on aphasia) and in language acquisition as a means of shedding light on the evolution of language (e.g., Darwin's work on the evolution of man).

Throughout their chapter, Hellal and Lorch explore themes that preoccupied early researchers yet also resonate strongly today: the relationship between brain and behaviour, the changing nature of classification and diagnostic labels, the extent to which verbal and non-verbal abilities can be differentially impaired, issues regarding which comparison groups to use when assessing areas of impairment, the need for interdisciplinary collaborations, the embracing of new technologies, and how best to translate theoretical understanding into effective remediation. The authors make a strong case for how considering the study of developmental disorders can, in their words, "throw into relief our own theoretical assumptions and research agendas".

Finally, **Roberto Filippi and Annette Karmiloff-Smith** consider what developmental disorders can teach us about *typical* development. Models of typical development are undoubtedly strengthened when they can account for cases of atypical development. The authors review studies from various developmental disorders to show how developmental processes that typically develop in concert can be pulled apart in atypical development, so revealing the dynamic interactions that take place between genes, brain, cognition, behaviour, and environment. They caution, however, that atypical development can only help us understand typical development when studies are truly developmental in design.

The study of developmental disorders over the past few decades can roughly be characterised as follows: on the one hand are researchers who argue that the uneven cognitive profiles exhibited in different developmental disorders provide evidence for the modularity of cognitive processes from the child's earliest days; on the other hand are those who argue that they do not. Modularists are inspired by adult cognitive neuropsychology, a framework in which certain cognitive mechanisms can be considered impaired while others are essentially intact. By extension, they argue that developmental disorders provide evidence for domain-specific cognitive processes in the developing child. The alternative, domain-relevant, approach (termed "Neuroconstructivism") proposes that the dichotomy between "impaired" and "unimpaired" is not supported by the data, and that although certain cognitive processes become domain-specific over developmental time, they do not start that way. WS and SLI have been studied extensively by both sides in this debate, and they are the focus of Filippi and Karmiloff-Smith's chapter. Cross-disorder studies of WS, FXS, DS, and ASD are also discussed.

Despite the theoretical disputes highlighted in this chapter, there can be little doubt that research into how to *teach* children with developmental disorders has actually taught us a great deal about how to educate typically developing children. This is particularly true for the teaching of reading. As Lloyd and Hallahan (2005) discuss, teachers of children with dyslexia were advocating systematic phonics instruction in the 1970s and 1980s when other educators were using holistic "look and say" methods. The dyslexia specialists were right – contemporary reading research highlights the benefits of phonics for *all* children. Even longer ago (at the end of the 19th century), Maria Montessori set up a class for children with intellectual disabilities (Montessori, 1948/1988). The system of multisensory, play-based learning that she developed was successful not only with those children, but, as she later showed, with children of all abilities. Montessori's teaching methods (including phonics) are now incorporated into pre-school and primary-school curricula world-wide, and beyond the schools that carry her name.

Final thoughts

The title of the book is "current issues in developmental disorders", and although the year of writing is 2011, the issues it covers look set to be relevant for many years to come. I wish you all a stimulating and rewarding read of the eight chapters that follow. Let us remember that for all our shared theoretical interest in developmental disorders, what matters most is the young people themselves and their families. Article 29 1a of UNICEF's Convention on the Rights of the Child (1989) states that "The education of the child shall be directed to the development of the child's personality, talents and mental and physical abilities to their fullest potential." Too little of current educational and social policy rests on an evidence base. It is our responsibility as developmental psychologists to provide that evidence base and to disseminate it to policy makers, educators, and other relevant professionals, so that they are in a better position to aid all children to reach their full potential.

Chloë R. Marshall
London, December 2011

References

Benasich, A. A., Choudhury, N., Friedman, J. T., Realpe Bonilla, T., Chojnowska, C., & Gou, Z. (2006). Infants as a prelinguistic model for language learning impairments: Predicting from event-related potentials to behavior. *Neuropsychologia, 44*, 396–411.

Bercow, J. (2008). *Bercow Review of Services for Children and Young People (0–19) with Speech, Language and Communication Needs* (DCSF-00632–2008). Nottingham, UK: DCSF Publications.

Bishop, D. V. M., & Edmundson, A. (1987). Language-impaired four-year-olds: Distinguishing transient from persistent impairment. *Journal of Speech and Hearing Disorders, 52*, 156–173.

Bongiovanni, A. M., Eberlein, W. R., & Jones, I. T. (1957). Idiopathic hypercalcemia of infancy, with failure to thrive: Report of three cases, with a consideration of the possible etiology. *New England Journal of Medicine, 257*, 951–958.

Brock, J. (2007). Language abilities in Williams syndrome: A critical review. *Development and Psychopathology, 19*, 97–127.

Byrne, B., Shankweiler, D., & Hine, D. (2008). Reading development in children at risk for dyslexia. In M. Mody & E. Silliman (Eds.), *Brain, behavior, and learning in language and reading disorders* (pp. 240–270). New York, NY: Guilford Press.

Cairns, P., & Jarrold, C. (2005). Exploring the correlates of impaired nonword repetition in Down syndrome. *British Journal of Developmental Psychology, 23*, 401–416.

Carroll, J. M., Maughan, B., Goodman, R., & Meltzer, H. (2005). Literacy difficulties and psychiatric disorders: Evidence for comorbidity. *Journal of Child Psychology and Psychiatry, 46*, 524–532.

Castles, A., & Coltheart, M. (1993). Varieties of developmental dyslexia. *Cognition, 47*, 149–180.

Charman, T., Pickles, A., Chandler, S., Wing, L., Bryson, S., Simonoff, E., . . . Baird, G. (2009). Commentary: Effects of diagnostic thresholds and research vs service and administrative diagnosis on autism prevalence. *International Journal of Epidemiology, 38*, 1234–1238.

Coady, J., & Evans, J. L. (2008). Uses and interpretations of non-word repetition tasks in children with and without specific language impairments (SLI). *International Journal of Language & Communication Disorders, 43*, 1–40.

Croen, L. A., Grether, J. K., & Selvin, S. (2001). The epidemiology of mental retardation of unknown cause. *Pediatrics, 107*, E86.

Durkin, M. S., Maenner, M. J., Meaney, F. J., Levy, S. E., DiGuiseppi, C., Nicholas, J. S., . . . Schieve, L. A. (2010). Socioeconomic inequality in the prevalence of autism spectrum disorder: Evidence from a U.S. cross-sectional study. *PLoS ONE 5*(7): e11551. doi:10.1371/journal.pone.0011551

Durkin, M. S., Schupf, N., Stein, Z. A., & Susser, M. W. (2007) Childhood cognitive disability. In R. B. Wallace(Ed.), *Public health and preventive medicine* (15th ed., pp. 1173–1184). Hightstown, NJ: McGraw-Hill.

Eaves, L. C., & Ho, H. H. (2004). The very early identification of autism: Outcome to age 4½–5. *Journal of Autism and Developmental Disorders, 34*, 367–378.

Friedmann, N., &Novogrodsky, R. (2011). Which questions are most difficult to understand? The comprehension of Wh questions in three subtypes of SLI. *Lingua, 121*, 367–382.

Frith, U. (2003). *Autism: Explaining the enigma* (2nd ed.). Oxford, UK: Blackwell.

Gathercole, S. E., & Baddeley, A. (1990). Phonological memory deficits in language-disordered children. *Journal of Memory and Language, 29*, 336–360.

Guttorm, T. K., Leppänen, P. H. T., Hämäläinen J. A., Eklund, K. M., & Lyytinen, H. (2010). Newborn event-related potentials predict poorer pre-reading skills in children at-risk for dyslexia. *Journal of Learning Disabilities*, *43*, 391–401.

Hasson N., & Joffe V. (2007). The case for dynamic assessment in speech and language therapy. *Child Language Teaching and Therapy*, *23*, 9–25.

Hulme, C., & Snowling, M. (2009). *Developmental disorders of language, learning and cognition*. Chichester, UK: Wiley-Blackwell.

Kanner, L. (1943). Autistic disturbances of affective contact. *Nervous Child*, *2*, 217–250.

Lai, C. S., Fisher, S. E., Hurst, J. A., Vargha-Khadem, F., & Monaco, A. P. (2001). A forkhead-domain gene is mutated in a severe speech and language disorder. *Nature*, *413*(6855), 519–523.

LeCouteur, A., Lord, C., & Rutter, M. (2003). *The Autism Diagnostic Interview – Revised (ADI-R)*. Los Angeles, CA: Western Psychological Services.

Lenhoff, H. M. (1999). A real-world source for the "little people". In G. Westfahl & G. E. Slusser (Eds.), *Nursery realms: Children in the worlds of science fiction, fantasy and horror* (pp. 150–170). Athens, GA: University of Georgia Press.

Leonard, L. B. (1998). *Children with specific language impairment*. Cambridge, MA: MIT Press.

Leung, P. W. L., Luk, S. L., Ho, T. P., Taylor, E., Lieh Mak, F., & Bacon-Shone, J. (1996). The diagnosis and prevalence of hyperactivity in Chinese schoolboys. *British Journal of Psychiatry*, *168*, 486–496.

Lindsay, G. (2011). The collection and analysis of data on children with speech, language and communication needs: The challenge to education and health services. *Child Language Teaching and Therapy*, *27*, 135–150.

Lindsay, G., Dockrell, J. E., Mackie, C., & Letchford, B. (2005). The role of specialist provision for children with specific speech and language difficulties in England and Wales: A model for inclusion? *Journal of Research in Special Educational Needs*, *5*, 88–96.

Lloyd, J. W., & Hallahan, D. P. (2005). Going forward: How the field of learning disabilities has and will contribute to education. *Learning Disability Quarterly*, *28*, 133–136.

Lord, C., Risi, S., Lambrecht, L., Cook, E. Leventhal, B., DiLavore, B., . . . & Rutter, M. (2000). The Autism Diagnostic Observation Schedule—Generic: A standard measure of social and communication deficits associated with the spectrum of autism. *Journal of Autism and Developmental Disorders*, *30*, 205–224.

Lotter, V. (1966). Epidemiology of autistic conditions in young children: I. Prevalence. *Social Psychiatry*, *1*, 124–137.

Luan, H. (2005). *The role of morphological awareness among Mandarin-speaking and Cantonese-speaking children*. Unpublished doctoral dissertation. The University of Hong Kong, Hong Kong.

Marshall, C. R., Mann, W., & Morgan, G. (2011). Short term memory in signed languages: Not just a disadvantage for serial recall. *Frontiers in Psychology*, *2*, 102.

Marshall, C. R., & van der Lely, H. K. J. (2009). Effects of word position and stress on onset cluster production: Evidence from typical development, SLI and dyslexia. *Language*, *85*, 39–57.

Mason, K., Rowley, K., Marshall, C. R., Atkinson, J. R., Herman, R., Woll, B., & Morgan, G. (2010). Identifying SLI in Deaf children acquiring British Sign Language: Implications for theory and practice. *British Journal of Developmental Psychology*, *28*, 33–49.

Messaoud-Galusi, S., & Marshall, C. R. (2010). Introduction to this special issue. The overlap between SLI and dyslexia: The role of phonology. *Scientific Studies of Reading*, *14*, 1–7.

Montessori, M. (1988). *The discovery of the child.* Oxford, UK: Clio Press. (Original work published 1948)

Peña, E., Reséndiz, M., & Gillam, R. B. (2007). The role of clinical judgements of modifiability in the diagnosis of language impairment. *Advances in Speech-Language Pathology, 9,* 332–345.

Penrose, L. S. (1967). The effects of change in maternal age distribution upon the incidence of mongolism. *Journal of Mental Deficiency Research, 11,* 54–57.

Price, C. (2011). *Dyslexia and the brain.* [The 6th Nata Goulandris Memorial Lecture]. University College London, UK, 20 June 2011.

Reichenberg, A., Gross, R., Weiser, M., Bresnahan, M., Silverman, J., Harlap, S., . . . Susser, E. (2006). Advancing paternal age and autism. *Archives of General Psychiatry, 63,* 1026–1032.

Rutter, M. (2009). Commentary: Fact and artefact in the secular increase in the rate of autism. *International Journal of Epidemiology, 38,* 1238–1239.

Schacter, J., & Jo, B. (2005). Learning when school is not in session: A reading summer day-camp intervention to improve the achievement of exiting first-grade students who are economically disadvantaged. *Journal of Research in Reading, 28,* 158–169.

Stewart, L. (2011). Characterising congenital amusia. *Quarterly Journal of Experimental Psychology, 64,* 625–638.

Stokes, S. F., Wong, A. M.-Y., Fletcher, P., & Leonard, L. B. (2006). Nonword repetition and sentence repetition as clinical markers of SLI: The case of Cantonese. *Journal of Speech, Language and Hearing Research, 49,* 219–236.

Stothard, S. E., Snowling, M. J., Bishop, D. V. M., Chipchase, B., & Kaplan, C. (1998). Language-impaired pre-schoolers: A follow-up in adolescence. *Journal of Speech, Language and Hearing Research, 41,* 407–418.

Tomblin, B. (2011). Co-morbidity of autism and SLI: Kinds, kin and complexity. *International Journal of Language and Communication Disorders, 46,* 127–137.

van der Lely, H. K. J., Rosen, S., & McClelland, A. (1998). Evidence for a grammarspecific deficit in children. *Current Biology, 8,* 1253–1258.

Whitehouse, A. J. O., Barry, J. G., & Bishop, D. V. M. (2008). Further defining the language impairment of autism: Is there a specific language impairment subtype? *Journal of Communication Disorders, 41,* 319–336.

Williams, D., Payne, H., & Marshall, C. R. (2012). Non-word repetition impairment in autism and specific language impairment: Evidence for distinct underlying neuro-cognitive causes. In press, *Journal of Autism and Developmental Disorders.*

Ziegler, J. C., Bertrand, D., Tóth, D., Csépe, V., Reis, A., Faísca, L., . . . Blomert, L. (2010). Orthographic depth and its impact on universal predictors of reading: A cross-language investigation. *Psychological Science, 21,* 551–559.

Part I

Current issues in the study of developmental disorders

1 Comorbidity and diagnosis of developmental disorders

David M. Williams and Sophie E. Lind

Introduction

This chapter explores two main themes in two separate sections. The first section explores some of the challenges involved in the diagnosis of complex developmental disorders such as specific language impairment (SLI), developmental dyslexia, attention deficit hyperactivity disorder (ADHD), and autism spectrum disorder (ASD). The second section considers the issue of comorbidity between developmental disorders, and discusses the various models that have been proposed to explain potential overlap.

Part I: Issues in the diagnosis of developmental disorders

Many developmental disorders that affect cognition and behaviour, such as Down syndrome, Fragile X syndrome, and Turner syndrome, have a known genetic basis. Some of these disorders also involve specific physical abnormalities, such as short stature or particular facial features that are characteristic of a particular disorder. The presence of testable genetic markers and outward physical signs mean that such disorders are relatively straightforward to diagnose. Williams syndrome (WS) is a case in point.

Phenotypically, WS is characterised by particular physical abnormalities, including facial dysmorphology ("elfin-like" appearance) and heart disease (most commonly, supravalvular aortic stenosis – narrowing of the aorta). Individuals with WS typically show "hyper-social" personalities but tend to lack skills in social judgement. On the cognitive level, WS is characterised by mental retardation (full-scale IQs usually in the range of 50–60), alongside a somewhat uneven cognitive profile, with relative strengths in expressive language and face processing, and particular weaknesses in visuo-spatial abilities (Karmiloff-Smith, 2008; Martens, Wilson, & Reutens, 2008; see also Filippi & Karmiloff-Smith, this volume).

WS is caused by a deletion of approximately 26 genes on the long arm of one copy of chromosome 7q11 (Peoples et al., 2000). Most significantly, 96 percent of individuals with classic WS show a deletion of one *ELN* allele (Lowery et al., 1995). The *ELN* gene codes for elastin, a structural protein found in connective tissue in multiple organs. Hemizygous *ELN* deletion is thought to result in abnormal elastin production and to ultimately cause the supravalvular aortic stenosis that affects individuals with WS. However, given that *ELN* is expressed only negligibly in the human brain, its deletion is unlikely to account for the cognitive characteristics of WS (Frangiskakis et al., 1996). Even though *ELN* deletion cannot completely account for the full WS phenotype, it nevertheless provides a useful genetic marker for the disorder.

ELN deletion can be detected using a chromosomal screening technique called fluorescent in situ hybridization (FISH), which utilises fluorescent probes to detect particular DNA sequences. As is true of virtually all developmental disorders, there is considerable variation in the expression of the WS phenotype. Some cases of WS, in which all the classic clinical signs are clearly apparent, are relatively easy to diagnose on the basis of the clinical phenotype. However, subtler, more difficult-to-diagnose cases in which, for example, facial abnormalities are not obvious or cardiac problems are mild, are not uncommon. FISH screening is particularly useful in such instances and provides an invaluable tool for confirming a diagnosis of WS.

The example of WS clearly illustrates the importance of genetic screening in the diagnosis of particular developmental disorders. However, such techniques can only be utilised when disorders have an established genetic basis. Indeed, there are numerous heritable developmental disorders for which genetic basis is yet to be established. For such disorders, diagnoses must be made purely on the basis of phenotypic characteristics. Although the phenotypic characteristics of some developmental disorders may include outwardly observable physical signs, many disorders involve no such diagnostic clues. Thus, diagnoses must be made on the basis of neurobiological, cognitive, or behavioural markers of the disorder. Dyslexia, ADHD, SLI and ASD are each an example of such disorders. These disorders can be more challenging to diagnose, given that they have no characteristic physical manifestations and no known set of necessary and sufficient genes to allow objective genetic confirmation of a diagnosis.

SLI

SLI is diagnosed among individuals who, despite no frank sensory or neurological dysfunction, and no significant ASD features, achieve scores on standardised tests of language significantly below that expected on the basis of their age and non-verbal abilities. For example, the International Classification of Diseases (ICD-10; World Health Organisation, 1993) specifies that language ability must fall more than 2 *SD*s below that expected for the individual's chronological age and at least 1 *SD* below their non-verbal ability. The SLI consortium (2004) specified that either receptive or expressive language skills should be at least 1.5 *SD*s below that expected for chronological age and that non-verbal IQ should be at least 80. In a large epidemiological study of SLI, Tomblin et al. (1997) specified that for a diagnosis of SLI, performance on at least two measures of (receptive or expressive) language should be at least 1.25 *SD*s below the mean (i.e., a standard score ≤ 80), with non-verbal IQ in the normal range (i.e., ≥ 85).

In reality, SLI is substantially heterogeneous, and has several empirically-derived subtypes defined according to profiles of ability across comprehension and expression, and according to the degree to which phonology, grammar, semantics and pragmatics are affected (see Leonard, 2000). However, SLI is a useful umbrella term and a substantial proportion (around 50 percent) of pre-school and school-aged children with SLI present with a common profile of language difficulties, which is characterised by problems in language production and comprehension. Moreover, deficits in phonology and syntax are more severe than are deficits in higher order, lexical, or pragmatic language skills.

Although there are differences between studies and between diagnostic manuals in terms of how severely language must be impaired in order to receive a diagnosis of SLI, agreement is almost universal that language ability must be discrepant from non-verbal ability. However, this can create problems for the detection and diagnosis of SLI, and some have questioned the validity of the criteria. Firstly, although language-impaired children with normal non-verbal IQ (NVIQ) tend to have better outcomes than language-impaired children with depressed NVIQ (e.g., Bishop & Edmundson, 1987; Stothard, Snowling, Bishop, Chipchase, & Kaplan, 1998), this does not show that the language impairment in the former case is qualitatively different from the language impairment in the latter case. Rather, high NVIQ may allow some children to compensate for their language problems, a route not open to those with low NVIQ.

Second, nonverbal ability appears to decline over time among people with SLI, with several studies reporting a drop in NVIQ of 10 points or more across development (Botting, 2005; Mawhood, Howlin, & Rutter, 2000; Tomblin, Freese, & Records, 1992). Therefore, receiving a diagnosis of SLI depends, in part, on the age at which an individual is assessed. A child may be referred at 5 years of age and have a NVIQ of 85, thus meeting criteria for SLI. If the same child had been referred at 8 years of age, their NVIQ could have dropped to 75 and thus they would not meet criteria for the diagnosis.

Related to both of these issues, language impairment in SLI is highly heritable, but the discrepancy between verbal and non-verbal ability appears not to be (Bishop, North, & Donlan, 1995). In twin studies, the heritability of a given trait (i.e., the proportion of variation in a trait that is accounted for by genes) is established by exploring the relative similarity of identical (monozygotic; MZ) and non-identical (dizygotic; DZ) twins on that trait. The basic logic here is that, for a given trait, the greater the degree of similarity between MZ twins (who share 100 percent of genes) relative to the degree of similarity between DZ twins (who share only 50 percent of genes, on average), the greater the contribution of genes to variation in that trait. The size of the difference between MZ and DZ twins is used to calculate the univariate heritability of the trait in question (DeFries & Fulker, 1985, 1988). To illustrate, imagine that one member of an MZ twin pair (the "proband") and one member of a DZ twin pair each has SLI and each scores 2 *SD*s below the typical mean on a test of language. Now imagine that the co-twin of the MZ proband also scores 2 *SD*s below the mean on the same language test, whereas the co-twin of the DZ proband only scores 1 *SD* below the mean.

This would give a heritability estimate for language ability of one (i.e., 100 percent of the variance in language ability is due to genetic variation). Now, in the twin study of SLI by Bishop et al., the heritability of language scores was very high (indeed, depending on which measure of language ability was used, it was close to one), whereas the heritability of the discrepancy between language scores and scores on a test of nonverbal ability was close to zero. This suggests that reference to NVIQ may not be essential when diagnosing SLI, given that language impairment has the same aetiology in SLI as it does in "non-specific" language impairment.

Given the difficulties associated with defining SLI (and other complex developmental disorders; see below), Bishop (e.g., 2006, p. 1153) has argued that we could "cut loose from conventional clinical criteria for diagnosing disorders and to focus instead on measures of underlying cognitive mechanisms. Psychology can inform genetics by clarifying what the key dimensions are for heritable phenotypes". For the purposes of conducting genetic studies of SLI (and other disorders) and for remediating the core language impairment in the disorder, perhaps defining SLI according to its cognitive endophenotype would be more productive. Generally-accepted criteria for an endophenotype (or "cognitive marker") are that it is associated with the disorder in question, is present at all stages of the disorder (even if superficial behavioural difficulties have resolved), is heritable, and is present in non-affected family members at levels greater than would be expected by chance (e.g., Gottesman & Gould, 2003). The most promising candidate for a cognitive marker of SLI is diminished nonsense word repetition (NWR). In a NWR test, the participant listens to non-words spoken by the tester, and repeats each immediately after hearing it. It is well established among typically developing (TD) individuals that NWR skills are strongly associated with structural language ability (Baddeley, Gathercole, & Papagno, 1998; Service, 1992), independent of NVIQ (e.g., Conti-Ramsden, Botting, & Faragher, 2001).

Critically, poor NWR distinguishes children with SLI from TD children in over 80 percent of cases (Conti-Ramsden et al., 2001) and even characterises "resolved cases" of SLI who receive an early clinical diagnosis, but who perform in the normal range on broad standardised language measures later in life (Bishop et al., 1995; Conti-Ramsden et al., 2001). Moreover, diminished NWR runs in the families of individuals with SLI (including among non-affected relatives; e.g., Lindgren, Folstein, Tomblin, & Tager-Flusberg, 2009) and is highly heritable (e.g., Barry, Yasin, & Bishop, 2007). Importantly, the inclusion in molecular genetic studies of NWR as a marker of SLI has become routine, and has led to significant advances in our understanding of the aetiology of the disorder (e.g., SLI Consortium, 2002, 2004).

Reading disorder

Reading disorder is diagnosed when an individual's "reading achievement, as measured by individually administered standardized tests of reading accuracy or comprehension, is substantially below that expected given the person's chronological age, measured intelligence, and age-appropriate education" (American Psychiatric Association, 2000). A major difficulty with this definition is that no distinction is drawn between distinct aspects of reading, namely reading accuracy and reading comprehension. An individual with "reading disorder" may be able to decode only a small fraction of printed words that they are exposed to, but may understand all of the words they can decode. In contrast, an individual might be able to decode the majority of printed material they encounter, but understand very little of the meaning of the material. The former kind of reading disorder is termed developmental dyslexia, whereas the latter is termed reading comprehension impairment. We'll focus our discussion on dyslexia, which is defined by the National Institute of Neurological Disorders and Stroke (http://www.ninds.nih.gov/disorders/dyslexia/dyslexia.htm) as,

> a brain-based type of learning disability that specifically impairs a person's ability to read. These individuals typically read at levels significantly lower than expected despite having normal intelligence. Although the disorder varies from person to person, common characteristics among people with dyslexia are difficulty with spelling, phonological processing (the manipulation of sounds) and/or rapid visual-verbal responding.

Using a criterion of scoring more than 2 *SD*s below the mean on a measure of reading accuracy, plus normal IQ, Rutter et al. (2004) found that between 3 percent and 6 percent of children in the UK could be classified as having dyslexia. However, as with the diagnosis of SLI, relying on discrepancy scores (in this case between IQ and reading ability) may obscure the underlying problem in dyslexia. Indeed, there is little evidence that greater gains in reading accuracy are made by poor readers with high IQ than poor readers with low IQ (e.g., Hatcher & Hulme, 1999). Nonetheless, as with SLI, it is possible to diagnose dyslexia on the basis of objective performance on standardised measures. Diagnosis of the two disorders that we consider next is rather more complicated.

ADHD

ADHD is defined as a "persistent pattern of inattention and/or hyperactivity-impulsivity that is more frequent and severe than is typically observed in individuals at a comparable level of development" (American Psychiatric Association, 2000). Specifically, a diagnosis requires that an individual shows six or more signs of inattention (e.g., not listening when spoken to directly; being forgetful in daily activities), hyperactivity/impulsivity (e.g., fidgeting; blurting out answers before questions have been completed), or both, for a period of at least six months. Three subtypes of ADHD have been identified: predominantly inattentive; predominantly hyperactive-impulsive; and combined inattentive/hyperactive-impulsive.

ADHD is diagnosed largely on the basis of behavioural signs. This is challenging not only because of the subjective nature of making judgements about behaviour, but also because ADHD features characteristically fluctuate over time and across contexts (see Byrne, Olson, & Samuelsson, this volume). Thus, a single behavioural assessment at one time point in one setting is insufficient for making a diagnosis; information from multiple sources must be obtained. Diagnostically relevant information is typically gathered through direct observation at school, at home, or in a clinical setting, as well as through the reports of parents, teachers and the affected individual. Detailed semi-structured parental interviews, such as the Parental Account of Children's Symptoms (Taylor, Schachar, Thorley, & Wieselberg, 1986), may be used. Information may also be gathered by asking the parent, teacher, or child themselves to complete standardised questionnaires, such as the Strengths and Difficulties Questionnaire (Goodman, 1997), which involves items that focus on ADHD-relevant aspects of behaviour (e.g., "Restless, overactive, cannot stay still for long: not true/somewhat true/certainly true").

The fact that behavioural reports and clinical observations are inherently subjective – opinions can potentially vary considerably between parent, teacher, clinician and the individual themselves – is a limitation in current diagnostic methods. Such difficulties have prompted researchers to try to identify reliable cognitive markers that may potentially be used to aid diagnosis of ADHD. For example, executive dysfunction has been suggested as a possible candidate. Executive function is an umbrella term for a set of abilities, related to frontal lobe functioning, which are involved in the flexible control of action by allowing disengagement from the immediate environment (see Part II, below, for further discussion). It is clear is that children with ADHD perform poorly on certain tasks (especially those assessing inhibitory control and working memory) that fall under the umbrella of executive functioning (e.g., Stuss & Knight, 2002), and performance on these tasks is associated with severity of ADHD features (e.g., Thorell & Wåhlstedt, 2006). Moreover, recent evidence suggests that executive dysfunction in ADHD meets a further criterion for an endophenotype/cognitive marker, in that unaffected family members also appear to show diminished executive functioning (Gau & Shang, 2010). It is not yet clear that executive dysfunction meets the remaining criteria for a cognitive marker of ADHD, but this finding is nevertheless promising. Indeed, it is possible that tests of executive functioning may eventually be used routinely in the differential diagnosis of ADHD.

ASD

The Diagnostic and Statistical Manual of Mental Disorders – Fourth Edition (*DSM-IV*; American Psychiatric Association, 2000) identifies five discrete "pervasive developmental disorders": (1) autistic disorder; (2) Rett's disorder; (3) childhood disintegrative disorder; (4) Asperger's disorder; and (5) pervasive developmental disorder–not otherwise specified (PDDNOS). According to *DSM-IV*, autistic disorder (autism) is characterised by impairments in three discrete domains: qualitative impairment in social interaction (e.g., poor eye contact; lack of social or emotional reciprocity); qualitative impairment in communication (e.g., delay or lack of spoken language; failure to initiate or sustain conversation); and restricted repetitive and stereotyped patterns of behaviour, interests and activities (e.g., motor mannerisms; inflexible adherence to specific, non-functional routines or rituals).

However, the validity of the pervasive developmental disorder categories has been called into question. Research shows that they cannot be reliably distinguished from each other, and presentation is unstable over time. For example, in our view, there is no conclusive evidence for any qualitative difference in the presentation or outcome of intellectually high-functioning autistic disorder and Asperger's disorder (e.g., Macintosh & Dissanayake, 2004). Indeed, the only distinction between these two diagnostic categories is the age at which first words/ phrases were spoken – a feature that is not core to the syndrome. Moreover, studies have shown that many children who meet PDDNOS criteria at one time point meet autistic disorder criteria at a later time point (Eaves & Ho, 2004; Stone et al., 1999). These issues have been recognised by many researchers for a number of years. Indeed, following Wing and Gould (1979), many have started to take a more dimensional view, widely adopting the term, "autism spectrum disorder" to encompass autistic disorder, Asperger's disorder and PDDNOS. This research is now being acknowledged by the American Psychiatric Association (2011), which has suggested that *DSM-IV* pervasive developmental disorder distinctions can be considered "equivalent to trying to 'cleave meatloaf at the joints'". Thus, a series of proposed changes, to be implemented in *DSM-5*, have recently been published online (American Psychiatric Association, 2011).

DSM-5 will adopt the new category "autism spectrum disorder" (ASD), which will subsume each of the pervasive developmental disorders listed in *DSM-IV*, except for Rett's syndrome. Most notably, the three domains of impairment that previously characterised autistic disorder in *DSM-IV* will be reduced to two, which will be used to diagnose ASD: (1) social-communication impairments (which must include deficits in social-emotional reciprocity, nonverbal communicative behaviours used for social interaction; and in developing and maintaining relationships, appropriate to developmental level); and (2) fixated interests and repetitive behaviours (which must include at least two of the following: stereotyped or repetitive speech, motor movements, or use of objects; excessive adherence to routines, ritualised patterns of verbal or nonverbal behaviour, or excessive resistance to change; highly restricted, fixated interests that are abnormal in intensity or focus; hyper-or hypo-reactivity to sensory input or unusual interest in sensory aspects of environment). This change reflects implicit recognition that social and communicative abilities are inextricably linked, which potentially poses a challenge to those researchers who claim that the genes underlying each aspect are different (Ronald et al., 2006). Rather than different genes contributing to two *components* of ASD (social abilities and communicative abilities), it seems more logical, perhaps, to suggest that multiple genes underlie one *aspect* (social-communication).

For a number of reasons, ASD is one of the most challenging developmental disorders to diagnose. Although a small proportion of ASD cases can be attributed to specific genetic syndromes such as Fragile X syndrome or tuberous sclerosis, the majority of ASD cases are idiopathic (arising from unknown causes). Although there is substantial evidence that the disorder has a (largely, but not exclusively) genetic basis (see Rutter, 2005), molecular genetic studies have, thus far, failed to establish a set of necessary and sufficient genes that underlie ASD (see Newbury, this volume, for a more detailed discussion).

Given the lack of clear cognitive, neurobiological, or genetic markers for ASD, the disorder can currently only be diagnosed on the basis of its behavioural characteristics. A number of standardised instruments have been developed to aid in the diagnosis of ASD for clinical and research purposes. These include checklists/ questionnaires, observational schedules and structured interviews. Checklists/ questionnaires such as the Social Responsiveness Scale (Constantino, 2002) and the Social Communication Questionnaire (Rutter et al., 2003) are usually completed by an informant (typically a parent or teacher), and generally stipulate a certain threshold, scores above which are said to be indicative of ASD. They have the advantage of being quick and cheap to administer. However, they rely on the judgements of untrained individuals who may have limited knowledge of whether particular behaviours should be considered normal or abnormal. Such measures are extremely useful in screening for ASD or for research purposes, but they cannot be used in isolation to establish a clinical diagnosis.

In clinical settings, it is considered good practice to use both an observational instrument and a parental interview to gain an insight into current behaviour, as well as developmental history. The most widely used observational instrument is the Autism Diagnostic Observation Schedule-Generic (ADOS-G; Lord et al., 2000). The ADOS-G is a semi-structured, standardised assessment of communication, social interaction and play/imaginative use of materials. It consists of four alternative modules, each of which is designed for individuals with particular verbal abilities and developmental level. ADOS-G diagnostic algorithms are based on *DSM-IV* and ICD-10 criteria and have thresholds for autism (autistic disorder) as well as broader ASD. However, the ADOS-G assesses social and communication impairments only – not restricted repetitive and stereotyped patterns of behaviour. Thus, the ADOS cannot be used without additional diagnostic checks. Given this limitation, the ADOS-G is frequently used alongside another standardised diagnostic tool, the Autism Diagnostic Interview-Revised (ADI-R; LeCouteur, Lord, & Rutter, 2003). The ADI-R is a semi-structured interview conducted with a parent, consisting of 93 items, which focus on behaviours relating to the three domains of impairment set out in *DSM-IV*.

The ADOS-G and ADI-R are frequently heralded as the "gold standard" tools for diagnosing ASD. However, each has significant disadvantages over other tools. One of the most significant limitations of the ADI-R concerns the development of the diagnostic algorithm. As Bishop (2011) points out, rather than using statistical analyses to establish a set of items that most accurately distinguishes between individuals with and without ASD, the algorithm items were simply selected on the basis of their match to clinical descriptions of ASD. This means that poorly discriminating items could unknowingly be included in the algorithm, leading to inaccurate diagnoses in complex/borderline cases. This raises serious questions about whether the ADI-R in its current form should be used in either clinical or research settings. Indeed, it is not clear that the ADI-R is a better diagnostic tool than shorter, cheaper alternatives that, unlike the ADI-R, require no special training. For example, Berument, Rutter, Lord, Pickles, and Bailey (1999) found that the Autism Screening Questionnaire, a 40-item questionnaire that takes just a few minutes to complete, was just as discriminating as the ADI-R.

In addition to the concerns raised above, the ADOS-G and ADI-R have been shown to have a surprisingly low specificity. In the largest study of its kind (involving around 1500 cases), Risi et al. (2006) found that, if used in isolation, the specificity of each measure was less than 50 percent. Indeed, they each identify around 29 percent of non-spectrum children as having autism. If used together, specificity is improved, but in over 15 percent of cases the instruments disagree on spectrum vs. non-spectrum diagnoses. Ultimately, in many cases, therefore, an ASD diagnosis comes down to expert clinical judgement.

Part II: Comorbidity between developmental disorders

In medicine, the term "comorbidity" was originally introduced to describe situations where two discrete diseases or disorders co-occur concurrently or across time (Feinstein, 1970). Applying this concept to the case of developmental psychopathology yields some striking statistics. Between 1/3 and 1/2 of all children/adolescents with a primary diagnosis of ADHD have a comorbid conduct disorder or oppositional defiance disorder (e.g., Anderson, Williams, McGee, & Silva, 1987). Some 13 percent of those with ADHD have a comorbid major depressive disorder and approximately the same percentage have an anxiety disorder (e.g., Velez, Johnson, & Cohen, 1989). Among children/adolescents with a primary diagnosis of major depressive disorder, between 1/3 and 1/2 have a comorbid anxiety disorder (e.g., Costello, Farmer, Angold, Burns, & Erkanli, 1997). Among individuals with ASD, some 70 percent have at least one comorbid disorder (most commonly social anxiety disorder), and over 40 percent have two or more such disorders (Simonoff et al., 2008). This list could be extended significantly, but is sufficiently long to illustrate the point that comorbidity in developmental psychopathology is apparently the rule, rather than the exception.

Such high levels of comorbidity between developmental/psychological disorders have led some to question whether the term can be meaningfully applied in this field, and indeed in any field outside of somatic medicine (e.g., van Praag, 1996, 2000). The extent of comorbidity in developmental psychopathology may call into question whether the current diagnostic systems laid down in the *DSM-IV* and ICD-10 can maintain the notion that psychopathology consists of discrete disease entities. Alternatively, there may exist discrete disorders, but the boundaries between them are not accurately drawn by the current diagnostic systems (Maj, 2005). Regardless, it is widely accepted that there are multiple competing explanations for comorbidity (see Neale & Kendler, 1995). In this chapter, we will focus on what we take to be one of the most important issues in this debate. This issue concerns whether comorbidity is real in a given case, or whether it is merely apparent or superficial. Put another way, the issue concerns whether the disorder identified as comorbid (e.g., social anxiety disorder) with the primary diagnosis (e.g., ASD) really represents the same clinical entity (with the same underlying causes) as that diagnosed in isolation from the primary diagnosis. This issue is captured perfectly by Maj (2005, p. 183) in his discussion of the relation between panic disorder and schizophrenia:

> But are we sure that the occurrence of panic attacks in a person with schizophrenia should be conceptualised as the "comorbidity of panic disorder and schizophrenia"? Is the panic of someone with agoraphobia, of a person with major depression, and of a person with schizophrenia the *same* psychopathological entity that simply "co-occurs" with the other three? (emphasis added)

In this example, it would be of great importance for our understanding of agoraphobia, schizophrenia and depression, for their diagnosis and for their clinical management, if the same "panic disorder" was associated with each disorder. However, if superficially similar presentation of panic across the disorders has a different underlying cause in each case (i.e., if the similarity in panic across the disorders is only apparent and does not reflect "panic disorder" in each case), then describing panic disorder as comorbid with each disorder not only distorts our understanding of the primary disorders themselves, but could also lead to the employment of ineffective forms of treatment to remediate the panic associated with each. Bishop (2010) uses the term "phenomimicry" to describe the situation where the causes of one disorder (e.g., schizophrenia) produce signs/features that resemble those of a separate disorder (e.g., panic disorder). Unlike the more common term "phenocopy", which refers to an environmentally-caused disorder resembling a genetically-caused disorder, the term phenomimicry does not make assumptions about aetiology, so we will continue to use this term throughout the chapter.

In order to establish empirically whether any two apparently co-occurring disorders are truly co-morbid, or whether one of the two is merely a phenomimic of another disorder, one needs to dig below the surface of behaviour and explore the underlying causes and correlates of behavioural impairment at the levels of cognition, neurobiology and genetics (Morton & Frith, 1995; Morton, 2004). Thus, disorders can potentially be comorbid at the levels of cognition, neurobiology and/or genetics. In our view, however, what is not sufficient from an empirical perspective (even if it may be justified from a clinical perspective), is to claim comorbidity merely on the basis of similarity in behavioural presentation of disorders. Quite simply, there are many different possible causal routes to the same behaviour, and so it is imprudent to assume that superficially similar behavioural presentations reflect the same clinical entity. Although the causal chain between genes and behaviour, via neurobiology and cognition, is undoubtedly complex and multifactorial, it seems reasonable to suggest that if comorbidity between disorders is real rather than apparent, then the signs/features of the disorder in that instance (e.g., social anxiety in people with ASD) have at least partially the same causal route as they do in the case of someone receiving a single diagnosis (i.e., social anxiety disorder in the absence of ASD). The search for causal pathways within and across developmental disorders is essential and we hope will be the focus of intense research activity in coming years.

Below, we will discuss two prominent cases where comorbidity between developmental disorders has been postulated. The first case concerns the relation between ASD and SLI. The second case concerns the relation between ADHD and developmental dyslexia. These cases provide an interesting contrast because, in our view, the former case is substantially more likely to represent an example of phenomimicry than the latter case. The point in this discussion is not to draw firm conclusions about comorbidity in either case, but to highlight the kind of evidence and critical analysis that is useful in coming to a decision about whether comorbidity is real or apparent.

The case of language impairment in ASD: comorbid SLI or phenomimic of SLI?

Around half of individuals with ASD manifest a clinically significant impairment in structural language (phonology/grammar/semantics), and this impairment can occur independently of any diminution of nonverbal IQ (NVIQ; e.g., Baird et al., 2006). In this way, language impairment in ASD can resemble SLI, which has led some to suggest that the two disorders are fundamentally related, and that language impairment in ASD represents comorbid SLI (e.g., Tager-Flusberg, 2004). Thus, according to this model, language-impaired individuals with ASD (henceforth ALI) have inherited both ASD and SLI (i.e., ALI = ASD + SLI). This model has been challenged by some researchers, who argue the available evidence suggests that language impairment in ASD is merely a phenomimic of SLI (e.g., Whitehouse, Barry, & Bishop, 2008; Williams, Botting, & Boucher, 2008). The debate regarding comorbidity between the two disorders continues abound. As discussed above, to answer any question regarding comorbidity, we need to dig below surface behaviour and explore the cognitive, neurobiological and aetiological causes of language impairment in each disorder.[1]

Neurocognitive underpinnings

When discussing cognition, we mean the mental operations or functions of the brain. Unlike neurobiology or behaviour, cognition is not directly observable, but has to be inferred from patterns of behaviour. However, as Morton (2004) points out, cognition is not merely a re-description of behaviour. It provides a mechanism for understanding and explaining behaviour, and leads to specific predictions that can be tested empirically.

---

1 Mainly because of space constraints, we will focus in this chapter on cognition and genetics, rather than neurobiology (but see Williams et al., 2008).

Several cognitive theories of SLI have been built on the basis that poor perform-ance on certain cognitive tasks serves as a clinical marker for SLI. As discussed above, the majority of individuals with SLI perform at least 1.25 *SD*s below the typical mean on tests of nonsense word repetition (NWR) and grammatical tense marking (Rice, Wexler, & Cleave, 1995). The test performance itself is merely an example of behaviour (Morton, 2004), but the specific *patterns* of difficulty shown by individuals with SLI on these tasks (or specific profiles of performance on different tasks) are suggestive of the underlying cognitive deficit in the disor-der. For example, the seminal finding that difficulty with NWR is seen only when items are 3 syllables or more in length (along with the finding that most children with SLI have a reduced digit span) fuelled the hypothesis that SLI results prima-rily from an underlying deficit in short-term memory (Gathercole & Baddeley, 1990). This theory has been challenged by other results, such as the finding that it is not just the length of the items to be repeated (i.e., the amount of material to be stored in short-term memory), but also the structure of the items. Hence, Marshall and van der Lely (2009) recently found that children with SLI found it disproportionately more difficult to repeat consonant clusters that were located medially in a nonsense word (e.g., *kadrepa*), as opposed to at the beginning of the word (e.g., *drepaka*). Marshall and van der Lely argued that the primary cogni-tive deficit in SLI was with the structure of underlying phonological representa-tions, which leads to a secondary limitation in the storage of novel phonological information. While the debate about the exact underlying cognitive impairment in SLI continues, the key issue for the current chapter is whether similar patterns of NWR performance are seen in children with ALI. If similar (atypical) patterns and levels of performance were evident, then this would provide solid evidence that the cognitive underpinnings of language impairment in ALI were partially the same as those underlying SLI. In this instance, we could be more confident that the similarities in language impairment in ALI and SLI were not merely a case of phenomimicry.

In fact, evidence is mounting that the neurocognitive underpinnings of lan-guage impairment in ALI are not the same as the neurocognitive underpinnings of language impairment in SLI. Children with ALI show impaired NWR relative to similar aged peers, whereas children with ASD who have unimpaired struc-tural language do not show diminished NWR (e.g., Kjelgaard & Tager-Flusberg, 2001). This finding was taken initially as supporting the notion the "ALI = ASD + SLI" model. However, several studies have reported patterns of NWR perform-ance among children with ALI that do not resemble those seen in SLI. Studies by Whitehouse et al. (2008) and Riches, Loucas, Baird, Charman, and Simonoff (2010) found a significantly greater effect of stimulus length (i.e., increasing number of syllables in a nonsense word) in SLI than in ALI, which both studies attributed to a primary problem with short-term memory in SLI, but not ALI. Such qualitative differences in NWR performance between the groups led Riches et al. to the same conclusion as Whitehouse et al., that "the claim for a phenotypic over-lap between SLI and ALI may have been overstated" (Riches et al., 2010, p. 10). More recently, Williams, Payne, and Marshall (2012) confirmed that NWR was impaired among children with ALI relative to typical age-matched peers. How-ever, their performance was remarkably similar in terms of levels and patterns of performance to typically developing children who were matched for *verbal men-tal age* (VMA), suggesting that NWR is only delayed in ALI, whereas it is deviant in SLI. Both the ALI group and the VMA-matched typical group were affected in an equivalent way by the length of the stimuli, as well as by the structure of the stimuli (i.e., the position in the nonsense word of a consonant cluster). In contrast, participants with SLI (who were matched with ALI participants for age, language abilities – including profile of language impairment – and non-verbal intelligence) showed unique patterns of performance, as well as patterns of error, and performed significantly less well than all other groups.

Similar to the findings regarding NWR, children with ALI and SLI also appear to show qualitatively different patterns of performance on tests of tense marking (for a review, see Williams et al., 2008). Together, these findings present convinc-ing evidence that the underlying neurocognitive cause of language impairment in ALI is not the same as that in SLI. Next, we consider whether ALI and SLI could be comorbid at the aetiological level.

Genetics

In our view, when researchers and clinicians suggest that two disorders are comor-bid, they are probably implying that surface level similarities between two disor-ders reflect overlapping aetiology. There are several types of data that are relevant to this issue. Firstly, family studies can establish the familial aggregation of each disorder. Secondly, twin studies can be used to establish the heritability of each disorder. In this regard, the data with respect to ASD and SLI are clear; ASD runs in families (e.g., Jorde et al., 1990) and is highly heritable (e.g., Bailey et al., 1995). Likewise, SLI runs in families (e.g., Conti-Ramsden, Falcaro, Simkin, & Pickles, 2007) and is highly heritable (e.g., Barry, Yasin, & Bishop, 2007; Bishop, North, & Donlan, 1995).

However, the critical issue to consider here is not just whether ASD and SLI are themselves familial and heritable, but also whether any covariance in features between the two disorders is familial/heritable. If two disorders, X and Y, are aeti-ologically related, then there should be increased incidence of disorder Y among the relatives of individuals with a diagnosis of X, and vice versa. With respect to ALI and SLI, again the family data is clear; family studies of language impairment in ASD have consistently failed to find evidence suggesting that structural lan-guage impairment is familial/heritable in this disorder, unlike in SLI (e.g., Lind-gren et al., 2009; for a review see Williams et al., 2008). Of central importance, are the findings that the NWR deficit characteristically observed in SLI is highly familial in this disorder (e.g., Barry, Yasin, & Bishop, 2007), but shows no signs of familial aggregation in ALI (Bishop et al., 2004; Lindgren et al., 2009).

To our knowledge, only one study has explored the distribution of ASD features and formal diagnoses of ASD among the families of individuals with SLI (Tomb-lin, Hafeman, & O'Brien, 2003). Compared to comparison families of typically developing children, Tomblin et al. found the families of children with SLI were not (a) significantly more likely to contain a member with an ASD diagnosis,[2] or (b) show elevated ASD features. Thus, family studies provide no support for the notion that ALI and SLI are comorbid at the aetiological level.

In order to establish the heritability (as opposed to familiality) of any apparent comorbidity between two disorders, a twin design can be used in which a so-called "cross-twin cross-trait" analysis is conducted. The basic logic of the twin method can be extended using this analysis to explore the heritability of *covariance* between two traits (bivariate heritability) by comparing the score of one member of a twin pair (the proband) on trait A (e.g., ASD features) with the score of the other member of the pair (the co-twin) on trait B (e.g., language ability). Bivariate heritability provides an estimate of the extent to which variation in trait A and variation in trait B have common genetic causes. In turn, univariate and bivariate heritability values can be used to derive a genetic correlation between the two traits. Using a variant of this technique, Dworzynski et al. (2008) found little evidence in support of the notion that ASD and SLI are genetically comorbid. From a large population-based twin sample (the Twins Early Development Study), Dworzynski et al. selected probands who achieved a score on an ASD screening measure that indicated a significant risk of ASD, and explored the (parent-reported) language abilities of their co-twins. The genetic correlation between the core social features of ASD and language abilities was negligible (r_g = .12). The genetic correlation between repetitive and restricted behaviours, and language abilities was even smaller (r_g = .10). Finally, the genetic correlation between language abilities and the final ASD feature, communication difficulties, was larger than the above correlations, but still modest (r_g = .36). Moreover, this latter correlation could have been artificially inflated, given that several of the items on the communication subscale of the ASD screening measure employed by Dworzynski et al. concerned structural language abilities, rather than necessarily communicative abilities (e.g., "Does s/he sometimes say 'you' or s/he' when s/he means 'I'?"; "Does s/he sometimes lose the listener because of not explaining what s/he is talking about?").

In short, family and twin studies suggest strongly that ASD and SLI are not overlapping disorders, and that language impairment in ASD is merely a phenomimic of SLI. However, the data from molecular genetic studies muddies the water somewhat. Several chromosomal regions have been identified as containing candidate genes for susceptibility to SLI, including 16q, 19q, and 7q (SLI Consortium, 2002, 2004). Numerous chromosomal regions have been implicated in ASD, although potential overlap with SLI is seen reliably at only one site. This

---

2 Cases of ASD in the families of individuals with SLI were significantly higher than the population estimate, however. Nonetheless, this could easily be a sampling artefact, considering only a very small number of ASD cases were discovered (*n* = 3). Indeed, the point of employing a comparison group is, presumably, to control for the possibility of such an artefact. Therefore, the fact that the two groups of families did not differ in rates of ASD is the most important result.

site, on chromosome 7q, contains a gene (*CNTNAP2*) that codes for neurexin, a protein that binds neurons at the synapse in the brain. Certain, not uncommon, variations in the DNA sequence of *CNTNAP2* are associated with a small but reliable decrease in language abilities among the typical population (e.g., White-house, Bishop, Ang, Pennell, & Fisher, 2011). Furthermore, polymorphisms of *CNTNAP2* have been implicated in SLI and, in particular, in the NWR deficits that are a cognitive marker of the disorder (Vernes et al., 2008). One key concept to bear in mind here is that SLI is unlikely to result from a mutation of a single gene that has a large detrimental effect on language ability. Rather, SLI is probably the consequence of inheriting particular variants of several genes, each of which alone has only a small effect on language ability, but when inherited in combination result (through additive and/or interactive effects) in a clinically significant language disorder. Thus, a particular variant of *CNTNAP2* is likely to contribute to SLI, but will be only one part of a complex causal chain.

Now, of critical importance to the debate about comorbidity of ALI and SLI, polymorphisms of *CNTNAP2* have also been implicated in ASD (Arking et al., 2008), and the association is seen most clearly among samples of language-impaired individuals with ASD (i.e., ALI; Alarcon et al., 2008). This creates a confusing scenario, in which a variation in a gene could contribute to language disorder in ALI, as well as in SLI, but (on the basis of family studies) appear heritable in the latter disorder only. Bishop (2010) offers a potential solution to this puzzle in terms of interactions between genes. The scenario she paints is this: Imagine there are 5 genes involved in SLI (genes 1, 2, 3, 4, & 5) and 5 genes involved in ASD (genes 6, 7, 8, 9, & 10). Now imagine that gene 1 is pleiotropic, meaning that it influences multiple phenotypic traits (in this case both ASD features and language). Imagine further that a risk variant of pleiotropic gene 1 has its (negative) effect on language abilities magnified when it occurs in the presence of certain combinations of ASD risk genes (e.g., genes 6 & 7, or genes 9 & 10, but no other combinations). In this case, gene 1 would be "epistatic", meaning that its expression has been modified by other genes. In the scenario presented by Bishop, a first-degree relative of an individual with ALI could carry certain risk variants for ASD (e.g., genes 8 and 10), which result in some sub-clinical features of ASD (the broad autism phenotype). The relative could also carry the risk variant for language impairment (gene 1), but this would not be expressed in the absence of the specific *combination* of ASD risk variants. Thus, language impairment would not appear heritable in ASD, despite having a genetic basis (and, indeed, a genetic basis that also contributes to SLI). In a computational model constructed by Bishop, this scenario produced results that parallel (relatively closely, although not exactly) real-world data on prevalence and severity of language impairment, as well as its familial transmission, in ALI and SLI.

Bishop's (2010) model supports the notion that ALI and SLI share partially overlapping aetiology, which lends weight to calls to consider the two disorders comorbid. Bishop is admirably cautious in reminding the reader that "the fact a simulation can fit a pattern in the observed data does not mean that the model is correct. Phenomimicry could also be involved" (p. 626). However, if we assume for a moment that the model is correct, does this really support the theoretical position that ALI = ASD + SLI? According to Bishop's model, language impairment in ASD arises from the inheritance of one genetic risk variant for SLI (of many risk variants that contribute to SLI), which has its phenotypic effects magnified by the presence of ASD risk variants that play no role in pure SLI. Thus, in Bishop's model, four (out of five) genes that contribute to SLI do *not* contribute to ALI. Furthermore, the single gene that does contribute to both disorders has a different consequence in SLI than in ALI (because of specific epistatic effects in ALI). We elaborate on this discussion in the conclusion below, but for now, we turn our attention to a case of comorbidity between two disorders that, in our view, more clearly merits the term.

The case of ADHD and dyslexia: a more likely example of true comorbidity?

Despite the fact that ADHD and dyslexia each affects only around 3–5 percent of the population, some 20–40 percent of individuals with a diagnosis of either disorder also manifest clinically significant signs of the other disorder (e.g., Willcutt & Pennington, 2000). In particular, dyslexia and the inattentive subtype of ADHD are thought to be more clearly comorbid than dyslexia and the hyperactive-impulsive ADHD subtype. Are these signs phenomimics or evidence of genuine underlying comorbidity?

Neurocognitive underpinnings

Many researchers believe that dyslexia involves a core cognitive deficit in phonological decoding (i.e., translating printed words into appropriate sounds). Although some researchers have argued for a multiple deficit account of dyslexia (e.g., Pennington, 2006), many researchers agree that an underlying deficit in phonological decoding/phonological awareness is the most proximal cognitive cause of dyslexia. As discussed above, many see executive dysfunction as the core underlying neurocognitive cause of ADHD. The key issue with respect to comorbidity between the two disorders concerns whether similar patterns of neurocognitive dysfunction are common to both disorders. (See also Byrne et al., this volume, for a longitudinal perspective on the comorbidity of dyslexia and ADHD.)

One early study by Pennington, Groisser, and Welsh (1993) provided support for the notion that ADHD in children with dyslexia was merely phenomimicry. They assessed children with pure ADHD, children with pure dyslexia, and a "comorbid" group (who had clinically significant features of both disorders) on a battery of executive functioning tasks and a battery of phonological processing tasks. Children with ADHD performed poorly on the former, but not the latter. Vice versa, children with pure dyslexia showed impaired phonological skills, but undiminished executive functioning. Crucially, the performance of the comorbid group paralleled that of the dyslexia group, but not that of the ADHD group. This suggested that the ADHD features in the comorbid group had a different underlying cognitive cause to the ADHD features in the pure form of the disorder, implying phenomimicry. Since the publication of Pennington et al.'s study, however, several studies have failed to support the phenomimic hypothesis. Rather, these studies have found that children with dyslexia who also have ADHD features perform poorly on measures of executive functioning, as well as on measures of phonological awareness (e.g., Willcutt et al., 2001).

More importantly, a meta-analysis of neurocognitive studies of ADHD and dyslexia suggested that deficits in processing speed might represent a shared neurocognitive deficit in ADHD and dyslexia (Willcutt, Sonuga-Barke, Nigg, & Sergeant, 2008). Recently, McGrath et al. (2011) supported this in a large-scale study involving 614 typically developing children/adolescents and children/adolescents with ADHD/dyslexia. Participants were tested using a large battery of tasks, including measures of phonological awareness, verbal working memory, inhibition, naming speed and processing speed. Structural equation modelling indicated that inhibition was uniquely related to measures of ADHD (both inattention and hyperactivity-impulsivity) and phonological awareness was uniquely related to measures of dyslexia (single word reading). Critically, however, processing speed was significantly associated with measures of reading, inattention and hyperactivity-impulsivity even after all other variables were accounted for. Associations between processing speed and reading and inattention were larger than with hyperactivity-impulsivity, supporting the notion that the inattentive subtype of ADHD may be more likely comorbid with dyslexia. This provides solid evidence in support of the notion that ADHD and dyslexia are linked at a level deeper than mere behaviour, and that they may have partially overlapping neurocognitive causes.

The crucial point here is that comorbidity between dyslexia and ADHD (at the neurocognitive level) is not suggested merely because children with features of both disorders perform poorly on measures of executive functioning and phonological awareness. As Morton (2004) highlights, performance on a test is merely a behaviour, not a sign of underlying cognition in itself. Rather, neurocognitive comorbidity is suggested because children with a primary diagnosis of dyslexia who also have ADHD features show a very similar *profile* of performance on executive functioning and phonological processing tasks to children with pure ADHD. This similarity in profile suggests that the underlying neurocognitive system is "damaged" in a similar way in comorbid cases as it is in pure cases, and that this damage contributes to the behavioural deficits in both kinds of case. Indeed, evidence for such an overlap is strengthened by findings from studies of the genetics of ADHD and dyslexia.

Genetics

As is the case with ASD and SLI, both ADHD and dyslexia run in families and are heritable. The heritability estimate for ADHD is approximately .76 (see Faraone et al., 2005), and approximately .50 for dyslexia (e.g., DeFries, Fulker, & LaBuda, 1987), although the heritability estimate for dyslexia is higher among the most severe cases of the disorder (Bishop, 2001). As with the cases of ASD and SLI discussed above, the critical issue to consider here is not just whether ADHD and dyslexia are themselves familial and heritable, but also whether any covariance in phenotypic features between the two disorders has a common genetic basis. Several studies have suggested that it does.

Friedman, Chhabildas, Budhiraja, Willcutt, and Pennington (2003) compared rates of ADHD in children of parents who had a history of (pure) reading impairment (i.e., reading difficulties in the absence of any ADHD features) to the rates of ADHD in the children of control parents who had no history of reading difficulties. They found that significantly more families with a reading disabled parent contained a child with ADHD (35 percent) than did control families in which parents had no history of ADHD or dyslexia (15 percent). As such, ADHD appears to run in the families of people with dyslexia. However, it is important to note that Friedman et al. found weaker evidence of the opposite pattern of familial aggregation, namely that of dyslexia running in families containing a parent with ADHD. Over half (51 percent) of families containing a parent with pure ADHD contained a reading disabled child. Although a smaller percentage (39 percent) of control families contained a child with reading difficulties, the between-group difference was non-significant. Thus, although it is clear from these results that ADHD aggregates in the families of people with reading difficulties, it is not as obvious that reading difficulties aggregate in the families of people with ADHD. Twin studies provide more robust evidence that genetic influences on ADHD and dyslexia are bidirectional, however.

As part of the Colorado Learning Disabilities Research Center Twin Study, Willcutt, Pennington, Olson, and DeFries (2007) assessed the genetic correlations between reading ability and ADHD features. Probands met criteria for either ADHD or dyslexia (and some probands met criteria for both). Co-twin scores on measures of reading ability and ADHD features were then investigated. Willcutt et al. found a substantial genetic correlation between (objectively assessed) reading ability and (parent- & teacher-assessed) ADHD features. The correlation between reading ability and inattention ($r_g = .72$) was larger than between reading and hyperactivity-impulsivity ($r_g = .40$), underscoring the close neurocognitive link between the inattentive ADHD subtype and dyslexia.

Willcutt et al.'s (2007) findings were closely replicated by Paloyelis, Rijsdijk, Wood, Asherson, and Kuntsi (2010) who employed a different sample (from the Twins Early Development Study), and different measures of ADHD and reading ability to Willcutt et al. Paloyelis et al. found a large genetic correlation between (parent-reported) reading difficulties and (parent-reported) inattention ($r_g = .60$). This correlation was more than double the size of that observed between reading difficulties and hyperactivity-impulsivity, again supporting the hypothesised link between the inattentive ADHD subtype and dyslexia.

Arguably the most convincing evidence that ADHD and dyslexia share aetiological causes, rather than being phenomimics of one another, comes from a recent study by Willcutt et al. (2010). Again employing a sample of twins from the Colorado Learning Disabilities Research Center Twin Study, Willcutt et al. extended their previous investigations of the aetiology of behavioural similarities between the two disorders by exploring potential shared genetic influences on neurocognition. Participants had completed a large battery of cognitive tasks, assessing cognitive domains such as working memory, processing speed, inhibition and phonological awareness (phenotypic analysis of these variables was conducted by McGrath et al., 2011; see above). Using a specific type of structural equation modelling (a genetic Cholesky decomposition analysis), Willcutt et al. found that a single genetic factor accounted for significant covariance between processing speed, reading ability, inattention and hyperactivity-impulsivity. Indeed, after controlling for the shared genetic influences with processing speed, there was no additional significant genetic influence on either reading ability or ADHD features. This suggests that apparent comorbidity between ADHD and dyslexia is due to shared genetic influences that lead to diminished processing speed in each disorder. Furthermore, recent studies have suggested a specific molecular genetic link between the two disorders.

As with most molecular genetic studies of developmental disorders, linkage studies of both ADHD and dyslexia have implicated a large number of chromosomal regions as harbouring susceptibility genes, with few results replicated (for reviews of the genetics of ADHD, see Faraone et al., 2005; for reviews of the genetics of dyslexia, see Paracchini, Scerri, & Monaco, 2007). However, the most replicated region of linkage to dyslexia is on chromosome 6p (e.g., Cardon et al., 1994). This region (and, indeed, polymorphism of a specific gene on 6p22) has been implicated in dyslexia in independent samples (Cope et al., 2005; Harold et al., 2006; Rice, Smith, & Gayan, 2009). Critically, this region has also been implicated in ADHD in independent studies (Wilcutt et al., 2002; Couto et al., 2009). In the study by Willcutt et al., this site showed strong linkage to both dyslexia phenotypes and ADHD phenotypes, independently. This suggests that a gene in this region has pleiotropic effects, contributing to both ADHD and reading disorders. Furthermore, two other regions, on chromosomes 14q and 20q, have been identified as harbouring genes that are potentially pleiotropic for both ADHD and dyslexia phenotypes (Gayan et al., 2005). What remains important for future research to assess is whether variations in the genes at these loci are associated with processing speed in ADHD and dyslexia. Potentially, however, we have a complete causal model to account for the comorbidity between the two disorders, with specific pleiotropic genes contributing to diminished processing speed, which in turn contributes to the behavioural phenotype of both ADHD and dyslexia.

Conclusion

We discussed some of the difficulties in diagnosing developmental disorders. Disorders such as ADHD and ASD present particular diagnostic challenges not only because there are no genetic tests but because there are currently no objective cognitive tests. When discussing comorbidity between disorders we considered at what level(s) of explanation disorders need to overlap in order for them to be considered comorbid, and what evidence can be used to establish such comorbidity (or lack thereof). We highlighted that, for many, the ultimate source of comorbidity is at the aetiological level. We suspect that in the coming years, molecular genetic studies will reveal many "generalist genes" that contribute to multiple disorders (e.g., Butcher, Kennedy, & Plomin, 2006). *CNTNAP2*, discussed above with respect to ASD and SLI, possibly represents one such generalist gene. Indeed, given that *CNTNAP2* is involved in the formation of synapses, it seems distinctly possible that it will be implicated in learning disorders other than ASD and SLI.

Ultimately, however, our concern is whether our understanding of each disorder is best served by focusing on "comorbidity" at this level of analysis. In order to understand developmental disorders (and have realistic hope of remediating them), we require an understanding of the causal chain between genes and behaviour, via neurobiology and cognition. Now, what appears clear from the studies cited above is that even if ALI and SLI, for instance, share partial aetiological causes, the effects on neurocognition (and, indeed, behaviour) are quite different in each disorder. For example, in SLI, polymorphisms of *CNTNAP2* are quite possibly linked to specific "damage" to the neurocognitive system that underpins NWR. However, as discussed above, it appears that the neurocognitive cause of NWR *impairment* in SLI is largely distinct from the underlying neurocognitive cause of NWR *delay* in ALI. Thus, even if there turns out to be a reliable overlap in the aetiology of ALI and SLI, the causal pathway to behaviour is almost certain to be different in each disorder. Therefore, in our view, to talk of language impairment in ASD *being SLI* is misleading.

This is not to say that genetic studies cannot inform psychology and vice versa (see Bishop, 2006, for a compelling argument in favour of "developmental cognitive genetics"), or that the discovery of generalist genes is not important. Our point is that, we must not ignore the critical differences between the disorders in the expression (at neurocognitive and behavioural levels) of that aetiology. More important, if such generalist genes are discovered then focusing on comorbidity (rather than difference) between disorders may be more appropriate in some cases than others. For example, if an attempt was made to remediate language impairment in ALI and in SLI, it would be counterintuitive to focus efforts on supporting the same neurocognitive system in each case, given that all the evidence points to different causal pathways in each disorder. On the other hand, treatment of ADHD with methylphenidate (MPH) not only remediates the core features of ADHD (see Wilens & Spencer, 2000), but also possibly improves reading ability (and basic phonological decoding skills) among children with ADHD and dyslexia features (e.g., Bental & Tirosh, 2008; Keulers, et al., 2007). Indeed, treatment with MPH may increase activity in neural networks associated with executive/attentional functioning (Shafritz, Marchione, Gore, Shaywitz, & Shaywitz, 2004). Perhaps, therefore, only when "comorbid" disorders share similar causal pathways will a focus on comorbidity lead to successful remediation of both disorders.

References

Alarcon, M., Abrahams, B. S., Stone, J. L., Duvall, J. A., Perederiy, J. V., Bomar, J. M., . . . Geschwind, D. H. (2008). Linkage, association and gene-expression analyses identify CNTNAP2 as an autism-susceptibility gene. *American Journal of Human Genetics, 82*, 150–159.

American Psychiatric Association. (2000). *Diagnostic and Statistical Manual of Mental Disorders* (4th ed., text revised). Washington DC: American Psychiatric Association.

American Psychiatric Association (2011). *American Psychiatric Association DSM-5 development. A 09 autism spectrum disorder > Proposed revisions.* Retrieved from http://www.dsm5.org/ProposedRevisions/Pages/proposedrevision.aspx?rid=94#

Anderson, J. C., Williams, S., McGee, R., & Silva, P. A. (1987). DSM-III disorders in pre-adolescent children: Prevalence in a large sample from the general-population. *Archives of General Psychiatry, 44*, 69–76.

Arking, D. E., Cutler, D. J., Brune, C. W., Teslovich, T. M., West, K., Ikeda, M., . . . Chakravarti, A. (2008). A common genetic variant in the neurexin superfamily member CNTNAP2 increases familial risk of autism. *American Journal of Human Genetics, 82*, 160–164.

Baddeley, A., Gathercole, S. E., & Papagno, C. (1998). The phonological loop as a language learning device. *Psychological Review, 105*, 158–173.

Bailey, A., Le Couteur, A. Gottesman, I., Bolton, P., Simonoff, E., Yuzda, E., & Rutter, M. (1995). Autism as a strongly genetic disorder: Evidence from a British twin study. *Psychological Medicine, 25*, 63–77.

Baird , G., Simonoff, E., Pickles, A., Chandler, S., Loucas, T., Meldrum, D., & Charman T. (2006). Prevalence of disorders of the autism spectrum in a population cohort of children in South Thames: The Special Needs and Autism Project (SNAP). *Lancet, 368*, 210–215.

Barry, J. G., Yasin, I., & Bishop, D. V. M. (2007). Heritable risk factors associated with language impairments. *Genes, Brain and Behavior, 6*, 66–76.

Bental, B., & Tirosh, E. (2008). The effects of methylphenidate on word decoding accuracy in boys with attention-deficit/hyperactivity disorder. *Journal of Clinical Psychopharmacology, 28*, 89–92.

Berument, S. K., Rutter, M., Lord, C., Pickles, A., & Bailey, A. (1999). Autism screening questionnaire: Diagnostic validity. *The British Journal of Psychiatry, 175*, 444–451.

Bishop, D. V. M. (2001). Genetic influences on language impairment and literacy problems in children: Same or different? *Journal of Child Psychology and Psychiatry, 42*, 189–198.

Bishop, D. V. M. (2006). Developmental cognitive genetics: How psychology can inform genetics. *Quarterly Journal of Experimental Psychology, 59*, 1153–1168.

Bishop, D. V. M. (2010). Overlaps between autism and language impairment: Phenomimicry or shared etiology? *Behavior Genetics, 40*, 618–629.

Bishop, D. V. M. (2011). Are our 'gold standard' autism diagnostic instruments fit for purpose? [Web log message] Retrieved May 30, 2011, from http://deevybee.blogspot.com/2011/05/are-our-gold-standard-autism-diagnostic.html

Bishop, D. V. M., & Edmundson, A. (1987). Specific language impairment as a maturational lag: Evidence from longitudinal data on language and motor development. *Developmental Medicine and Child Neurology, 29*, 442–459.

Bishop, D. V. M., Maybery, M., Wong, D., Maley, A., Hill, W., & Hallmayer, J. (2004). Are phonological processing deficits part of the broad autism phenotype? *American Journal of Medical Genetics Part B-Neuropsychiatric Genetics, 128B*(1), 54–60.

Bishop, D. V. M., North, T., & Donlan, C. (1995). Genetic basis of specific language impairment: Evidence from a twin study. *Developmental Medicine and Child Neurology, 37,* 56–71.

Botting, N. (2005). Non-verbal cognitive development and language impairment. *Journal of Child Psychology and Psychiatry, 46,* 317–326.

Butcher, L. M., Kennedy, J. K. J., & Plomin, R. (2006). Generalist genes and cognitive neuroscience. *Current Opinion in Neurobiology, 16,* 145–151.

Cardon, L. R., Smith, S. D., Fulker, D. W., Kimberling, W. J., Pennington, B. F., & DeFries, J. C. (1994). Quantitative trait locus for reading-disability on chromosome-6. *Science 266,* 276–279.

Constantino, J. N. (2002). *The Social Responsiveness Scale.* Los Angeles, CA: Western Psychological Services.

Constantino, J. N., & Todd, R. D. (2003). Autistic traits in the general population: A twin study. *Archives of General Psychiatry, 60,* 524–530.

Conti-Ramsden, G., Botting, N., & Faragher, B. (2001). Psycholinguistic markers for specific language impairment (SLI). *Journal of Child Psychology and Psychiatry, 42,* 741–748.

Conti-Ramsden, G., Falcaro, M., Simkin, Z., & Pickles, A. (2007). Familial loading in specific language impairment: Patterns of differences across proband characteristics, gender and relative type. *Genes Brain and Behavior, 6,* 216–228.

Cope, N., Harold, D., Hill, G., Moskvina, V., Stevenson, J., Holmans, P., . . . Williams, J. (2005). Strong evidence that KIAA0319 on chromosome 6p is a susceptibility gene for developmental dyslexia. *American Journal of Human Genetics, 76,* 581–591.

Costello, E. J., Farmer, E. M. Z., Angold, A., Burns, B. J., & Erkanli, A. (1997). Psychiatric disorders among American Indian and white youth in Appalachia: The Great Smoky Mountains Study. *American Journal of Public Health, 87,* 827–832.

Couto, J. M., Gomez, L., Wigg, K., Ickowicz, A., Pathare, T., Malone, M., . . . Barr, C. L. (2009). Association of attention-deficit/hyperactivity disorder with a candidate region for reading disabilities on chromosome 6p. *Biological Psychiatry, 66,* 368–375.

DeFries, J. C., & Fulker, D. W. (1985). Multiple-regression analysis of twin data. *Behavior Genetics, 15,* 467–473.

DeFries, J. C., & Fulker, D. W. (1988). Multiple-regression analysis of twin data: Etiology of deviant scores versus individual-differences. *Acta Geneticae Medicae et Gemellologiae, 37,* 205–216.

DeFries, J. C., Fulker, D. W., & LaBuda, M. C. (1987). Evidence for a genetic etiology in reading-disability of twins. *Nature, 329,* 537–539.

Dworzynski, K., A., Ronald, A., Hayiou-Thomas, M. E., McEwan, F., Happé, F., Bolton, P., & Plomin, R. (2008). Developmental path between language and autistic-like impairments: A twin study. *Infant and Child Development, 17,* 121–136.

Eaves, L. C., & Ho, H. H. (2004). The very early identification of autism: Outcome to age 4½–5. *Journal of Autism and Developmental Disorders, 34,* 367–378.

Faraone, S. V., Perlis, R. H., Doyle, A. E., Smoller, J. W., Goralnick, J. J., Holmgren, M. A., & Sklar, P. (2005). Molecular genetics of attention-deficit/hyperactivity disorder. *Biological Psychiatry, 57,* 1313–1323.

Feinstein, A. R. (1970). The pre-therapeutic classification of co-morbidity in chronic disease. *Journal of Chronic Disease, 23,* 455–468.

Frangiskakis, J. M., Ewart, A. K., Morris, C. A., Mervis, C. B., Bertrand, J., Robinson, B. F., . . . Keating, M. T. (1996). *LIM-kinase1* hemizygosity implicated in impaired visuospatial constructive cognition. *Cell, 86,* 59–69.

Friedman, M. C., Chhabildas, N., Budhiraja, N., Willcutt, E. G., & Pennington, B. F. (2003). Etiology of the comorbidity between RD and ADHD: Exploration of the non-random mating hypothesis. *American Journal of Medical Genetics Part B-Neuropsychiatric Genetics, 120B,* 109–115.

Gathercole, S. E., & Baddeley, A. D. (1990). Phonological memory deficits in language disordered children: Is there a causal connection? *Journal of Memory and Language, 29,* 336–360.

Gau, S. S., & Shang, C. (2010). Executive functions as endophenotypes in ADHD: Evidence from the Cambridge Neuropsychological Test Battery (CANTAB). *Journal of Child Psychology and Psychiatry, 51,* 838–849.

Gayan, J., Willcutt, E. G., Fisher, S. E., Francks, C., Cardon, L. R., Olson, R. K., . . . DeFries, J. C. (2005). Bivariate linkage scan for reading disability and attention-deficit/hyperactivity disorder localizes pleiotropic loci. *Journal of Child Psychology and Psychiatry, 46,* 1045–1056.

Goodman, R. (1997). The Strengths and Difficulties Questionnaire. *Journal of Child Psychology and Psychiatry, 38,* 581–586.

Gottesman, I. I., & Gould, T. D. (2003). The endophenotype concept in psychiatry: Etymology and strategic intentions. *American Journal of Psychiatry, 160,* 636–645.

Harold, D., Paracchini, S., Scerri, T., Dennis, M., Cope, N., Hill, G., . . . Monaco, A. P. (2006). Further evidence that the KIAA0319 gene confers susceptibility to developmental dyslexia. *Molecular Psychiatry, 11,* 1085–1091.

Hatcher, P. J., & Hulme, C. (1999). Phonemes, rhymes, and intelligence as predictors of children's responsiveness to remedial reading instruction: Evidence from a longitudinal intervention study. *Journal of Experimental Child Psychology, 72,* 130–153.

Jorde, L. B, Mason-Brothers, A., Waldmann, R., Ritvo, E. R., Freeman, B. J., Pingree, C., . . . Mo, A. (1990). The UCLA University of Utah epidemiologic survey of autism: Genealogical analysis of familial aggregation. *American Journal of Medical Genetics, 36,* 85–88.

Karmiloff-Smith, A. (2008). Research into Williams Syndrome: The state of the art. In C. A. Nelson & M. Luciana (Eds.), *Handbook of developmental cognitive neuroscience* (pp. 691–700). Cambridge, MA: MIT Press.

Keulers, E. H. H., Hendriksen, J. G. M., Feron, F. J. M., Wassenberg, R., Wuisman-Frerker, M. G. F., Jolles, J., & Vles, S. H. (2007). Methylphenidate improves reading performance in children with attention deficit hyperactivity disorder and comorbid dyslexia: An unblinded clinical trial. *European Journal of Paediatric Neurology, 11,* 21–28.

Kjelgaard, M. M., & Tager-Flusberg, H. (2001). An investigation of language impairment in autism: Implications for genetic subgroups. *Language and Cognitive Processes, 16,* 287–308.

LeCouteur, A., Lord, C., & Rutter, M. (2003). *The Autism Diagnostic Interview – Revised (ADI-R).* Los Angeles, CA: Western Psychological Services.

Leonard, L. B. (2000). *Children with specific language impairment.* Cambridge, MA: MIT Press.

Lindgren, K. A., Folstein, S. E., Tomblin, J. B., & Tager-Flusberg, H. (2009). Language and reading abilities of children with autism spectrum disorders and specific language impairment and their first-degree relatives. *Autism Research, 2,* 22–38.

Lord, C., Risi, S., Lambrecht, L., Cook, E., Leventhal, B., DiLavore, B., . . . Rutter, M. (2000). The Autism Diagnostic Observation Schedule – Generic: A standard measure of social and communication deficits associated with the spectrum of autism. *Journal of Autism and Developmental Disorders, 30,* 205–224.

Lowery, M. C., Morris, C. A., Ewart, A. K., Brothman, L., Zhu, X. L., Leonard, C. O., . . . Brothman, A. R. (1995). Strong correlation of elastin deletions, detected by FISH, with Williams syndrome: Evaluation of 235 patients. *American Journal of Human Genetics, 57,* 49–53.

Macintosh, K. E., & Dissanayake, C. (2004). The similarities and differences between autistic disorder and Asperger's disorder: A review of the empirical evidence. *Journal of Child Psychology and Psychiatry, 45,* 421–434.

Maj, M. (2005). 'Psychiatric comorbidity': An artefact of current diagnostic systems? *British Journal of Psychiatry, 186,* 182–184.

Martens, M. A., Wilson, S. J., & Reutens, D. C. (2008). Research Review: Williams syndrome: A critical review of the cognitive, behavioral, and neuroanatomical phenotype. *Journal of Child Psychology and Psychiatry, 49,* 576–608.

Marshall, C. R., & van der Lely, H. K. J. (2009). Effects of word position and stress on onset cluster production: Evidence from typical development, specific language impairment, and dyslexia. *Language, 85,* 39–57.

Mawhood, L., Howlin, P., & Rutter, M. (2000). Autism and developmental receptive language disorder – A comparative follow-up in early adult life: I. Cognitive and language outcomes. *Journal of Child Psychology and Psychiatry, 41,* 547–559.

McGrath, L. M., Pennington, B. F., Shanahan, M. A., Santerre-Lemmon, L. E., Barnard, H. D., Willcutt, E. G., . . . Olson, R. K. (2011). A multiple deficit model of reading disability and attention-deficit/hyperactivity disorder: Searching for shared cognitive deficits. *Journal of Child Psychology and Psychiatry, 52,* 547–557.

Morton, J. (2004). *Understanding developmental disorders: A causal modelling approach.* Malden, MA: Blackwell.

Morton, J., & Frith, U. (1995). Causal modelling: A structural approach to developmental psychopathology. In D. Cicchetti & D. J. Cohen (Eds.), *Developmental psychopathology: Vol. 1. Theory and methods* (pp. 357–390). New York, NY: Wiley.

Neale, M. C., & Kendler, K. S. (1995). Models of comorbidity for multifactorial disorders. *American Journal of Human Genetics, 57,* 935–953.

Paloyelis, Y., Rijsdijk, F., Wood, A. C., Asherson, P., & Kuntsi, J. (2010). The genetic association between ADHD symptoms and reading difficulties: The role of inattentiveness and IQ. *Journal of Abnormal Child Psychology, 38,* 1083–1095.

Paracchini, S., Scerri, T., & Monaco, A. P., (2007). The genetic lexicon of dyslexia. *Annual Review of Genomics and Human Genetics, 8,* 57–79.

Pennington, B. F. (2006). From single to multiple deficit models of developmental disorders. *Cognition, 101,* 385–413.

Pennington, B. F., Groisser, D., & Welsh, M. C. (1993). Contrasting cognitive deficits in attention deficit hyperactivity disorder versus reading disability. *Developmental Psychology, 29,* 511–523.

Peoples, R., Franke, Y., Wang, Y., Perez-Jurado, L., Paperna, T., Cisco, M., & Francke, U. (2000). A physical map, including a BAC/PAC clone contig, of the Williams–Beuren syndrome deletion region at 7q11.23. *American Journal of Human Genetics, 66,* 47–68.

Rice, M. L., Wexler, K., & Cleave, P. L. (1995). Specific language impairment as a period of extended optional infinitive. *Journal of Speech and Hearing Research, 38,* 850–863.

Rice, M. L., Smith, S. D., & Gayan, J. (2009). Convergent genetic linkage and associations to language, speech, and reading measures in families of probands with specific language impairment. *Journal of Neurodevelopmental Disorders, 1,* 264–282.

Riches, N. G., Loucas, T., Baird, G., Charman, T., & Simonoff, E. (2010). Non-word repetition in adolescents with specific language impairment and autism plus language impairments: A qualitative analysis. *Journal of Communication Disorders, 44*, 23–36.

Risi, S., Lord, C., Gotham, K., Corsello, C., Chrysler, C., Szatmari, P., . . . Pickles, A. (2006). Combining information from multiple sources in the diagnosis of autism spectrum disorder. *Journal of the American Academy of Child and Adolescent Psychiatry, 45*, 1094–1103.

Ronald, A., Happé, F., Bolton, P., Butcher, L. M., Price, T. S., Wheelwright, S., . . . Plomin, R. (2006). Genetic heterogeneity between the three components of the autism spectrum: A twin study. *Journal of the American Academy of Child and Adolescent Psychiatry, 45*, 691–699.

Rutter, M. (2005). Aetiology of autism: Findings and questions. *Journal of Intellectual Disability Research, 49*, 231–238.

Rutter, M., Bailey, A., Berument, S. K., LeCouteur, A., Lord, C., & Pickles, A. (2003). *Social Communication Questionnaire*. Los Angeles, CA: Western Psychological Services.

Rutter, M., Caspi, A., Fergusson, D., Horwood, L. J., Goodman, R., Maughan, B., . . . Carroll, J. (2004). Sex differences in developmental reading disability: New findings from 4 epidemiological studies. *Journal of the American Medical Association, 291*, 2007–2012.

Service, E. (1992). Phonology, working memory, and foreign-language learning. *Quarterly Journal of Experimental Psychology, 45A*, 21–50.

Shafritz, K. M., Marchione, K. E., Gore, J. C., Shaywitz, S. E., & Shaywitz, B. A. (2004). The effects of methylphenidate on neural systems of attention in attention deficit hyperactivity disorder. *American Journal of Psychiatry, 161*, 1990–1997.

Simonoff, E., Pickles, A., Charman, T., Chandler, S., Loucas, T., & Baird, G. (2008). Psychiatric disorders in children with autism spectrum disorders: Prevalence, comorbidity, and associated factors in a population-derived sample. *Journal of the American Academy of Child and Adolescent Psychiatry, 47*, 921–929.

SLI Consortium. (2002). A genome-wide scan identifies two novel loci involved in specific language impairment. *American Journal of Human Genetics, 70*, 384–398.

SLI Consortium. (2004). Highly significant linkage to the *SLI1* locus in an expanded sample of individuals affected by specific language impairment. *American Journal of Human Genetics, 74*, 1225–1238.

Stone, W. L., Lee, E. B., Ashford, L., Brissie, J., Hepburn, S. L., Coonrod, E. E., & Weiss, B. H. (1999). Can autism be diagnosed accurately in children under 3 years? *Journal of Child Psychology and Psychiatry, 40*, 219–226.

Stothard, S. E., Snowling, M. J., Bishop, D. V. M., Chipchase, B. B., & Kaplan, C. A. (1998). Language-impaired preschoolers: A follow-up into adolescence. *Journal of Speech Language and Hearing Research, 41*, 407–418.

Stuss, D. T., & Knight, R. T. (2002). *Principles of frontal lobe function*. Oxford, UK: Oxford University Press.

Tager-Flusberg, H. (2004). Strategies for conducting research on language in autism. *Journal of Autism and Developmental Disorders, 34*, 75–80.

Taylor, E., Schachar, R., Thorley, G., & Wieselberg, M. (1986). Conduct disorder and hyperactivity: I. Separation of hyperactivity and antisocial conduct in British child psychiatric patients. *British Journal of Psychiatry, 149*, 760–768.

Thorell, L. B., & Wåhlstedt, C. (2006). Executive functioning deficits in relation to symptoms of ADHD and/or ODD in preschool children. *Infant and Child Development, 15*, 503–518.

Tomblin, J. B., Freese, P. R., & Records, N. L. (1992). Diagnosing specific language impairment in adults for the purpose of pedigree analysis. *Journal of Speech and Hearing Research, 35*, 832–843.

Tomblin, J. B., Records, N. L., Buckwalter, P., Zhang, X. Y., Smith, E., & O'Brien, M. (1997). Prevalence of specific language impairment in kindergarten children. *Journal of Speech Language and Hearing Research, 40*, 1245–1260.

Tomblin, J. B., Hafeman, L. L., & O'Brien, M. (2003). Autism and autism risk in siblings of children with specific language impairment. *International Journal of Language & Communication Disorders, 38*, 235–250.

Velez, C. N., Johnson, J., & Cohen, P. (1989). A longitudinal analysis of selected risk-factors for childhood psychopathology. *Journal of the American Academy of Child and Adolescent Psychiatry, 28*, 861–864.

van Praag, H. M. (1996). Comorbidity (psycho) analysed. *British Journal of Psychiatry, 168*(Suppl. 30), 129–134.

van Praag, H. M. (2000). Nosologomania: A disorder of psychiatry. *World Journal of Biological Psychiatry, 1*, 151–158.

Vernes, S. C., Newbury, D. F., Abrahams, B. S, Winchester, L., Nicod, J., Groszer, M., . . . Fisher, S. E. (2008). A functional genetic link between distinct developmental language disorders. *New England Journal of Medicine, 359*, 2337–2345.

Whitehouse, A. J. O., Barry, J. G., & Bishop, D. V. M. (2008). Further defining the language impairment of autism: Is there a specific language impairment subtype? *Journal of Communication Disorders, 41*, 319–336.

Whitehouse, A. J. O., Bishop, D. V. M., Ang, Q. W., Pennell, C. E., & Fisher, S. E. (2011). CNTNAP2 variants affect early language development in the general population. *Genes, Brain, and Behavior, 10*, 451–456.

Willcutt, E. G., & Pennington, B. F. (2000). Psychiatric comorbidity in children and adolescents with reading disability. *Journal of Child Psychology and Psychiatry, 41*, 1039–1048.

Willcutt, E. G., Pennington, B. F., Boada, R., Ogline, J. S., Tunick, R. A., Chhabildas, N. A., & Olson, R. K. (2001). A comparison of the cognitive deficits in reading disability and attention-deficit/hyperactivity disorder. *Journal of Abnormal Psychology, 110*, 157–172.

Willcutt, E. G., Pennington, B. F., Smith, S. D., Cardon, L. R., Gayan, J., Knopik, V. S., . . . DeFries, J. C. (2002). Quantitative trait locus for reading disability on chromosome 6p is pleiotropic for attention-deficit hyperactivity disorder. *American Journal of Medical Genetics, 114*, 260–268.

Willcutt, E. G., Pennington, B. F., Olson, R. K., & DeFries, J. C. (2007). Understanding comorbidity: A twin study of reading disability and attention-deficit/hyperactivity disorder. *American Journal of Medical Genetics Part B-Neuropsychiatric Genetics, 144B*, 709–714.

Willcutt, E. G., Sonuga-Barke, E. J. S., Nigg, J. T., & Sergeant, J. A. (2008). Recent developments in neuropsychological models of childhood psychiatric disorders. In *Advances in Biological Psychiatry, 24*, 195–226.

Wilens, T. E., & Spencer, T. J. (2000). The stimulants revisited. *Child and Adolescent Psychiatric Clinics of North America, 9*, 573–603.

Williams, D., Botting, N., & Boucher, J. (2008). Language in autism and specific language impairment: Where are the links? *Psychological Bulletin, 134*, 944–963.

Williams, D., Payne, H., & Marshall, C. R. (2012). Non-word repetition impairment in autism and specific language impairment: Evidence for distinct underlying neurocognitive causes. In press, *Journal of Autism and Developmental Disorders*.

Wing, L., & Gould, J. (1979). Severe impairments of social-interaction and associated abnormalities in children: Epidemiology and classification. *Journal of Autism and Developmental Disorders, 9,* 11–29.

World Health Organisation (1993). *International classification of mental and behavioural disorders: Clinical descriptions and diagnostic guidelines* (10th ed.). Geneva, Switzerland: World Health Organisation.

2 The genetics of developmental disorders

Dianne Newbury

Introduction

Genetic effects are thought to play a causal role in susceptibility to many developmental disorders. However, this genetic contribution is expected to be complex in nature and involve interactions between multiple genetic and environmental factors. In the past decade, our understanding of the nature of these genetic factors has increased greatly. Genetic risk variants have been identified for several developmental disorders providing us with a window into the molecular basis of these disorders.

In this chapter I discuss the genetic techniques used to identify genes for complex disorders and the kinds of genetic effects that have been identified as risk factors for developmental disorders. I consider the role of common genetic variations, chromosome abnormalities and copy number variants (CNVs) and specific gene mutations in developmental disorders and consider how new genetic advances might progress our understanding of the genetic basis of developmental disorders.

Genes and genetic variation

The human genome project

The human genome is a string of approximately 3 billion copies of the four nucleotide bases, adenine (A), guanine (G), thymine (T) and cytosine (C), arranged across 23 chromosomes (chromosomes 1–22 and the sex chromosomes X and Y). In 2003, the human genome project completed the transcription of this sequence, from base 1 of chromosome 1 through to base 57,772,954 of chromosome Y (Lander et al., 2001; Venter et al., 2001). Although a significant technical achievement, the publication of the human genome did not answer all our questions regarding human genetics. Instead it revealed just how complex the human genome is and spawned a whole fresh set of questions and a new era of research. The human genome project allowed us to position approximately 25,000 gene sequences within the DNA sequence and to identify conserved regulatory, functional and structural motifs but we still have very little understanding about the purpose of a large proportion of the sequence that lies between genes. Furthermore, the sequences themselves can vary between individuals, genes can be switched on and off across time points and proteins can exist in alternative formats between tissues.[1] Thus the real secrets of the human genome do not lie in the sequence itself but rather in the way that these individual gene sequences can interact in complex networks and pathways to build a dynamic and responsive machinery that meets the needs of an individual over time and between environments.

Genetic variation

A large area of modern genomic research focuses upon the variations in DNA sequences between individuals, and the way that these variations contribute, not only to disease and disorders, but also to normal variation and behaviour. For example, if we sequenced the entire genome of a single individual, we might see that at position 5,204,808 of chromosome 11 they carried a thymine base (T). Bio-informatic analyses of this sequence would tell us that it lies in a section of DNA which encodes the haemoglobin beta gene. Nonetheless, this single sequence read in a single individual does not tell us much beyond this. However, if we sequenced this section in 1,000 individuals, we would soon find that whilst the majority of individuals have a T at this position, a small proportion have an adenine (A). Thus we can tell that this base is variant between individuals and has two different possible 'alleles': T and A. Further investigations would reveal that those individuals with the A allele are likely to have African ancestry and those with two copies of the A allele have sickle cell anaemia. In this way, the investigation of DNA sequence variations across a number of individuals can yield important information about the function of the sequence and its relevance to disease. Accordingly, efforts are now underway to sequence the entire genomes of thousands of individuals to enable the cataloguing of human sequence variants and the study of their contribution to disease.

Types of genetic variation

Genetic variations come in many different forms. In the example above, the sequence variant involved a single base that fell within a gene. The presence of an A allele at this base altered the protein coding sequence in a deleterious way. By definition, these changes are labelled mutations. The majority of classical genetic diseases involve mutations, but variations in genetic sequences need not alter protein properties. They may retain the meaning of the amino acid sequence (synonymous mutations), or may alter an amino acid in a region of the protein that is not structurally or functionally important. Alternatively, they may lie outside of

---

1 In this chapter, we will focus upon sequence variations underlying susceptibility to developmental disorders. Note, however, that the function of genes can also be modulated by changes outside of the DNA sequence, or so-called epigenetic mechanisms. (For a review of epigenetic effects in learning and memory processes, see Roth, Roth, & Sweatt, 2010.)

gene coding sequences altogether. Variants may affect only a single base (called single nucleotide polymorphisms, or SNPs, when it is a commonly recognised site of variation) or may involve the deletion or duplication of small stretches of DNA (indels) or more extensive structural rearrangements (copy number variations, or CNVs). Recent research indicates that these kinds of small-scale genetic variations are much more common than previously thought. In a recent pilot study, the 1,000 genomes project catalogued 14.4 million SNPs, 1.3 million indels and over 20,000 CNVs (Durbin et al., 2010). They estimated that the DNA sequence of any given individual is likely to differ from the human genome reference sequence at approximately 3 million bases. Approximately 10,000 of these variations will result in an amino acid coding change and 250 will be predicted to result in a loss of protein function. Genetic variants which fall outside of coding sequences were more common than those occurring within coding sequences. This is thought to be because these kinds of variants are less likely to have a directly deleterious effect upon the individual and so are more likely to be maintained within a population. Nonetheless, the fact that a variant falls in a non-coding region or is synonymous does not necessarily indicate that it is not relevant to disease. Common genetic variations can subtly affect the way in which genes and proteins function and interact through the modulation of regulatory and structural DNA sequences. Such effects are thought to be particularly important in the genetic basis of common diseases. Under the 'common disease–common variant' hypothesis, individual variants do not cause disease themselves but certain combinations of variants may place particular individuals at risk of the development of a given disorder through subtle effects upon relevant biological pathways. What is clear is that the level of inter-individual genetic variation is enormous and the task of identifying a relatively small set of variants contributing to any single given disorder will be immense.

SNPs and developmental disorders

Linkage and association

Under the common disease–common variant hypothesis, the majority of non-syndromic developmental disorders are proposed to involve multiple common non-coding variants, each with a relatively small individual effect size, and, as such, are labelled 'genetically complex' disorders. Over the last decade, numerous studies have attempted to identify the variants that contribute to such disorders, focussing primarily upon autism, Specific Language Impairment (SLI), dyslexia and Attention Deficit Hyperactivity Disorder (ADHD). This chapter does not aim to give a comprehensive catalogue of every study performed but rather, to give an overview of the field using examples of such studies to illustrate relevant concepts and issues. For a list of suggested in-depth reviews, please see 'further reading' at the end of this chapter.

The majority of genetic studies of developmental disorders have relied upon linkage techniques, which compare genetic markers between hundreds of sibling pairs and search for regions of the genome where there is a correlation between the genetic similarity and the phenotypic identity of the siblings. Following developments in genetic typing technologies, it is now more common to utilise genome-wide association-based methods, but these have yet to be extensively applied to developmental disorders. In association studies, single nucleotide polymorphisms (SNPs) are characterised in thousands of unrelated affected and unaffected individuals to allow the identification of genetic variants that are significantly more common in cases than controls.

On a case-by-case basis, linkage and association studies of developmental disorders have met with varied success. While many have identified chromosome segments (loci) that are linked to impairment or genetic variants that are significantly associated with disorder, an equal number have failed to yield significant results, and the replication between studies has often been poor. Nonetheless, if one looks at the field as a whole, these studies have enabled the identification of consistent genetic risk loci for most disorders and have provided a better understanding of the kinds of genetic effects that contribute to such disorders.

Sample selection

A large amount of the inter-study variation for developmental disorders can be explained by differences between subject ascertainment or assessment and by the relatively small sample sizes employed. For example, to date, three independent whole genome linkage studies of SLI have been completed (Bartlett et al., 2002; SLI Consortium, 2002; Villanueva et al., 2011). Between them, they have found significant linkage to chromosomes 7 (Villanueva et al., 2011), 13 (Bartlett et al., 2002), 16 (SLI Consortium, 2002) and 19 (SLI Consortium, 2002). Each of these linkages has now been replicated by targeted genetic analyses, or has support from investigations of alternative disorders (Bartlett et al., 2004; Falcaro et al., 2008; SLI Consortium, 2004; Vernes et al., 2008), but upon initial appraisal, the disparity between the results of these three genome-wide studies is stark. In this instance, it is possible that a large amount of divergence can be accounted for by differences in study design. One study investigated large American families and assessed language impairment on the basis of spoken language and reading ability (Bartlett et al., 2002). The second studied small British families and used continuous measures of language ability as a marker of impairment (SLI Consortium, 2002). The final study involved an isolated Chilean population and employed tests of grammar and phonology to define affected individuals (Villanueva et al., 2011). These overt differences in study design are typical in genetic investigations of developmental disorders and often make it difficult to directly compare data across studies or to comment on similarities or differences between studies.

Qualitative and quantitative measures

These studies of SLI neatly illustrate the importance of standardised ascertainment and assessment criteria in genetic studies. However, since many developmental disorders do not have globally accepted diagnostic criteria (see Williams & Lind, this volume), variable definitions of affection status are perhaps unavoidable. Some researchers choose to apply a binary or qualitative definition of affection status, defining all participants as affected or unaffected. This approach may rely upon standard questionnaires and diagnostic guidelines, for example, the Autism Diagnostic Observation Schedule (ADOS) or the Autism Diagnostic Interview (ADI) in autism. Alternatively qualitative studies may employ a threshold method of affection definition, where all individuals meeting pre-defined criteria are classified as affected. For disorders like dyslexia or SLI, however, the unambiguous derivation of a binary affection status can be problematic. Diagnostic criteria often vary between sites, and within any given sample, there will usually be individuals who are borderline to diagnosis. Because of this, continuous behavioural measures (phenotypes) are commonly used as an indication of an individual's ability in a relevant area (for example, reading measures in the study of dyslexia). These quantitative trait studies negate the need to label individuals as affected or unaffected and instead rely upon the identification of chromosome segments or genetic variants that are correlated with performance on the task in hand. Thus they not only allow the inclusion of both affected and unaffected individuals from a family unit but also enable a certain level of phenotype dissection. Nonetheless, quantitative analyses can bring their own complications with regard to the interpretation of what a given behavioural test actually measures. In addition, the use of multiple quantitative tests is often desirable to capture different aspects of disability. This greatly increases the number of tests performed and hence the likelihood of false positives. Another area that is often overlooked in molecular genetic studies but which is particularly pertinent to developmental disorders is the longitudinal consideration of the disorder. This topic is discussed by Byrne, Olson, and Samuelsson in this volume.

Trait dissection

An example of the complexities of relating genetic linkage to behavioural measures is given by dyslexia. An early study of dyslexia found significant linkage between chromosome 6 and measures of phonological awareness and chromosome 15 and a test of single word reading (Grigorenko et al., 1997). On the basis of these results, it was suggested that these two alternative genetic loci may contribute to distinct components of reading-related skills (Grigorenko et al., 1997). However, subsequent linkage studies did not replicate this specificity, instead reporting linkage to multiple measures of reading including reading, spelling, phonology and orthographics across both loci (Deffenbacher et al., 2004; Fisher et al., 1999; Schulte-Korne et al., 1998). Thus although attractive from a theoretical perspective, it is now accepted as unlikely that single genetic regions or variants will map to specific components or behavioural traits. Indeed, as more genetic data has become available from increasingly large studies, the reverse seems to be true. Many genetic loci are not only linked, or associated, with multiple traits within a single disorder population, but also with multiple traits across related disorders. For example, the regions of chromosome 6 and 15 identified in the above study have also been linked to speech sound disorder (Smith, Pennington, Boada, & Shriberg, 2005), verbal IQ (Posthuma et al., 2005), and ADHD (Bakker et al., 2003; Wigg et al., 2008). Variants in dyslexia candidate genes have also been associated with ADHD (Couto et al., 2009) and spoken language disorder (Newbury et al., 2011; Rice, Smith, & Gayan, 2009). Thus many researchers now propose that risk variants are likely to contribute to shared developmental processes across related disorders. From a biological perspective, this is perhaps more congruent, as it is hard to see how one would expect genes and proteins to exclusively contribute to specific processes or restricted disorders that are apparently closely related at the behavioural level.

Multivariate genetic analyses

A more detailed picture of genetic effects and the relationships between behavioural measures can be achieved by multivariate analyses. While univariate quantitative methods assume that each trait is independent, multivariate techniques consider the covariance between traits within a genetic model. By applying multivariate methods to a linkage analysis of dyslexia, Marlow et al. demonstrated that joint effects across multiple reading- and language-related traits contributed to the locus on chromosome 6 (Marlow et al., 2003). Similar investigations of SLI loci indicate that the chromosome 13 linkage is predominantly driven by poor readers with low language ability (Simmons et al., 2010). Chromosome 16 is thought to contribute equally to phonological short-term memory, reading and spelling traits while chromosome 19 influences primarily language-related phenotypes (Monaco, 2007). Targeted association studies of the region of linkage on chromosome 16 have since led to the identification of common non-coding variants in the *ATP2C2* and *CMIP* genes that are associated with reduced phonological short-term memory in language-impaired individuals (Newbury et al., 2009).

Sample sizes and the winner's curse

Another factor that can cause increased rates of false positive results and reduced replication between studies is sample size. The majority of genetic studies of developmental disorders to date have relied upon linkage analyses involving less than 100 families, which are unlikely to provide adequate power to detect genetic variants of small effect sizes. It must be remembered that linkage and association methods are statistical in nature and only provide a likelihood that a given genetic region or variant has an effect upon the disorder, given the data in hand. Thus if a study is performed with a small sample, the chances of a false positive result will be increased. Note that the number of tests involved in a genome-wide association study means that the chances of a false positive are already very high. For this reason, the threshold of significance in such studies is deliberately set very high (typically $p < 5 \times 10^{-8}$ for genome-wide significance). Since every study represents an independent selection of individuals from the disorder population, there will be some element of chance involved in the frequencies of genetic risk elements present in any given sample. While some genetic risk variants will be over-represented, if compared to the disorder population as a whole, others will be under-represented. Flipping this rationale on its head, we can say that if a genetic risk variant is identified within a sample, especially if the sample size is small, then it is likely to be because that specific variant happens to be over-represented within that sample, because of random selection variables. This phenomenon is known as the 'winner's curse' as it unfortunately means that subsequent selected samples are likely to have reduced power to replicate the findings of the original sample as the chances of an over-representation of the same locus in two subsequent samples is low (Kraft, 2008). In an ideal world, we would sample every single individual within a given disorder population but, of course this is not possible. Nonetheless, as the size of the selected sample increases, then these sampling effects diminish. Thus successful genome-wide association studies require sample sizes of thousands of individuals, which currently do not exist for developmental disorders such as SLI and dyslexia.

Meta-analyses

A way around the problem of small sample sizes, without collecting complete new cohorts, is the meta-analysis of data-sets from collaborative sites. This approach has proven successful for ADHD in which a meta-analysis was performed for seven moderately sized linkage studies, none of which had found significant linkage in isolation. This enabled the combined analysis of 2,084 cases selected from different sites using alternative diagnostic and selection criteria and yielded a significant linkage to chromosome 16q23 within the *CDH13* (Cadherin13) gene (Zhou et al., 2008). *CDH13* encodes a cadherin protein that plays a role in cell adhesion, neuronal migration and neurite outgrowth, and thus represents a good candidate gene for ADHD (Lesch et al., 2008). Similar meta-analyses of four genome-wide association studies of ADHD also supported the involvement of the *CDH13* gene, although not at a genome-wide significant level. In fact, even though this association meta-analysis included nearly 3,000 affected individuals, it did not yield any results of genome-wide significance ($p < 5 \times 10^{-8}$) reiterating the need for extremely large sample sizes in these kinds of studies. Thus, whilst meta-analyses such as these hold promise, it is likely that the success of future studies will hinge upon new large-scale sample collections with consistent and comprehensive assessment batteries.

Functional variants

Linkage studies tend to locate large chromosome regions, while association studies allow the identification of specific genetic variants that are associated with disorder. Both these techniques usually require some subsequent 'fine-mapping' to allow the refinement of the signal. However, once a certain resolution is reached, the genetic variants are all so highly correlated with each other that it can be difficult to distinguish between those which have a functional contributory role and those which are correlated with a functional variant simply because they happen to lie near by in the genetic sequence. Linkage and association methods both allow the identification of regions and variants of interest, but neither have the ability to definitively discern a functional variant. For example, the variants in *CDH13* gene associated with ADHD lie very close to those in the *ATP2C2* gene, which is associated with SLI. It is therefore theoretically possible that all of these associated variants are correlated with a single underlying functional variant which contributes to both ADHD and SLI. Equally, these data may represent the co-incidental identification of neighbouring risk genes for distinct developmental processes. For a causal relationship to be deduced, functional experiments must be used to provide a direct link between a specific sequence variation and the modulation of a relevant biological process.

Proof of causality

A good example of the importance of proof of functionality is given by the study of the dyslexia linkage locus on chromosome 6 (named DYX2). DYX2 was the one of first reported linkage regions for dyslexia and remains one of the most replicated (Cardon et al., 1994; Fisher et al., 1999; Gayan et al., 1999; Grigorenko et al., 1997; Grigorenko, Wood, Meyer, & Pauls, 2000; Kaplan et al., 2002). However, this locus covers several million base pairs of DNA and contains over 100 genes. Several groups therefore performed independent fine mapping experiments and associations were reported across several different genes including *DCDC2* (Doublecortin domain containing protein 2) (Lind et al., 2010; Meng et al., 2005; Schumacher et al., 2006) and *KIAA0319* (Cope et al., 2005; Francks et al., 2004; Ludwig et al., 2008), which lie just 150,000 base pairs apart on the chromosome. Each of these associations was replicated by independent groups and was statistically significant. The problem therefore lay in determining the functionality of each of the associated variants to establish the nature of the relationship between *DCDC2*, *KIAA0319* and dyslexia. There is now a growing amount of functional evidence to support the independent involvement of both of these genes in the aetiology of dyslexia. It was suggested that perhaps the reason that the chromosome 6 linkage was so robust was because it contained multiple genetic variants that contributed to dyslexia susceptibility (Meng et al., 2005). Indeed, a recent study suggests that, besides *KIAA0319* and *DCDC2*, there may be more even contributory genes yet to be discovered at this locus (Konig et al., 2011).

KIAA0319 and dyslexia

The correlations between variants contained within contiguous genetic sequences mean that significant SNPs can be spread cross quite large regions. The SNPs around the *KIAA0319* gene that are associated with dyslexia are actually spread across the coding regions of three adjacent genes; *KIAA0319*, *THEM2* and *TTRAP*, so initially it was unclear which of these genes represented the true candidate.

The comparison of gene expression between cells carrying risk variants against those with no risk variants showed that the expression of *KIAA0319* was significantly reduced in risk cells, whilst the expression of the other two genes remained unchanged (Paracchini et al., 2006). This experiment not only allowed the identification of a specific candidate gene but also demonstrated that the identified risk variants in this region had a functional effect upon the expression of that gene. The identified variants fall around the start of the *KIAA0319* gene, which is a common region for regulatory elements, but it was still unclear which of the multiple risk variants was causing this effect (Couto et al., 2011; Elbert et al., 2011; Paracchini et al., 2006). In-depth analyses of gene expression and regulation led to the identification of a single variant which directly alters the binding site of a regulatory protein (transcription factor) and is associated with reduced *KIAA0319* expression (Dennis et al., 2009). Thus it has been proposed that this single variant alters the regulation of *KIAA0319*, which contributes to dyslexia susceptibility (Dennis et al., 2009). *KIAA0319* is expressed in the brain, and the protein can exist in many different forms, presumably with different functions (Velayos-Baeza, Toma, da Roza, Paracchini, & Monaco, 2007; Velayos-Baeza, Toma, Paracchini, & Monaco, 2008). The prevention of *Kiaa0319* expression (known as 'knockout' when gene expression is completely obliterated, or 'knockdown' when the gene expression is reduced) in the rat cortex leads to altered neuronal migration, demonstrating that this protein is relevant to brain development (Paracchini et al., 2006). Knockdown of *Kiaa0319* caused pockets of neurons within the cortex that failed to migrate properly (periventricular heterotopias) (Peschansky et al., 2010), which fits with the findings of postmortem neuroanatomical studies of dyslexic patients (Galaburda, Sherman, Rosen, Aboitiz, & Geschwind, 1985).

DCDC2 and dyslexia

Investigation of the sequence surrounding the associated variants in *DCDC2* identified a deletion of 2,445 base pairs within the *DCDC2* gene that was significantly more common in people with dyslexia than in controls (Meng et al., 2005). This deletion was shown to cover some regulatory sequences and its presence reduces the expression of the *DCDC2* gene (Meng et al., 2011). Magnetic Resonance Imaging (MRI) of individuals carrying this deletion found significantly increased grey matter volumes in regions of the brain implicated in reading, language and symbol-decoding tasks, particularly in the left hemisphere (Meda et al., 2008). A recent morphometric study also found localised pockets of cortical grey matter in dyslexic individuals, but suggested that this may represent a technical anomaly of the automatised brain tissue classification system used in morphometric studies. They suggested that ectopias may be interpreted as local increases in grey matter tissue by this system (Silani et al., 2005). Interestingly, the knockdown of *Dcdc2* expression in developing rat cortex was also found to disrupt neuronal migration (Meng et al., 2005) and result in pockets of heterotopic neurons in the periventricular region (Burbridge et al., 2008). In mice, however, this effect was not found unless a second gene from the doublecortin family was also knocked out. This suggests that the lack of *Dcdc2* expression in mice can be compensated for by other related genes in the same family (Wang et al., 2011). We do not yet know whether this partial redundancy also occurs in humans.

DYX1C1 and neuronal migration

As well as *DCDC2* and *KIAA0319*, a third dyslexia candidate gene, *DYX1C1* (dyslexia susceptibility 1 candidate 1, also known as *EKN1*), has also been shown to be important in neuronal migration processes.

   DYX1C1, on chromosome 15 (at the DYX1 locus), was first identified as a dyslexia candidate gene by the breakpoint mapping of a chromosome translocation (t(2;15)(q11;q21)) that co-segregated with dyslexia in a single family (Nopola-Hemmi et al., 2000; Taipale et al., 2003). Further investigation of this region in other dyslexic individuals who did not have chromosome abnormalities, identified other rare sequence variations, with potentially functional effects, that were more common in dyslexic cases than controls or associated with quantitative reading-related measures (Bates et al., 2009; Dahdouh et al., 2009; Lim, Ho, Chou, & Waye, 2011; Taipale et al., 2003; Wigg et al., 2004). Like that reported for *Dcdc2* and *Kiaa0319*, the knockdown of *Dyx1c1* in rat cortex also resulted in cortical heteropia and disrupted neuronal migration (Rosen et al., 2007; Wang et al., 2006). Furthermore, these effects could be reversed by the reactivation of *Dyx1c1* expression (Wang et al., 2006). Behavioural analyses of rats with cortical heteroplasias found that they had impairments in spatial learning and auditory processing, further strengthening the evidence for *Dyx1c1* as a candidate gene (Szalkowski et al., 2011; Threlkeld et al., 2007).

Pathway analyses

As we have seen above, alternative results from seemingly conflicting studies can sometimes converge to provide a global overview of processes or pathways that might be important for disorders. An objective global approach that is often taken in the investigation of genome-wide association studies (often called GWAs) is that of pathway, or network, analyses. Genome-wide association studies can result in the identification of several significantly associated risk variants (called hits) at different loci across the genome. Pathway analyses attempt to draw out relevant biological pathways by considering the functional relationships between associated variants.

   To date, among the developmental disorders discussed here, genome-wide association analyses have only been completed for ADHD and autism. In ADHD, a pathway analysis of five independent genome-wide association studies found that 45 of the 85 top-ranked hits could be fitted together in a network involved in neurite development and outgrowth (Poelmans, Pauls, Buitelaar, & Franke, 2011).

Genome-wide studies of autism have tended to include large sample sizes, but yet have still met with relatively little success. Across four studies, only two identified variants have met genome wide significance levels ($p < 5 \times 10^{-8}$) (Anney et al., 2010; Ma et al., 2009; Wang et al., 2009; Weiss, Arking, Daly, & Chakravarti, 2009). These variants fall between the *CDH9* (Cadherin 9) and *CDH10* (Cadherin 10) genes on chromosome 5 (Ma et al., 2009; Wang et al., 2009), and coincide with the *MACROD2* (Macro-domain containing-2) and *FLRT3* (Fibronectin-like domain-containing leucine-rich transmembrane protein 3) genes on chromosome 20 (Anney et al., 2010). However, none of these associations were replicated across studies. Pathway analyses of autism GWA data have implicated genes in the cadherin pathway, which not only include *CDH9* and *CDH10* but also other autism candidate genes, such as *CNTNAP2* (Contactin-associated protein-like 2 precursor), as well as genes associated with related developmental disorders, such as the *CDH13* gene described above for ADHD (Wang et al., 2009). Additional pathway analyses of autism association data have found an enrichment of association in genes involved in the metabolism of pyruvate (which is a product of many metabolic processes), transcription factor activation, cell-signalling and cell-cycle regulation (Anney et al., 2011). Thus, although it may seem premature to be thinking about pathways when so few genome-wide significant results have been generated, these studies demonstrate the power of pathway analyses to identify higher-order global effects from borderline significant data by considering the underlying relationships between loci.

CNVs and developmental disorders

Chromosome rearrangements

It is an established fact that large-scale chromosome rearrangements can cause genetic disorders. These events can be detected by chromosome staining or Fluorescence In-Situ Hybridisation (FISH) techniques and typically involve the duplication, deletion, or rearrangement of large chromosome segments that affect a number of genes. Coding sequences that are contained within the rearranged segment will have altered dosage, and genes at the ends of rearrangements can be directly disrupted by break points. Chromosome rearrangements usually lead to severe syndromic disorders with characteristic, but variable, clinical features. For example, the deletion of a specific region of chromosome 22 (known as 22q11) causes DiGeorge or velocardiofacial syndrome, which is characterised by immune deficiency, cardiac defects and developmental delays (de la Chapelle, Herva, Koivisto, & Aula, 1981). The exact clinical characteristics of individuals with chromosome 22q11 deletions vary dramatically, as does the size of the deleted region. Although some researchers have attempted to relate the deletion of particular genes with specific clinical characteristics in DiGeorge syndrome (Meechan, Maynard, Tucker, & LaMantia, 2011), it appears that the underlying aetiology is often more complex than this simple correlation model allows.

Copy number variants (CNVs)

Recent advances in genomic technology have enabled the development of assays that allow the rapid screening of entire genomes and the detection of much smaller, submicroscopic, genomic deletions and duplications, known as copy number variants (CNVs). Whilst the presence of CNVs in the human genome is well-documented, the extent of their occurrence and their possible clinical relevance is only just beginning to be appreciated. Large-scale studies of control populations have identified over 10,000 sites at which copy number events commonly occur in the human genome, indicating that CNVs are likely to account for a large proportion of normal genetic variation (Craddock et al., 2010; Iafrate et al., 2004; Redon et al., 2006; Sebat et al., 2004). Although common copy number events lead to extra or depleted copies of genomic material, and often include gene coding sequences, they apparently have no negative side effects. However, recent studies have also indicated that rare CNVs may contribute to neuropsychiatric disorders such as schizophrenia (Guilmatre et al., 2009; Levinson et al., 2011; Stefansson et al., 2009), intellectual disability (Guilmatre et al., 2009), ADHD (Elia et al., 2009; Williams et al., 2010), and autism (Guilmatre et al., 2009; Marshall et al., 2008; Pinto et al., 2010; Sebat et al., 2007). In such cases, it is thought that disease-risk is increased through the disruption of coding sequences, the alteration of dosage sensitive genes, or via more subtle effects upon gene expression such as the interruption of regulatory sequences.

CNVs in autism

Genome-wide studies of copy number variants in autistic individuals indicate that between 5 and 10 percent of sporadic cases (i.e., affected individuals with no family history of autistic disorder) of autism are caused by large *de novo* (i.e., new CNVs that have not been transmitted from a parent) copy number events that cover a gene (Christian et al., 2008; Levy et al., 2011; Marshall et al., 2008; Sanders et al., 2011; Sebat et al., 2007). These studies have also detected a small, but consistent, number of autistic individuals who carry two or more *de novo* CNVs or have independently inherited two rare CNVs, one from each parent (Girirajan et al., 2010; Marshall et al., 2008; Pagnamenta et al., 2010; Pinto et al., 2010). These findings have led to the 'two-hit' model under which it is proposed that combinations of insults (which may take the form of rare or *de novo* CNVs, deleterious mutations or adverse environmental events) during development significantly increase the likelihood of severe paediatric disease, such as autism (Girirajan et al., 2010). In particular, this model has been applied to chromosome 16p11 rearrangements, which represent one of the most recurrent CNVs described in autism (Bijlsma et al., 2009; Fernandez et al., 2010; Girirajan et al., 2010; Levy et al., 2011; Marshall et al., 2008; Sanders et al., 2011; Shinawi et al., 2010; Weiss et al., 2008). Approximately one-third of individuals with 16p11 deletions or duplications are on the autistic spectrum. Many other carriers have alternative neurodevelopmental problems of variable severity but this CNV is also observed in normal controls (Girirajan et al., 2010; Hanson et al., 2010). Attempts to draw correlations between the size or extent of the deletion or duplication and distinct behavioural or clinical features have met with limited success (Fernandez et al., 2010). However, in general, deletions of this region tend to lead to more severe phenotypes, as do the presence of a second 'hit' (Fernandez et al., 2010; Girirajan et al., 2010). An interesting extension of the two-hit model is provided by a recent study which suggests that autistic females carry a higher frequency of large genic copy number variants than those observed in their male counterparts (Gilman et al., 2011; Levy et al., 2011). Autistic spectrum disorders have a characteristic male excess, with unknown aetiology. The authors of this study therefore suggest that females appear to be more resistant to genetic risk of autism and perhaps require more hits to cross an affection threshold (Levy et al., 2011).

Aside from 16p11, a few other CNVs have been found in multiple unrelated cases of autism. These include: duplications of 7q11 (Berg et al., 2007; Depienne et al., 2007; Gilman et al., 2011; Sanders et al., 2011; Van der Aa et al., 2009), which overlaps with the region commonly deleted in Williams syndrome, a complex developmental disorder that includes facial dysmorphology, heart defects and hyper-sociability (Beuren, Apitz, & Harmjanz, 1962; Williams, Barratt-Boyes, & Lowe, 1961); deletions or duplications of 15q13 in a region that overlaps with the Prader-Willi/Angelman syndrome locus (Helbig et al., 2009; Marshall et al., 2008; Pagnamenta et al., 2009; Sharp et al., 2008; Weiss et al., 2008); and deletions of the *NRXN1* gene on chromosome 2 (Ching et al., 2010; Zahir et al., 2008). Less frequent cases of duplications of 1q21, duplications of 16p13, and deletions of chromosome 16q23 have also been described (Levy et al., 2011; Sanders et al., 2011).

Pathway analyses

Although a handful of loci have been identified with recurrent events, the majority of *de novo* CNVs identified in autistic cases tend to be rare, or even private to a given individual. The main difficulty in these studies is therefore the proof of causality. If a given variant is only seen to occur, at most, in a handful of individuals, it will never be statistically significant and it is hard to draw conclusions regarding the relevance of the observed event. Many researchers have therefore turned to pathway or network analyses, similar to those described for genome-wide association analyses. Pathway analyses have increased confidence in the relevance of rare CNV events by demonstrating that they are significantly more likely to contain, or lie close to, genes that have previously been implicated in autism or other developmental disorders than events observed in controls (Glessner et al., 2009; Marshall et al., 2008; Roohi et al., 2009). Furthermore, pathway analyses have shown that the CNVs found in autistic individuals involve an enrichment of genes involved in cell and neuronal development and function including projection, motility and proliferation (Gilman et al., 2011; Pinto et al., 2010).

Mutations and developmental disorders

For the main part, syndromes caused by single gene mutations are rare and exceptionally severe disorders with characteristic features. In contrast, 'mainstream' nonsyndromic developmental disorders, such as autism, Specific Language Impairment, dyslexia and ADHD are usually considered to involve variants that modulate gene function, as opposed to mutations that impair gene function.

FOXP2

Occasionally, a rare coding mutation is found to cause a disorder that mimics a complex developmental disorder. Although such events are rare and usually involve a different genetic basis to the majority of mainstream disorders, they can provide vital information regarding the biological basis of developmental impairments. For example, the KE family are a large four-generation pedigree in which approximately half the members are affected by a distinctive form of verbal dyspraxia caused by a single coding mutation in the *FOXP2* (Forkhead box P2) gene on chromosome 7q (Fisher, Vargha-Khadem, Watkins, Monaco, & Pembrey, 1998; Lai, Fisher, Hurst, Vargha-Khadem, & Monaco, 2001). Although this gene is not thought to represent a general risk factor for speech and language impairments (Meaburn, Dale, Craig, & Plomin, 2002; Newbury et al., 2002; O'Brien, Zhang, Nishimura, Tomblin, & Murray, 2003), its mutation is causative in a small number of individuals, all of whom have syndromes that feature verbal dyspraxia (Feuk et al., 2006; Lennon et al., 2007; MacDermot et al., 2005; Pariani, Spencer, Graham, & Rimoin, 2009; Shriberg et al., 2006; Tomblin et al., 2009; Zeesman et al., 2006). The *FOXP2* gene encodes a transcription factor, which is responsible for the regulation of a large number of genes (300–400 neural genes) during development (Spiteri et al., 2007; Vernes et al., 2007). The study of these interactions and regulation pathways has allowed the identification of biological networks that are involved in speech and language acquisition processes. For example, one of the genes down-regulated by *FOXP2* is the contactin-associated protein *CNTNAP2*, which has not only been associated with autism (Alarcon et al., 2008; Arking et al., 2008; Bakkaloglu et al., 2008; Jackman, Horn, Molleston, & Sokol, 2009; Poot et al., 2009; Rossi et al., 2008), but with a wide range of additional neuropsychiatric disorders, including SLI (Vernes et al., 2008), Gilles de Tourette syndrome (Belloso et al., 2007; Verkerk et al., 2003), schizophrenia (Friedman et al., 2008; O'Dushlaine et al., 2010), epilepsy (Friedman et al., 2008; Mefford et al., 2010; Strauss et al., 2006), ADHD (Elia et al., 2009), intellectual disability (Zweier et al., 2009), selective mutism (Stein et al., 2011), and stuttering (Petrin et al., 2010). A second gene, known as *FOXP1* (Forkhead box P1), which is highly similar to and forms a binding partner for FOXP2, has also been found to be disrupted by both mutations and deletions, in individuals with verbal dyspraxia (Vernes, MacDermot, Monaco, & Fisher, 2009), autistic spectrum disorder (Hamdan et al., 2010; O'Roak et al., 2011), intellectual disability (Hamdan et al., 2010; Horn et al., 2010), and other developmental delays (Carr et al., 2010; Pariani et al.,

2009). Thus it is clear that members of gene cascades and networks regulated by *FOXP2* play a contributory role in developmental processes and disorders.

Coding mutations in autism

The investigation of rare coding mutations has also played an important role in our understanding of autistic spectrum disorders. Early single candidate gene screening in autistic cases often revealed mutations in a handful of cases within any single cohort, especially in sporadic individuals (Bonora et al., 2002; Bonora et al., 2005; Buxbaum, Cai, Chaste et al., 2007; Buxbaum, Cai, Nygren et al., 2007). Since they occurred at only a low level, many of these mutations were assumed not to be causative. However, as more data emerged, both from mutation studies and CNV investigations, it became clear that these rare coding mutations were not random but tended to occur in genes encoding synaptic and cell adhesion proteins (Betancur, Sakurai, & Buxbaum, 2009; Bourgeron, 2009), and overlapped with genes and regions hit by rare CNVs (see previous section). These include mutations in the neuroligin genes *NLGN3* (Neuroligin 3) and *NLGN4* (Neuroligin 4) (Daoud et al., 2009; Jamain et al., 2003; Laumonnier et al., 2004), the neurexin gene *NRXN1* (Neurexin 1) (Kim et al., 2008), the postsynaptic protein *SHANK3* (SH3 and multiple ankyrin repeat domains 3) (Durand et al., 2007; Gauthier et al., 2009) and the contactin-associated protein, *CNTNAP2* (Bakkaloglu et al., 2008). The synaptic function of these genes seems to fit in with the pathway analyses of CNV and genome-wide association data, and this is further supported by recent genome-wide investigations of gene expression levels (Voineagu et al., 2011), exome sequencing studies (O'Roak et al., 2011) and animal models (Etherton, Blaiss, Powell, & Sudhof, 2009; Jamain et al., 2008; Peca et al., 2011). Thus, there is a growing amount of converging evidence from CNV, mutation and functional studies that rare or private mutations with large effect sizes may be of more importance in autistic spectrum disorders than combinations of common variants, and that the disruption of genes involved in synaptic modulation and cell adhesion may be of particular relevance.

Summary

The study of human genetic variation, at the level of common single nucleotide polymorphism (SNPs), rare or *de novo* copy number variants (CNVs) and rare coding mutations in developmental disorders have transformed our understanding of the biological basis of these disorders.

The study of common variation has enabled the identification of risk loci and candidate genes for the developmental disorders Specific Language Impairment (SLI), dyslexia, ADHD and autistic spectrum disorders. Future genome-wide association analyses (GWAs) are likely to identify more contributory variants in these disorders but will require large sample sizes to achieve adequate power.

Much of the current genetic research focuses upon pathway analyses rather than the identification or functional characterisation of individual risk variants or genes. The process of neurite development and outgrowth is thought to play a role in the neuropathology of ADHD. Neuronal migration pathways are thought to be important in dyslexia, and synaptic modulation and cell adhesion seem to be of particular relevance to autistic spectrum disorders. Many genes or pathways have been found to contribute to related developmental disorders and it is likely that there are certain key pathways that contribute to crucial developmental processes. The disruption of these pathways may lead to varied outcomes depending on other factors that are specific to the individual, such as the genetic background and environmental effects.

The majority of developmental disorders are considered to follow the common disease – common variant model but recent evidence has suggested that, contrary to this hypothesis, rare copy number variants and mutations of large effect sizes may underlie the aetiology of autistic spectrum disorders.

As genomic technologies develop, the rate of data generation is growing exponentially. The challenge in human genetics over the next decade, therefore, lies in determining ways to apply and interpret this information in the study of complex and inter-related disorders.

Further reading

- For a review of the genetics of speech and language impairments see Newbury and Monaco (2010) and Kang and Drayna (2011).
- For a review of dyslexia genetics see Scerri and Schulte-Korne (2009).
- For a review of the role of genetics in ADHD see Faraone and Mick (2010).
- For a review of FOXP2 see Fisher and Scharff (2009).
- For a review of the genetics of autistic spectrum disorders see Abrahams and Geschwind (2010) and Toro et al. (2010).
- For a review of the role of copy number variants in disease see Stankiewicz and Lupski (2010).
- For a review of the role of copy number variants in cognitive disorders see Morrow (2010).
- For a review of the role of genetics in developmental disorders see Willcutt et al. (2010) and Bishop (2009).

References

Abrahams, B. S., & Geschwind, D. H. (2010). Connecting genes to brain in the autism spectrum disorders. *Archives of Neurology, 67*(4), 395–399.

Alarcon, M., Abrahams, B. S., Stone, J. L., Duvall, J. A., Perederiy, J. V., Bomar, J. M., et al. (2008). Linkage, association, and gene-expression analyses identify CNTNAP2 as an autism-susceptibility gene. *American Journal of Human Genetics, 82*(1), 150–159.

Anney, R., Klei, L., Pinto, D., Regan, R., Conroy, J., Magalhaes, T. R., et al. (2010). A genome-wide scan for common alleles affecting risk for autism. *Human Molecular Genetics, 19*(20), 4072–4082.

Anney, R. J., Kenny, E. M., O'Dushlaine, C., Yaspan, B. L., Parkhomenka, E., Buxbaum, J. D., et al. (2011). Gene-ontology enrichment analysis in two independent family-based samples highlights biologically plausible processes for autism spectrum disorders. *European Journal of Human Genetics, 19*(10), 1082–1089.

Arking, D. E., Cutler, D. J., Brune, C. W., Teslovich, T. M., West, K., Ikeda, M., et al. (2008). A common genetic variant in the neurexin superfamily member CNTNAP2 increases familial risk of autism. *American Journal of Human Genetics, 82*(1), 160–164.

Bakkaloglu, B., O'Roak, B. J., Louvi, A., Gupta, A. R., Abelson, J. F., Morgan, T. M., et al. (2008). Molecular cytogenetic analysis and resequencing of contactin associated protein-like 2 in autism spectrum disorders. *American Journal of Human Genetics, 82*(1), 165–173.

Bakker, S. C., van der Meulen, E. M., Buitelaar, J. K., Sandkuijl, L. A., Pauls, D. L., Monsuur, A. J., et al. (2003). A whole-genome scan in 164 Dutch sib pairs with attention-deficit/hyperactivity disorder: Suggestive evidence for linkage on chromosomes 7p and 15q. *American Journal of Human Genetics, 72*(5), 1251–1260.

Bartlett, C. W., Flax, J. F., Logue, M. W., Smith, B. J., Vieland, V. J., Tallal, P., et al. (2004). Examination of potential overlap in autism and language loci on chromosomes 2, 7, and 13 in two independent samples ascertained for specific language impairment. *Human Heredity, 57*(1), 10–20.

Bartlett, C. W., Flax, J. F., Logue, M. W., Vieland, V. J., Bassett, A. S., Tallal, P., et al. (2002). A major susceptibility locus for specific language impairment is located on 13q21. *American Journal of Human Genetics, 71*(1), 45–55.

Bates, T. C., Lind, P. A., Luciano, M., Montgomery, G. W., Martin, N. G., & Wright, M. J. (2009). Dyslexia and DYX1C1: Deficits in reading and spelling associated with a missense mutation. *Molecular Psychiatry,15*(12), 1090–1096 .

Belloso, J. M., Bache, I., Guitart, M., Caballin, M. R., Halgren, C., Kirchhoff, M., et al. (2007). Disruption of the CNTNAP2 gene in a t(7;15) translocation family without symptoms of Gilles de la Tourette syndrome. *European Journal of Human Genetics, 15*(6), 711–713.

Berg, J. S., Brunetti-Pierri, N., Peters, S. U., Kang, S. H., Fong, C. T., Salamone, J., et al. (2007). Speech delay and autism spectrum behaviors are frequently associated with duplication of the 7q11.23 Williams-Beuren syndrome region. *Genetics in Medicine, 9*(7), 427–441.

Betancur, C., Sakurai, T., & Buxbaum, J. D. (2009). The emerging role of synaptic cell-adhesion pathways in the pathogenesis of autism spectrum disorders. *Trends in Neurosciences, 32*(7), 402–412.

Beuren, A. J., Apitz, J., & Harmjanz, D. (1962). Supravalvular aortic stenosis in association with mental retardation and a certain facial appearance. *Circulation, 26,* 1235–1240.

Bijlsma, E. K., Gijsbers, A. C., Schuurs-Hoeijmakers, J. H., van Haeringen, A., Fransen van de Putte, D. E., Anderlid, B. M., et al. (2009). Extending the phenotype of recurrent rearrangements of 16p11.2: Deletions in mentally retarded patients without autism and in normal individuals. *European Journal of Medical Genetics, 52*(2–3), 77–87.

Bishop, D. V. (2009). Genes, cognition, and communication: Insights from neurodevelopmental disorders. *Annals of the New York Academy of Sciences, 1156,* 1–18.

Bonora, E., Bacchelli, E., Levy, E. R., Blasi, F., Marlow, A., Monaco, A. P., et al. (2002). Mutation screening and imprinting analysis of four candidate genes for autism in the 7q32 region. *Molecular Psychiatry, 7*(3), 289–301.

Bonora, E., Lamb, J. A., Barnby, G., Sykes, N., Moberly, T., Beyer, K. S., et al. (2005). Mutation screening and association analysis of six candidate genes for autism on chromosome 7q. *European Journal of Human Genetics, 13*(2), 198–207.

Bourgeron, T. (2009). A synaptic trek to autism. *Current Opinion in Neurobiology, 19*(2), 231–234.

Burbridge, T. J., Wang, Y., Volz, A. J., Peschansky, V. J., Lisann, L., Galaburda, A. M., et al. (2008). Postnatal analysis of the effect of embryonic knockdown and overexpression of candidate dyslexia susceptibility gene homolog Dcdc2 in the rat. *Neuroscience, 152*(3), 723–733.

Buxbaum, J. D., Cai, G., Chaste, P., Nygren, G., Goldsmith, J., Reichert, J., et al. (2007). Mutation screening of the PTEN gene in patients with autism spectrum disorders and macrocephaly. *American Journal of Medical Genetics B Neuropsychiatric Genetics, 144B*(4), 484–491.

Buxbaum, J. D., Cai, G., Nygren, G., Chaste, P., Delorme, R., Goldsmith, J., et al. (2007). Mutation analysis of the NSD1 gene in patients with autism spectrum disorders and macrocephaly. *BMC Medical Genetics, 8*, 68.

Cardon, L. R., Smith, S. D., Fulker, D. W., Kimberling, W. J., Pennington, B. F., & DeFries, J. C. (1994). Quantitative trait locus for reading disability on chromosome 6. *Science, 266*(5183), 276–279.

Carr, C. W., Moreno-De-Luca, D., Parker, C., Zimmerman, H. H., Ledbetter, N., Martin, C. L., et al. (2010). Chiari I malformation, delayed gross motor skills, severe speech delay, and epileptiform discharges in a child with FOXP1 haploinsufficiency. *European Journal of Human Genetics, 18*, 1216–1220.

Ching, M. S., Shen, Y., Tan, W. H., Jeste, S. S., Morrow, E. M., Chen, X., et al. (2010). Deletions of NRXN1 (neurexin-1) predispose to a wide spectrum of developmental disorders. *American Journal of Medical Genetics B Neuropsychiatric Genetics, 153B*(4), 937–947.

Christian, S. L., Brune, C. W., Sudi, J., Kumar, R. A., Liu, S., Karamohamed, S., et al. (2008). Novel submicroscopic chromosomal abnormalities detected in autism spectrum disorder. *Biological Psychiatry, 63*(12), 1111–1117.

Cope, N., Harold, D., Hill, G., Moskvina, V., Stevenson, J., Holmans, P., et al. (2005). Strong evidence that KIAA0319 on chromosome 6p is a susceptibility gene for developmental dyslexia. *American Journal of Human Genetics, 76*(4), 581–591.

Couto, J. M., Gomez, L., Wigg, K., Ickowicz, A., Pathare, T., Malone, M., et al. (2009). Association of attention-deficit/hyperactivity disorder with a candidate region for reading disabilities on chromosome 6p. *Biological Psychiatry, 66*(4), 368–375.

Couto, J. M., Livne-Bar, I., Huang, K., Xu, Z., Cate-Carter, T., Feng, Y., et al. (2011). Association of reading disabilities with regions marked by acetylated H3 histones in KIAA0319. *American Journal of Medical Genetics B Neuropsychiatric Genetics, 153B*(2), 447–462.

Craddock, N., Hurles, M. E., Cardin, N., Pearson, R. D., Plagnol, V., Robson, S., et al. (2010). Genome-wide association study of CNVs in 16,000 cases of eight common diseases and 3,000 shared controls. *Nature, 464*(7289), 713–720.

Dahdouh, F., Anthoni, H., Tapia-Paez, I., Peyrard-Janvid, M., Schulte-Korne, G., Warnke, A., et al. (2009). Further evidence for DYX1C1 as a susceptibility factor for dyslexia. *Psychiatric Genetics, 19*(2), 59–63.

Daoud, H., Bonnet-Brilhault, F., Vedrine, S., Demattei, M. V., Vourc'h, P., Bayou, N., et al. (2009). Autism and nonsyndromic mental retardation associated with a de novo mutation in the NLGN4X gene promoter causing an increased expression level. *Biological Psychiatry, 66*(10), 906–910.

de la Chapelle, A., Herva, R., Koivisto, M., & Aula, P. (1981). A deletion in chromosome 22 can cause DiGeorge syndrome. *Human Genetics, 57*(3), 253–256.

Deffenbacher, K. E., Kenyon, J. B., Hoover, D. M., Olson, R. K., Pennington, B. F.,

DeFries, J. C., et al. (2004). Refinement of the 6p21.3 quantitative trait locus influencing dyslexia: Linkage and association analyses. *Human Genetics, 115*(2), 128–138.

Dennis, M. Y., Paracchini, S., Scerri, T. S., Prokunina-Olsson, L., Knight, J. C., Wade-Martins, R., et al. (2009). A common variant associated with dyslexia reduces expression of the KIAA0319 gene. *PLoS Genetics, 5*(3), e1000436.

Depienne, C., Heron, D., Betancur, C., Benyahia, B., Trouillard, O., Bouteiller, D., et al. (2007). Autism, language delay and mental retardation in a patient with 7q11 duplication. *Journal of Medical Genetics, 44*(7), 452–458.

Durand, C. M., Betancur, C., Boeckers, T. M., Bockmann, J., Chaste, P., Fauchereau, F., et al. (2007). Mutations in the gene encoding the synaptic scaffolding protein SHANK3 are associated with autism spectrum disorders. *Nature Genetics, 39*(1), 25–27.

Durbin, R. M., Abecasis, G. R., Altshuler, D. L., Auton, A., Brooks, L. D., Gibbs, R. A., et al. (2010). A map of human genome variation from population-scale sequencing. *Nature, 467*(7319), 1061–1073.

Elbert, A., Lovett, M. W., Cate-Carter, T., Pitch, A., Kerr, E. N., & Barr, C. L. (2011). Genetic variation in the KIAA0319 5' region as a possible contributor to dyslexia. *Behavior Genetics, 41*(1), 77–89.

Elia, J., Gai, X., Xie, H. M., Perin, J. C., Geiger, E., Glessner, J. T., et al. (2009). Rare structural variants found in attention-deficit hyperactivity disorder are preferentially associated with neurodevelopmental genes. *Molecular Psychiatry, 15*(6), 637–646.

Etherton, M. R., Blaiss, C. A., Powell, C. M., & Sudhof, T. C. (2009). Mouse neurexin-1alpha deletion causes correlated electrophysiological and behavioral changes consistent with cognitive impairments. *Proceedings of the National Academy of Sciences of the United States of America, 106*(42), 17998–18003.

Falcaro, M., Pickles, A., Newbury, D. F., Addis, L., Banfield, E., Fisher, S. E., et al. (2008). Genetic and phenotypic effects of phonological short-term memory and grammatical morphology in specific language impairment. *Genes Brain and Behavior, 7*(4), 393–402.

Faraone, S. V., & Mick, E. (2010). Molecular genetics of attention deficit hyperactivity disorder. *Psychiatric Clinics of North America, 33*(1), 159–180.

Fernandez, B. A., Roberts, W., Chung, B., Weksberg, R., Meyn, S., Szatmari, P., et al. (2010). Phenotypic spectrum associated with de novo and inherited deletions and duplications at 16p11.2 in individuals ascertained for diagnosis of autism spectrum disorder. *Journal of Medical Genetics, 47*(3), 195–203.

Feuk, L., Kalervo, A., Lipsanen-Nyman, M., Skaug, J., Nakabayashi, K., Finucane, B., et al. (2006). Absence of a paternally inherited FOXP2 gene in developmental verbal dyspraxia. *American Journal of Human Genetics, 79*(5), 965–972.

Fisher, S. E., Marlow, A. J., Lamb, J., Maestrini, E., Williams, D. F., Richardson, A. J., et al. (1999). A quantitative-trait locus on chromosome 6p influences different aspects of developmental dyslexia. *American Journal of Human Genetics, 64*(1), 146–156.

Fisher, S. E., & Scharff, C. (2009). FOXP2 as a molecular window into speech and language. *Trends in Genetics, 25*(4), 166–177.

Fisher, S. E., Vargha-Khadem, F., Watkins, K. E., Monaco, A. P., & Pembrey, M. E. (1998). Localisation of a gene implicated in a severe speech and language disorder. *Nature Genetics, 18*(2), 168–170.

Francks, C., Paracchini, S., Smith, S. D., Richardson, A. J., Scerri, T. S., Cardon, L. R., et al. (2004). A 77–kilobase region of chromosome 6p22.2 is associated with dyslexia in families from the United Kingdom and from the United States. *American Journal of Human Genetics, 75*(6), 1046–1058.

Friedman, J. I., Vrijenhoek, T., Markx, S., Janssen, I. M., van der Vliet, W. A., Faas,

B. H., et al. (2008). CNTNAP2 gene dosage variation is associated with schizophrenia and epilepsy. *Molecular Psychiatry, 13*(3), 261–266.

Galaburda, A. M., Sherman, G. F., Rosen, G. D., Aboitiz, F., & Geschwind, N. (1985). Developmental dyslexia: Four consecutive patients with cortical anomalies. *Annals of Neurology, 18*(2), 222–233.

Gauthier, J., Spiegelman, D., Piton, A., Lafreniere, R. G., Laurent, S., St-Onge, J., et al. (2009). Novel de novo SHANK3 mutation in autistic patients. *American Journal of Medical Genetics B Neuropsychiatric Genetics, 150B*(3), 421–424.

Gayan, J., Smith, S. D., Cherny, S. S., Cardon, L. R., Fulker, D. W., Brower, A. M., et al. (1999). Quantitative-trait locus for specific language and reading deficits on chromosome 6p. *American Journal of Human Genetics, 64*(1), 157–164.

Gilman, S. R., Iossifov, I., Levy, D., Ronemus, M., Wigler, M., & Vitkup, D. (2011). Rare de novo variants associated with autism implicate a large functional network of genes involved in formation and function of synapses. *Neuron, 70*(5), 898–907.

Girirajan, S., Rosenfeld, J. A., Cooper, G. M., Antonacci, F., Siswara, P., Itsara, A., et al. (2010). A recurrent 16p12.1 microdeletion supports a two-hit model for severe developmental delay. *Nature Genetics, 42*(3), 203–209.

Glessner, J. T., Wang, K., Cai, G., Korvatska, O., Kim, C. E., Wood, S., et al. (2009). Autism genome-wide copy number variation reveals ubiquitin and neuronal genes. *Nature, 459*(7246), 569–573.

Grigorenko, E. L., Wood, F. B., Meyer, M. S., Hart, L. A., Speed, W. C., Shuster, A., et al. (1997). Susceptibility loci for distinct components of developmental dyslexia on chromosomes 6 and 15. *American Journal of Human Genetics, 60*(1), 27–39.

Grigorenko, E. L., Wood, F. B., Meyer, M. S., & Pauls, D. L. (2000). Chromosome 6p influences on different dyslexia-related cognitive processes: Further confirmation. *American Journal of Human Genetics, 66*(2), 715–723.

Guilmatre, A., Dubourg, C., Mosca, A. L., Legallic, S., Goldenberg, A., Drouin-Garraud, V., et al. (2009). Recurrent rearrangements in synaptic and neurodevelopmental genes and shared biologic pathways in schizophrenia, autism, and mental retardation. *Archives of General Psychiatry, 66*(9), 947–956.

Hamdan, F. F., Daoud, H., Rochefort, D., Piton, A., Gauthier, J., Langlois, M., et al. (2010). De novo mutations in FOXP1 in cases with intellectual disability, autism, and language impairment. *American Journal of Human Genetics, 87*(5), 671–678.

Hanson, E., Nasir, R. H., Fong, A., Lian, A., Hundley, R., Shen, Y., et al. (2010). Cognitive and Behavioral Characterization of 16p11.2 Deletion Syndrome. *Journal of Developmental and Behavioral Pediatrics, 31*(8), 649–657.

Helbig, I., Mefford, H. C., Sharp, A. J., Guipponi, M., Fichera, M., Franke, A., et al. (2009). 15q13.3 microdeletions increase risk of idiopathic generalized epilepsy. *Nature Genetics, 41*(2), 160–162.

Horn, D., Kapeller, J., Rivera-Brugues, N., Moog, U., Lorenz-Depiereux, B., Eck, S., et al. (2010). Identification of FOXP1 deletions in three unrelated patients with mental retardation and significant speech and language deficits. *Human Mutation, 31*(11), E1851–E1860.

Iafrate, A. J., Feuk, L., Rivera, M. N., Listewnik, M. L., Donahoe, P. K., Qi, Y., et al. (2004). Detection of large-scale variation in the human genome. *Nature Genetics, 36*(9), 949–951.

Jackman, C., Horn, N. D., Molleston, J. P., & Sokol, D. K. (2009). Gene associated with seizures, autism, and hepatomegaly in an Amish girl. *Pediatric Neurology, 40*(4), 310–313.

Jamain, S., Quach, H., Betancur, C., Rastam, M., Colineaux, C., Gillberg, I. C., et al.

(2003). Mutations of the X-linked genes encoding neuroligins NLGN3 and NLGN4 are associated with autism. *Nature Genetics, 34*(1), 27–29.

Jamain, S., Radyushkin, K., Hammerschmidt, K., Granon, S., Boretius, S., Varoqueaux, F., et al. (2008). Reduced social interaction and ultrasonic communication in a mouse model of monogenic heritable autism. *Proceedings of the National Academy of Sciences of the United States of America, 105*(5), 1710–1715.

Kang, C., & Drayna, D. (2011). Genetics of Speech and Language Disorders. *Annual Review of Genomics and Human Genetics, 12*, 145–164.

Kaplan, D. E., Gayan, J., Ahn, J., Won, T. W., Pauls, D., Olson, R. K., et al. (2002). Evidence for linkage and association with reading disability on 6p21.3–22. *American Journal of Human Genetics, 70*(5), 1287–1298.

Kim, H. G., Kishikawa, S., Higgins, A. W., Seong, I. S., Donovan, D. J., Shen, Y., et al. (2008). Disruption of neurexin 1 associated with autism spectrum disorder. *American Journal of Human Genetics, 82*(1), 199–207.

Konig, I. R., Schumacher, J., Hoffmann, P., Kleensang, A., Ludwig, K. U., Grimm, T., et al. (2011). Mapping for dyslexia and related cognitive trait loci provides strong evidence for further risk genes on chromosome 6p21. *American Journal of Medical Genetics B Neuropsychiatric Genetics, 156B*(1), 36–43.

Kraft, P. (2008). Curses – winner's and otherwise – in genetic epidemiology. *Epidemiology, 19*(5), 649–651; discussion 657–648.

Lai, C. S., Fisher, S. E., Hurst, J. A., Vargha-Khadem, F., & Monaco, A. P. (2001). A forkhead-domain gene is mutated in a severe speech and language disorder. *Nature, 413*(6855), 519–523.

Lander, E. S., Linton, L. M., Birren, B., Nusbaum, C., Zody, M. C., Baldwin, J., et al. (2001). Initial sequencing and analysis of the human genome. *Nature, 409*(6822), 860–921.

Laumonnier, F., Bonnet-Brilhault, F., Gomot, M., Blanc, R., David, A., Moizard, M. P., et al. (2004). X-linked mental retardation and autism are associated with a mutation in the NLGN4 gene, a member of the neuroligin family. *American Journal of Human Genetics, 74*(3), 552–557.

Lennon, P. A., Cooper, M. L., Peiffer, D. A., Gunderson, K. L., Patel, A., Peters, S., et al. (2007). Deletion of 7q31.1 supports involvement of FOXP2 in language impairment: clinical report and review. *American Journal of Medical Genetics A, 143*(8), 791–798.

Lesch, K. P., Timmesfeld, N., Renner, T. J., Halperin, R., Roser, C., Nguyen, T. T., et al. (2008). Molecular genetics of adult ADHD: converging evidence from genome-wide association and extended pedigree linkage studies. *Journal of Neural Transmission, 115*(11), 1573–1585.

Levinson, D. F., Duan, J., Oh, S., Wang, K., Sanders, A. R., Shi, J., et al. (2011). Copy number variants in schizophrenia: confirmation of five previous findings and new evidence for 3q29 microdeletions and VIPR2 duplications. *American Journal of Psychiatry, 168*(3), 302–316.

Levy, D., Ronemus, M., Yamrom, B., Lee, Y. H., Leotta, A., Kendall, J., et al. (2011). Rare de novo and transmitted copy-number variation in autistic spectrum disorders. *Neuron, 70*(5), 886–897.

Lim, C. K., Ho, C. S., Chou, C. H., & Waye, M. M. (2011). Association of the rs3743205 variant of DYX1C1 with dyslexia in Chinese children. *Behavioral and Brain Functions, 7*(1), 16.

Lind, P. A., Luciano, M., Wright, M. J., Montgomery, G. W., Martin, N. G., & Bates, T.

C. (2010). Dyslexia and DCDC2: Normal variation in reading and spelling is associated with DCDC2 polymorphisms in an Australian population sample. *European Journal of Human Genetics, 18*, 668–673.

Ludwig, K. U., Roeske, D., Schumacher, J., Schulte-Korne, G., Konig, I. R., Warnke, A., et al. (2008). Investigation of interaction between DCDC2 and KIAA0319 in a large German dyslexia sample. *Journal of Neural Transmission, 115*(11), 1587–1589.

Ma, D., Salyakina, D., Jaworski, J. M., Konidari, I., Whitehead, P. L., Andersen, A. N., et al. (2009). A genome-wide association study of autism reveals a common novel risk locus at 5p14.1. *Annals of Human Genetics, 73*(Pt 3), 263–273.

MacDermot, K. D., Bonora, E., Sykes, N., Coupe, A. M., Lai, C. S., Vernes, S. C., et al. (2005). Identification of FOXP2 truncation as a novel cause of developmental speech and language deficits. *American Journal of Human Genetics, 76*(6), 1074–1080.

Marlow, A. J., Fisher, S. E., Francks, C., MacPhie, I. L., Cherny, S. S., Richardson, A. J., et al. (2003). Use of multivariate linkage analysis for dissection of a complex cognitive trait. *American Journal of Human Genetics, 72*(3), 561–570.

Marshall, C. R., Noor, A., Vincent, J. B., Lionel, A. C., Feuk, L., Skaug, J., et al. (2008). Structural variation of chromosomes in autism spectrum disorder. *American Journal of Human Genetics, 82*(2), 477–488.

Meaburn, E., Dale, P. S., Craig, I. W., & Plomin, R. (2002). Language-impaired children: No sign of the FOXP2 mutation. *Neuroreport, 13*(8), 1075–1077.

Meda, S. A., Gelernter, J., Gruen, J. R., Calhoun, V. D., Meng, H., Cope, N. A., et al. (2008). Polymorphism of DCDC2 reveals differences in cortical morphology of healthy individuals: A preliminary voxel based morphometry study. *Brain Imaging and Behavior, 2*(1), 21–26.

Meechan, D. W., Maynard, T. M., Tucker, E. S., & LaMantia, A. S. (2011). Three phases of DiGeorge/22q11 deletion syndrome pathogenesis during brain development: patterning, proliferation, and mitochondrial functions of 22q11 genes. *International Journal of Developmental Neuroscience, 29*(3), 283–294.

Mefford, H. C., Muhle, H., Ostertag, P., von Spiczak, S., Buysse, K., Baker, C., et al. (2010). Genome-wide copy number variation in epilepsy: novel susceptibility loci in idiopathic generalized and focal epilepsies. *PLoS Genetics, 6*(5), e1000962.

Meng, H., Powers, N. R., Tang, L., Cope, N. A., Zhang, P. X., Fuleihan, R., et al. (2011). A dyslexia-associated variant in DCDC2 changes gene expression. *Behavior Genetics, 41*(1), 58–66.

Meng, H., Smith, S. D., Hager, K., Held, M., Liu, J., Olson, R. K., et al. (2005). DCDC2 is associated with reading disability and modulates neuronal development in the brain. *Proceedings of the National Academy of Sciences of the United States of America, 102*(47), 17053–17058.

Monaco, A. P. (2007). Multivariate linkage analysis of specific language impairment (SLI). *Annals of Human Genetics, 71*(5), 660–673.

Morrow, E. M. (2010). Genomic copy number variation in disorders of cognitive development. *Journal of the American Academy of Child and Adolescent Psychiatry, 49*(11), 1091–1104.

Newbury, D. F., Bonora, E., Lamb, J. A., Fisher, S. E., Lai, C. S., Baird, G., et al. (2002). FOXP2 is not a major susceptibility gene for autism or specific language impairment. *American Journal of Human Genetics, 70*(5), 1318–1327.

Newbury, D. F., & Monaco, A. P. (2010). Genetic advances in the study of speech and language disorders. *Neuron, 68*(2), 309–320.

Newbury, D. F., Paracchini, S., Scerri, T. S., Winchester, L., Addis, L., Richardson, A. J., et al. (2011). Investigation of dyslexia and SLI risk variants in reading- and language-impaired subjects. *Behavior Genetics, 41*(1), 90–104.

Newbury, D. F., Winchester, L., Addis, L., Paracchini, S., Buckingham, L. L., Clark, A., et al. (2009). CMIP and ATP2C2 modulate phonological short-term memory in language impairment. *American Journal of Human Genetics, 85*(2), 264–272.

Nopola-Hemmi, J., Taipale, M., Haltia, T., Lehesjoki, A. E., Voutilainen, A., & Kere, J. (2000). Two translocations of chromosome 15q associated with dyslexia. *Journal of Medical Genetics, 37*(10), 771–775.

O'Brien, E. K., Zhang, X., Nishimura, C., Tomblin, J. B., & Murray, J. C. (2003). Association of specific language impairment (SLI) to the region of 7q31. *American Journal of Human Genetics, 72*(6), 1536–1543.

O'Dushlaine, C., Kenny, E., Heron, E., Donohoe, G., Gill, M., Morris, D., et al. (2010). Molecular pathways involved in neuronal cell adhesion and membrane scaffolding contribute to schizophrenia and bipolar disorder susceptibility. *Molecular Psychiatry, 16*(3), 286–292.

O'Roak, B. J., Deriziotis, P., Lee, C., Vives, L., Schwartz, J. J., Girirajan, S., et al. (2011). Exome sequencing in sporadic autism spectrum disorders identifies severe de novo mutations. *Nature Genetics, 43*(6), 585–589.

Pagnamenta, A. T., Bacchelli, E., de Jonge, M. V., Mirza, G., Scerri, T. S., Minopoli, F., et al. (2010). Characterization of a family with rare deletions in CNTNAP5 and DOCK4 suggests novel risk loci for autism and dyslexia. *Biological Psychiatry, 68*(4), 320–328.

Pagnamenta, A. T., Wing, K., Akha, E. S., Knight, S. J., Bolte, S., Schmotzer, G., et al. (2009). A 15q13.3 microdeletion segregating with autism. *European Journal of Human Genetics, 17*(5), 687–692.

Paracchini, S., Thomas, A., Castro, S., Lai, C., Paramasivam, M., Wang, Y., et al. (2006). The chromosome 6p22 haplotype associated with dyslexia reduces the expression of KIAA0319, a novel gene involved in neuronal migration. *Human Molecular Genetics, 15*(10), 1659–1666.

Pariani, M. J., Spencer, A., Graham, J. M., Jr., & Rimoin, D. L. (2009). A 785kb deletion of 3p14.1p13, including the FOXP1 gene, associated with speech delay, contractures, hypertonia and blepharophimosis. *European Journal of Medical Genetics, 52*(2–3), 123–127.

Peca, J., Feliciano, C., Ting, J. T., Wang, W., Wells, M. F., Venkatraman, T. N., et al. (2011). Shank3 mutant mice display autistic-like behaviours and striatal dysfunction. *Nature, 472*(7344), 437–442.

Peschansky, V. J., Burbridge, T. J., Volz, A. J., Fiondella, C., Wissner-Gross, Z., Galaburda, A. M., et al. (2010). The effect of variation in expression of the candidate dyslexia susceptibility gene homolog Kiaa0319 on neuronal migration and dendritic morphology in the rat. *Cerebral Cortex, 20*(4), 884–897.

Petrin, A. L., Giacheti, C. M., Maximino, L. P., Abramides, D. V., Zanchetta, S., Rossi, N. F., et al. (2010). Identification of a microdeletion at the 7q33–q35 disrupting the CNTNAP2 gene in a Brazilian stuttering case. *American Journal of Medical Genetics A, 152A*(12), 3164–3172.

Pinto, D., Pagnamenta, A. T., Klei, L., Anney, R., Merico, D., Regan, R., et al. (2010). Functional impact of global rare copy number variation in autism spectrum disorders. *Nature, 466*(7304), 368–372.

Poelmans, G., Pauls, D. L., Buitelaar, J. K., & Franke, B. (2011). Integrated genome-wide association study findings: Identification of a neurodevelopmental network for attention deficit hyperactivity disorder. *American Journal of Psychiatry, 168*(4), 365–377.

Poot, M., Beyer, V., Schwaab, I., Damatova, N., Van't Slot, R., Prothero, J., et al. (2009). Disruption of CNTNAP2 and additional structural genome changes in a boy with speech delay and autism spectrum disorder. *Neurogenetics, 11*, 81–89.

Posthuma, D., Luciano, M., Geus, E. J., Wright, M. J., Slagboom, P. E., Montgomery, G. W., et al. (2005). A genomewide scan for intelligence identifies quantitative trait loci on 2q and 6p. *American Journal of Human Genetics, 77*(2), 318–326.

Redon, R., Ishikawa, S., Fitch, K. R., Feuk, L., Perry, G. H., Andrews, T. D., et al. (2006). Global variation in copy number in the human genome. *Nature, 444*(7118), 444–454.

Rice, M. L., Smith, S. D., & Gayan, J. (2009). Convergent genetic linkage and associations to language, speech and reading measures in families of probands with Specific Language Impairment. *Journal of Neurodevelopmental Disorders, 1*(4), 264–282.

Roohi, J., Montagna, C., Tegay, D. H., Palmer, L. E., DeVincent, C., Pomeroy, J. C., et al. (2009). Disruption of contactin 4 in three subjects with autism spectrum disorder. *Journal of Medical Genetics, 46*(3), 176–182.

Rosen, G. D., Bai, J., Wang, Y., Fiondella, C. G., Threlkeld, S. W., LoTurco, J. J., et al. (2007). Disruption of neuronal migration by RNAi of Dyx1c1 results in neocortical and hippocampal malformations. *Cerebral Cortex, 17*(11), 2562–2572.

Rossi, E., Verri, A. P., Patricelli, M. G., Destefani, V., Ricca, I., Vetro, A., et al. (2008). A 12Mb deletion at 7q33–q35 associated with autism spectrum disorders and primary amenorrhea. *European Journal of Medical Genetics, 51*(6), 631–638.

Roth, T. L., Roth, E. D., & Sweatt, J. D. (2010). Epigenetic regulation of genes in learning and memory. *Essays in Biochemistry, 48*(1), 263–274.

Sanders, S. J., Ercan-Sencicek, A. G., Hus, V., Luo, R., Murtha, M. T., Moreno-De-Luca, D., et al. (2011). Multiple recurrent de novo CNVs, including duplications of the 7q11.23 Williams Syndrome region, are strongly associated with autism. *Neuron, 70*(5), 863–885.

Scerri, T. S., & Schulte-Korne, G. (2009). Genetics of developmental dyslexia. *European Child and Adolescent Psychiatry, 19*(3), 179–197.

Schulte-Korne, G., Grimm, T., Nothen, M. M., Muller-Myhsok, B., Cichon, S., Vogt, I. R., et al. (1998). Evidence for linkage of spelling disability to chromosome 15. *American Journal of Human Genetics, 63*(1), 279–282.

Schumacher, J., Anthoni, H., Dahdouh, F., Konig, I. R., Hillmer, A. M., Kluck, N., et al. (2006). Strong genetic evidence of DCDC2 as a susceptibility gene for dyslexia. *American Journal of Human Genetics, 78*(1), 52–62.

Sebat, J., Lakshmi, B., Malhotra, D., Troge, J., Lese-Martin, C., Walsh, T., et al. (2007). Strong association of de novo copy number mutations with autism. *Science, 316*(5823), 445–449.

Sebat, J., Lakshmi, B., Troge, J., Alexander, J., Young, J., Lundin, P., et al. (2004). Large-scale copy number polymorphism in the human genome. *Science, 305*(5683), 525–528.

Sharp, A. J., Mefford, H. C., Li, K., Baker, C., Skinner, C., Stevenson, R. E., et al. (2008). A recurrent 15q13.3 microdeletion syndrome associated with mental retardation and seizures. *Nature Genetics, 40*(3), 322–328.

Shinawi, M., Liu, P., Kang, S. H., Shen, J., Belmont, J. W., Scott, D. A., et al. (2010). Recurrent reciprocal 16p11.2 rearrangements associated with global developmental delay, behavioural problems, dysmorphism, epilepsy, and abnormal head size. *Journal of Medical Genetics, 47*(5), 332–341.

Shriberg, L. D., Ballard, K. J., Tomblin, J. B., Duffy, J. R., Odell, K. H., & Williams, C. A.

(2006). Speech, prosody, and voice characteristics of a mother and daughter with a 7;13 translocation affecting FOXP2. *Journal of Speech, Language, and Hearing Research, 49*(3), 500–525.

Silani, G., Frith, U., Demonet, J. F., Fazio, F., Perani, D., Price, C., et al. (2005). Brain abnormalities underlying altered activation in dyslexia: A voxel based morphometry study. *Brain, 128*(Pt 10), 2453–2461.

Simmons, T. R., Flax, J. F., Azaro, M. A., Hayter, J. E., Justice, L. M., Petrill, S. A., et al. (2010). Increasing genotype-phenotype model determinism: Application to bivariate reading/language traits and epistatic interactions in language-impaired families. *Human Heredity, 70*(4), 232–244.

SLI Consortium. (2002). A genomewide scan identifies two novel loci involved in specific language impairment. *American Journal of Human Genetics, 70*(2), 384–398.

SLI Consortium. (2004). Highly significant linkage to the SLI1 locus in an expanded sample of individuals affected by specific language impairment. *American Journal of Human Genetics, 74*(6), 1225–1238.

Smith, S. D., Pennington, B. F., Boada, R., & Shriberg, L. D. (2005). Linkage of speech sound disorder to reading disability loci. *Journal of Child Psychology and Psychiatry and Allied Disciplines, 46*(10), 1057–1066.

Spiteri, E., Konopka, G., Coppola, G., Bomar, J., Oldham, M., Ou, J., et al. (2007). Identification of the transcriptional targets of FOXP2, a gene linked to speech and language, in developing human brain. *American Journal of Human Genetics, 81*(6), 1144–1157.

Stankiewicz, P., & Lupski, J. R. (2010). Structural variation in the human genome and its role in disease. *Annual Review of Medicine, 61*, 437–455.

Stefansson, H., Ophoff, R. A., Steinberg, S., Andreassen, O. A., Cichon, S., Rujescu, D., et al. (2009). Common variants conferring risk of schizophrenia. *Nature, 460*(7256), 744–747.

Stein, M. B., Yang, B. Z., Chavira, D. A., Hitchcock, C. A., Sung, S. C., Shipon-Blum, E., et al. (2011). A common genetic variant in the neurexin superfamily member CNTNAP2 is associated with increased risk for selective mutism and social anxiety-related traits. *Biological Psychiatry, 69*(9), 825–831.

Strauss, K. A., Puffenberger, E. G., Huentelman, M. J., Gottlieb, S., Dobrin, S. E., Parod, J. M., et al. (2006). Recessive symptomatic focal epilepsy and mutant contactin-associated protein-like 2. *New England Journal of Medicine, 354*(13), 1370–1377.

Szalkowski, C. E., Hinman, J. R., Threlkeld, S. W., Wang, Y., LePack, A., Rosen, G. D., et al. (2011). Persistent spatial working memory deficits in rats following in utero RNAi of Dyx1c1. *Genes Brain and Behavior, 10*(2), 244–252.

Taipale, M., Kaminen, N., Nopola-Hemmi, J., Haltia, T., Myllyluoma, B., Lyytinen, H., et al. (2003). A candidate gene for developmental dyslexia encodes a nuclear tetratricopeptide repeat domain protein dynamically regulated in brain. *Proceedings of the National Academy of Sciences of the United States of America, 100*(20), 11553–11558.

Threlkeld, S. W., McClure, M. M., Bai, J., Wang, Y., LoTurco, J. J., Rosen, G. D., et al. (2007). Developmental disruptions and behavioral impairments in rats following in utero RNAi of Dyx1c1. *Brain Research Bulletin, 71*(5), 508–514.

Tomblin, J. B., O'Brien, M., Shriberg, L. D., Williams, C., Murray, J., Patil, S., et al. (2009). Language features in a mother and daughter of a chromosome 7;13 translocation involving FOXP2. *Journal of Speech, Language, and Hearing Research, 52*(5), 1157–1174.

Toro, R., Konyukh, M., Delorme, R., Leblond, C., Chaste, P., Fauchereau, F., et al. (2010).

Key role for gene dosage and synaptic homeostasis in autism spectrum disorders. *Trends in Genetics, 26*(8), 363–372.

Van der Aa, N., Rooms, L., Vandeweyer, G., van den Ende, J., Reyniers, E., Fichera, M., et al. (2009). Fourteen new cases contribute to the characterization of the 7q11.23 microduplication syndrome. *European Journal of Medical Genetics, 52*(2–3), 94–100.

Velayos-Baeza, A., Toma, C., da Roza, S., Paracchini, S., & Monaco, A. P. (2007). Alternative splicing in the dyslexia-associated gene KIAA0319. *Mammalian Genome, 18*(9), 627–634.

Velayos-Baeza, A., Toma, C., Paracchini, S., & Monaco, A. P. (2008). The dyslexia-associated gene KIAA0319 encodes highly N- and O-glycosylated plasma membrane and secreted isoforms. *Human Molecular Genetics, 17*(6), 859–871.

Venter, J. C., Adams, M. D., Myers, E. W., Li, P. W., Mural, R. J., Sutton, G. G., et al. (2001). The sequence of the human genome. *Science, 291*(5507), 1304–1351.

Verkerk, A. J., Mathews, C. A., Joosse, M., Eussen, B. H., Heutink, P., & Oostra, B. A. (2003). CNTNAP2 is disrupted in a family with Gilles de la Tourette syndrome and obsessive compulsive disorder. *Genomics, 82*(1), 1–9.

Vernes, S. C., MacDermot, K. D., Monaco, A. P., & Fisher, S. E. (2009). Assessing the impact of FOXP1 mutations on developmental verbal dyspraxia. *European Journal of Human Genetics, 17*(10), 1354–1358.

Vernes, S. C., Newbury, D. F., Abrahams, B. S., Winchester, L., Nicod, J., Groszer, M., et al. (2008). A functional genetic link between distinct developmental language disorders. *New England Journal of Medicine, 359*(22), 2337–2345.

Vernes, S. C., Spiteri, E., Nicod, J., Groszer, M., Taylor, J. M., Davies, K. E., et al. (2007). High-throughput analysis of promoter occupancy reveals direct neural targets of FOXP2, a gene mutated in speech and language disorders. *American Journal of Human Genetics, 81*(6), 1232–1250.

Villanueva, P., Newbury, D. F., Jara, L., De Barbieri, Z., Mirza, G., Palomino, H. M., et al. (2011). Genome-wide analysis of genetic susceptibility to language impairment in an isolated Chilean population. *European Journal of Human Genetics, 19*(6), 687–695.

Voineagu, I., Wang, X., Johnston, P., Lowe, J. K., Tian, Y., Horvath, S., et al. (2011). Transcriptomic analysis of autistic brain reveals convergent molecular pathology. *Nature, 474*(7351), 380–384.

Wang, K., Zhang, H., Ma, D., Bucan, M., Glessner, J. T., Abrahams, B. S., et al. (2009). Common genetic variants on 5p14.1 associate with autism spectrum disorders. *Nature, 459*(7246), 528–533.

Wang, Y., Paramasivam, M., Thomas, A., Bai, J., Kaminen-Ahola, N., Kere, J., et al. (2006). DYX1C1 functions in neuronal migration in developing neocortex. *Neuroscience, 143*(2), 515–522.

Wang, Y., Yin, X., Rosen, G., Gabel, L., Guadiana, S. M., Sarkisian, M. R., et al. (2011). Dcdc2 knockout mice display exacerbated developmental disruptions following knockdown of doublecortin. *Neuroscience, 190*, 398–408.

Weiss, L. A., Arking, D. E., Daly, M. J., & Chakravarti, A. (2009). A genome-wide linkage and association scan reveals novel loci for autism. *Nature, 461*(7265), 802–808.

Weiss, L. A., Shen, Y., Korn, J. M., Arking, D. E., Miller, D. T., Fossdal, R., et al. (2008). Association between microdeletion and microduplication at 16p11.2 and autism. *New England Journal of Medicine, 358*(7), 667–675.

Wigg, K. G., Couto, J. M., Feng, Y., Anderson, B., Cate-Carter, T. D., Macciardi, F., et al. (2004). Support for EKN1 as the susceptibility locus for dyslexia on 15q21. *Molecular Psychiatry, 9*(12), 1111–1121.

Wigg, K. G., Feng, Y., Crosbie, J., Tannock, R., Kennedy, J. L., Ickowicz, A., et al. (2008). Association of ADHD and the Protogenin gene in the chromosome 15q21.3 reading disabilities linkage region. *Genes Brain and Behavior, 7*(8), 877–886.

Willcutt, E. G., Pennington, B. F., Duncan, L., Smith, S. D., Keenan, J. M., Wadsworth, S., et al. (2010). Understanding the complex etiologies of developmental disorders: Behavioral and molecular genetic approaches. *Journal of Developmental and Behavioral Pediatrics, 31*(7), 533–544.

Williams, J. C., Barratt-Boyes, B. G., & Lowe, J. B. (1961). Supravalvular aortic stenosis. *Circulation, 24*, 1311–1318.

Williams, N. M., Zaharieva, I., Martin, A., Langley, K., Mantripragada, K., Fossdal, R., et al. (2010). Rare chromosomal deletions and duplications in attention-deficit hyperactivity disorder: A genome-wide analysis. *Lancet, 376*(9750), 1401–1408.

Zahir, F. R., Baross, A., Delaney, A. D., Eydoux, P., Fernandes, N. D., Pugh, T., et al. (2008). A patient with vertebral, cognitive and behavioural abnormalities and a de novo deletion of NRXN1alpha. *Journal of Medical Genetics, 45*(4), 239–243.

Zeesman, S., Nowaczyk, M. J., Teshima, I., Roberts, W., Cardy, J. O., Brian, J., et al. (2006). Speech and language impairment and oromotor dyspraxia due to deletion of 7q31 that involves FOXP2. *American Journal of Medical Genetics A, 140*(5), 509–514.

Zhou, K., Dempfle, A., Arcos-Burgos, M., Bakker, S. C., Banaschewski, T., Biederman, J., et al. (2008). Meta-analysis of genome-wide linkage scans of attention deficit hyperactivity disorder. *American Journal of Medical Genetics B Neuropsychiatric Genetics, 147B*(8), 1392–1398.

Zweier, C., de Jong, E. K., Zweier, M., Orrico, A., Ousager, L. B., Collins, A. L., et al. (2009). CNTNAP2 and NRXN1 are mutated in autosomal-recessive Pitt-Hopkins-like mental retardation and determine the level of a common synaptic protein in Drosophila. *American Journal of Human Genetics, 85*(5), 655–666.

3   The longitudinal perspective on developmental disorders

Brian Byrne, Richard K. Olson,
and Stefan Samuelsson

Introduction

In this chapter we use developmental dyslexia to exemplify the value of employing longitudinal designs in research on developmental disorders. We show that a full understanding of dyslexia, its characteristics, its causes, and its treatment, depends on studying it longitudinally, and failing to do so would lead to an impoverished account of the disorder. We also make reference to other disabilities as a way of testing the generality and value of our conclusions from dyslexia.

What kind of disorder is developmental dyslexia?

There are two main forms of dyslexia, *acquired* and *developmental*. Acquired dyslexia is impairment in reading and writing that results from brain injury or disease, often in adulthood and after literacy skills have been established. Developmental dyslexia is impairment that emerges during the course of learning to read and for which there appears to be no gross brain damage of the kind seen in the acquired form. Although researchers have explored the degree of similarity between the two forms (e.g., Coltheart, 2005), for this volume we restrict ourselves to developmental dyslexia, and refer to it simply as *dyslexia*.

We first consider issues surrounding the definition of dyslexia in order to place it more broadly within the variety of developmental disorders. To summarize in advance, we characterize dyslexia as a quantitative trait, the low end of a normal distribution, and one that is best studied in its own right rather than only when it is defined as a discrepancy between literacy levels and general intelligence. It may come in a variety of forms, or *subtypes*, though this is a contested issue.

Formal definitions

The current *Diagnostic and Statistical Manual of the American Psychiatric Association* (*DSM-IV-TR*) defines dyslexia (or "reading disorder" as it prefers) in part as follows:

> Reading achievement, as measured by individually administered standardized tests of reading accuracy or comprehension, is substantially below that

expected given the person's chronological age, measured intelligence, and age-appropriate education.

(American Psychiatric Association, 2000, p. 53)

The next edition of the manual, *DSM-5*, is currently being planned. It is proposed that the disorder be actually named *dyslexia*, "consistent with international use," with the following definition:

> Difficulties in accuracy or fluency of reading that are not consistent with the person's chronological age, educational opportunities, or intellectual abilities.
>
> Multiple sources of information are to be used to assess reading, one of which must be an individually administered, culturally appropriate, and psychometrically sound standardized measure of reading and reading-related abilities.

(American Psychiatric Association, 2012)

The primary change in the *DSM-5* draft is the exclusion of difficulties in reading comprehension, which do figure in *DSM-IV-TR*. Both versions agree that word reading ("decoding") is a key criterion, but additional notes supplied with the planned *DSM-5* definition assigns failures in reading comprehension to broader oral language impairments. This decision is motivated by a well-accepted framework supplied by Hoover and Gough's (1990) "simple view" of reading, which holds that reading comprehension, referred to as R, is the product of processes that support oral language comprehension, L (for language), and D (decoding): $R = L \times D$. This idea has proven robust in a great deal of research besides Hoover and Gough's original contribution (e.g., Keenan, Betjemann, Wadsworth, DeFries, & Olson, 2006).

For this chapter we will use the current (*DSM-IV-TR*) version, that is, include problems in reading comprehension. We mention the proposal to shed comprehension in *DSM-5*, however, because it demonstrates one advantage of adopting a longitudinal perspective on developmental disorders – provision of a more complete characterization of them. It turns out that a dissociation between decoding accuracy and fluency on the one hand and text comprehension on the other is only in evidence once children have advanced to more mature levels of word identification. In the earliest school grades variability in comprehension is almost fully determined by variability in decoding. It is only as decoding becomes relatively automatic that separate sources of variance in comprehension start to come into play (in fact, these are processes central to comprehension of oral language, such as working memory, mastery of grammatical structures, and vocabulary) (Keenan et al., 2006; Keenan, Betjemann, & Olson, 2008). So the complexities of reading difficulties, broadly defined as encompassing how successfully an individual extracts meaning from text, only become clear from a longitudinal perspective.

More generally, purely cross-sectional study of a disorder at a single age risks generating an inaccurate description of it, in the case of dyslexia, that decoding and text comprehension form a single construct. This, in turn, would likely underestimate the complexity of causes, in the case of dyslexia, that all problems stem from poor decoding, and point to a more restricted range of treatments than are actually needed, for dyslexia that only word-level (decoding) processes need be targeted.

There are other examples of developmental change. In attention deficit/hyperactivity disorder (ADHD), hyperactivity, but not inattention, actually declines in severity as children grow older (Ebejer et al., 2010; Rietveld, Hudziak, Bartels, van Beijsterveldt, & Boomsma, 2004; Smith, Barkley, & Shapiro, 2006). This observation might be relevant to a public perception that ADHD is "just" the "symptoms of childhood" (more likely in the case of hyperactivity), and offer some hope for families of young children showing signs of hyperactivity. The most convincing case for age-based changes comes from following the same children longitudinally, akin to the power and precision advantages of within-subject compared to between-subject designs in experimental psychology.

The discrepancy issue

We highlight one other difference between *DSM-IV-TR* and *DSM-5*: the change in wording about the "discrepancy" criterion. In *DSM-IV-TR*, for dyslexia to be diagnosed, reading must be "substantially below" intelligence (plus age and educational opportunities), in *DSM-5* this is relaxed to be "not consistent" with these factors. The rationale offered by the *DSM* development team is that "there is little evidence to support the *DSM-IV-TR* criterion of a substantial discrepancy between achievement and intellectual ability" (http://www.dsm5.org/Proposed Revision/Pages/proposedrevision.aspx?rid=84#). We concur with the decision. The pattern of reading performance and the pattern of associated cognitive deficits (apart from IQ itself) has not been found to differ much between groups of reading-impaired children with and without an IQ discrepancy (Stanovich, 1994; Stanovich & Siegel, 1994; Vellutino, Scanlan, & Lyon, 2000), and in a large-scale study of remediation the degree of discrepancy between IQ and reading scores did not predict how well children responded to intensive one-on-one daily tutoring (Vellutino & Fletcher, 2005).

The discrepancy question arises in other developmental disabilities defined by academic achievement, such as marked deficiencies in mathematics ("dyscalculia"). Should only those children who are at or above normal in IQ be included in the definition and, by extension, in research? We suggest that, broadly, decisions to exclude non-discrepant children will restrict the value of research, including longitudinal research where the relations between the disability and other mental constructs are the focus. With dyslexia, for example, it is known that with age the amount of reading that children engage in is likely to influence IQ measures, if only because vocabulary is part of most IQ tests and reading experience contributes to vocabulary growth (Anderson & Nagy, 1992). If the effect is cumulative, as is likely, then IQ and reading skill will become more closely aligned over time (again, better seen in longitudinal studies). But this change might appear larger in a group of disabled readers defined by discrepancy than in a group where discrepancy is not a selection criterion because the correlation will be lower in the first place for the discrepancy-defined group as a consequence of range restriction in the IQ scores. Hence there is more room for an increase with time. In general, definitions matter in developmental disabilities, not only for practice but also for research, perhaps particularly for longitudinal studies (for additional arguments against the discrepancy criterion, see Williams & Lind, this volume).

Quantitative versus qualitative traits

A further issue that needs to be considered is whether it is better to think of dyslexia as a qualitative trait, a distinct disability akin to measles that a person either has or does not have, or as a quantitative trait, a graded disability akin to obesity that differs from being somewhat overweight only by degree. We interpret the current consensus on this as favouring the quantitative trait stance. Scores on standardized tests of reading show a decidedly Gaussian distribution (no "lump" in the low tail; Rodgers, 1983). Evidence from behaviour-genetic research is so far consistent with the quantitative trait hypothesis (Kovas, Haworth, Dale, & Plomin, 2007; Plomin & Kovas, 2005), and among children with a familial risk for dyslexia (parents and/or siblings with the disorder) the risk liability is a continuous variable, not a categorical one (Snowling, Gallagher, & Frith, 2003).

This means that use of the term *dyslexia* is inappropriate to the degree that it implies a categorically distinct entity. If all that is meant is reading ability in the lowest 5 percent (or 10, or 15 percent . . .), then its use is less loaded with unwarranted assumptions. That is how we will use the term.

One advantage of a quantitative approach to dyslexia is that researchers and practitioners can draw on the large volume of research on reading ability across the full range. This includes the kind of longitudinal research into treatment that we will summarize later. To the degree that we understand the cognitive steps that children go through in learning to read (Byrne, 1998, 2005), we also begin to understand where the processes can fail, leading to reading disability. To the degree that we understand the best ways to tailor instruction to guide young learners through those steps, we also begin to understand how best to intervene in a preventative way or to remediate reading disability if it begins to establish.

As a quantitative trait, dyslexia is like some other developmental disabilities, such as mathematics learning difficulties, insofar as the causes are best thought of as continuous with those affecting normal-range variation. It is unlike others, such as mental retardation associated with chromosomal abnormalities, whose causes are likely to be categorically distinct from those affecting normal-range variation. Consequently, the advantages conferred by employing longitudinal approaches in research may apply more firmly to some than other disabilities. For example, intervention based on the idea that disability is best treated using (presumably more intensive) versions of normally successful teaching methods may not apply to qualitative traits. This, of course, is an open question, one that can only be answered empirically, but as a starting point it may be imprudent to assume transfer from one kind of trait to another.

Subtypes

Several researchers contend that dyslexia comes in different forms, defined by the kinds of deficits that sufferers exhibit. One distinction is due largely to Coltheart and his group (Castles & Coltheart, 1993; Coltheart, 2005) between "phonological" and "surface" dyslexia. Phonological dyslexics are troubled by nonwords such as *flub* and *pontflact* but read familiar words adequately, including irregular ones such as *once*, *yacht* and *knight*, and surface dyslexics show the opposite pattern – adequate decoding ability (reading nonwords) but deficient memorization skills for whole words, including irregular words. Other subtypes that have been proposed include one that differentiates problems in reading fluency versus reading accuracy (Lovett, 1984), and one that bears some similarity to Lovett's, due to Wolf and Bowers (1999).

There is considerable discussion about the utility of subtypes, particularly phonological versus surface dyslexia (e.g., Coltheart, 2005; Plaut, 2005). Vellutino and Fletcher (2005) summarize evidence that surface dyslexia does not appear to be stable across development, more prevalent in younger children. So it has been suggested that it may be a transient disorder, due to limited reading experience (Stanovich, 2000), with some supporting evidence from Zabell and Everatt (2002). However, the case for this subtype distinction is bolstered by the finding from Castles, Datta, Gayan, and Olson (1999) that the mix of genetic and environmental influences differs between the two types, with higher heritability for phonological dyslexia. It would take us too far afield to explore this question fully, but we mention it here as an example of an issue for which longitudinal data are particularly valuable, as they are in the case of hyperactivity – the stability or otherwise of particular developmental disabilities or of their proposed subtypes.

A similar set of issues arise for other developmental disabilities. ADHD has already been mentioned, with a distinction made between inattentive, hyperactive, and combined types (Barkley & Murphy, 1998). Autism, too, appears to segregate partly according to the dominance of communication, social integration, or behavioural (repetitiveness, restricted interests) aspects (Filipek et al., 1999). Longitudinal data that tracks the trajectory of the hypothesized variants would be of value on a number of grounds; differential long-term patterns, or differential outcomes in the face of treatments, for example, would tend to confirm the validity of the distinctions.

Prediction in developmental disability research

There are two types of situations in which prediction forms the basis of research: where the disability is not apparent at birth, and where it is important to know the likely developmental trajectory of the disability once it has been diagnosed. In both cases there is no substitute for longitudinal research. We have already referred to research that traces the course of developmental dyslexia, for example addressing the subtype issue. In this section we cover studies designed to predict the onset of impaired reading.

Predicting the onset of reading impairment

Reading impairment does not show up with certainty until literacy instruction has been instituted and a child begins to falter, generally at school. There are no tests that can be given to detect impending dyslexia analogous to fluorescent in situ hybridizationscreening for chromosomal abnormalities (see Williams & Lind, this volume). Nevertheless, there are factors that increase the liability for dyslexia. The primary one is a family history of reading difficulties. It has been known for over a hundred years that reading difficulties run in families (Thomas, 1905) with later, more substantial studies, providing additional evidence (e.g., Hallgren, 1950). Children in families where one or both parents are dyslexic have a much higher than normal likelihood of themselves experiencing reading difficulties (Gilger, Pennington, & DeFries, 1991), and relatives of children diagnosed with dyslexia are more likely than normal to exhibit reading difficulties (DeFries, Singer, Foch, & Lewitter, 1978).

Families share both genes and environments, but behaviour-genetic research, that can disambiguate genetic from environmental influence, has confirmed that genes are substantially responsible for familial aggregation of marked reading difficulties as well as for normal-range variability in reading, with estimates of the proportion of variability in marked impairment and normal-range reading ranging from about 50 percent to as high as 80 percent (Byrne, Fielding-Barnsley, & Ashley, 2000; Byrne et al., 2006, 2009; Olson, Byrne & Samuelsson, 2009; Pennington & Olson, 2005; Samuelsson et al., 2005).

Several research projects have attempted to identify the critical factors within the group of children at familial risk that lead to the actual emergence of reading impairment. This research is valuable not only for illuminating candidate causes but also for suggesting intervention strategies. It can also be applied to children where there is no known family history – reading difficulties emerge in these children too.

Scarborough (1989) pioneered this kind of longitudinal study, selecting children whose family members had experienced reading difficulties and following them over time. In Grade 2 two-thirds of the sample had become disabled readers, and almost all of the control sample (29/31 with no known family reading disability) had become normal readers. Testing conducted on the children at around 60 months showed that vocabulary, phonological awareness and letter identification (but not IQ, socioeconomic status, gender, or age) were also good predictors of subsequent reading status.

Perhaps the most ambitious project of this kind was initiated in Finland in 1992 with the selection of 107 mothers-to-be in risk families (one or both parents plus at least one close relative with marked reading difficulties) and 93 control mothers, with their children to be followed from birth to school entry and beyond. There is now a substantial body of research from this study (e.g., Guttorm et al., 2005; Lyytinen, Aro et al., 2006; Lyytinen, Erskine et al., 2006; Lyytinen et al., 2005). The data confirm that family history of dyslexia is indeed a risk factor, with around half of the children in that group showing signs of delayed reading (Lyytinen, Erskine et al., 2006). There were several trajectories into reading impairment, characterized by differing patterns on preliteracy measures over a wide variety of language and other cognitive tasks, collected between 12 months and 5 years of age. One group showed a general decline in most measures over time except for processing speed measured by rapid naming, while a second showed particular impairment in processing speed (and subsequently low reading fluency). In both of these groups, at-risk children predominated. A third group, with equal numbers of risk and non-risk children, showed an unexpectedly low level of letter-name knowledge, and the risk subgroup turned out to remain low in reading accuracy in school. In another study (Guttorm et al., 2005), it was shown that event-related potential (ERP) patterns for speech that typified at-risk children (compared to controls), in particular prolonged positivity to a /ga/ stimulus at around 600m sec in the right hemisphere, modestly predicted some language skills prior to school, indicating that neural responses in infancy might already announce possible language and literacy difficulties several years later.

Research by Hindson, Byrne, Fielding-Barnsley, Newman, Hine, and Shankweiler (2005) confirmed that at-risk children show a variety of deficiencies prior to school entry, particularly in vocabulary, phonological awareness, letter and print knowledge, and speed of phonological processing (articulation rate in this case). Nonverbal IQ was also compromised in these children. We report longitudinal aspects of this project later.

One message to be taken from these studies is that reading difficulties are preceded by signs of impairment in language and cognitive processes such as phonological awareness, print knowledge, vocabulary, and speed of phonological processing. The same processes are known to correlate with established reading levels in school-aged children and in adults (Bruck, 1992; Snowling, 2000), but the risk research helps establish that low levels of these cognitive and linguistic processes in dyslexia are not simply the consequence of impaired reading ability – they precede it – so they may be causal, or the two domains may be linked by shared variables.

Describing the developmental trajectory of developmental disabilities

Most research that we will review under this heading concerns how individuals react to various intervention strategies, and we will consider them in a later section. Here we mention one informative study that illustrates the value of combining longitudinal and neuroscientific research (Hoeft et al., 2011). This study followed a group of dyslexic children over 2.5 years. They measured initial brain function through functional magnetic resonance imaging (fMRI) while the children performed a rhyme judgement task, and white matter integrity through diffusion tensor magnetic imaging (DTI). They identified the right inferior frontal gyrus (IFG) through fMRI and the right superior longitudinal fasciculus (SLF) through DTI as regions that correlated with growth in word identification in the dyslexic group but not in normal control children. The neural measures were better predictors of reading progress than a variety of other cognitive ones, suggesting that "neuroprognosis" holds promise for prediction in developmental disabilities. This project also offers longitudinal confirmation that white matter integrity plays a role in dyslexia (Klingberg et al., 2000), now placing it as central to gains. It also suggests that right prefrontal mechanisms might be critical for improvement among reading-impaired children, and consequently that reading development depends on different processes than it does in typical children. Overall, therefore, this study offers a nice demonstration of the value of taking a longitudinal perspective along with other established methods of investigation, although the small sample size (25 or fewer participants with dyslexia in each analysis) and the possibility of chance findings when multiple brain regions are considered mean that replication of this result will be important.

Other quantitative traits

Many of the issues that arise in research and practice in developmental dyslexia are of interest within other quantitative traits; language delay and learning disabilities in various academic domains such as mathematics, for instance. Consequently, advantages conferred by a longitudinal perspective may apply to them as well. In mathematics there is debate about the distinction between generally low maths skills and "developmental dyscalculia" and about whether different forms exist – the subtype issue. As for dyslexia, research with longitudinal elements may help settle matters. For example, it would be of interest to determine if different intervention techniques are required to remediate different hypothesized subtypes (Butterworth, Varma, & Laurillard, 2011). However, Butterworth et al. describe dyscalculia as the "poor relation" of dyslexia research, and it is true that longitudinal studies are particularly sparse (for interesting exceptions, see Andersson, 2010, and Toll, Van der Ven, Kroesbergen, & Van Luit, 2011). But several of the "open questions" that Butterworth et al. identify in their recent review are precisely the kinds that require longitudinal research: whether neuroscience will furnish early risk indicators for dyscalculia as it has, they suggest, in the case of dyslexia (Lyytinen et al., 2005); whether neural changes over time can be detected following successful intervention, as have been shown to occur with dyslexia (see Frost et al., 2009); and whether cognitive and neural functions following intervention show up as compensatory mechanisms or as those typical of normal development. Dowker (2009) also identifies the need for longitudinal studies of remediation to evaluate the effectiveness of various approaches to mathematical underperformance in school students. We could also add that, as far as we are aware, no research has yet exploited familial risk for mathematics impairment as a longitudinal design, though the relatively high heritability of mathematics attainment (Kovas et al., 2007) indicates that, as for dyslexia, it could be informative. Hence, we can agree with the call from Butterworth et al. for a more concerted research effort focused on mathematical disabilities.

Longitudinal approaches in genetically-informative research designs

Developmental disabilities are often heritable. Some, such as the mental retardation associated with unmanaged phenylketonuria and neurofibromatosis Type 1, are the result of single-gene abnormalities that are transmitted in known, "Mendelian" ways (recessive and dominant respectively). Others, such as autism and attention deficit/hyperactivity disorder (ADHD), are likely the result of multiple genes, plus environmental influences, and although progress has been made in identifying the degrees to which these multiple-gene disorders are genetically as against environmentally influenced, to date attempts to identify the genes involved have had limited success. (Yet other disabilities, such as Angelman syndrome and Williams syndrome, are "genetic" in that they involve chromosomal abnormalities, but often these occur spontaneously in the formation of gametes rather than being passed down across the generations.) Newbury (this volume) provides an in-depth discussion of the genetics of developmental disorders.

Estimating the relative influence of genes and the environment on liability for a disorder is a valuable contribution to understanding it, but additional information can be garnered from adopting a longitudinal framework in genetic studies, particularly about genetic and environmental stability and change over time. We illustrate with reading impairment studied using the classic twin design.

Normal-range variation in reading and low-end performance levels (dyslexia) are substantially heritable. Most of the research demonstrating this comes from studies of twin children, with higher within-pair similarity for monozygotic (MZ) compared to dizygotic (DZ) pairs as the sign of genetic influence (see Williams & Lind, this volume, for an explanation of twin-study methodology). Typically, twin studies produce estimates of heritability (proportion of total variance attributable to genetic differences) for normal-range variation and for membership of the impaired-reader group of the order of .5–.8 (see Byrne, Khlentzos, Olson, & Samuelsson, 2010, and Pennington & Olson, 2005, for reviews). Further, reading disability appears to be relatively stable over time, such that children diagnosed as reading impaired generally retain the diagnosis across their school years and often into adulthood (Maughan, Hagell, Rutter, & Yule, 1994; Shaywitz et al., 1999; Wadsworth, DeFries, Olson, & Wilcutt, 2007). An appropriate question, therefore, is whether the stability is primarily genetically or environmentally mediated. Multivariate behaviour-genetic methods can help answer this question.

Wadsworth et al. (2007) report correlations of up to .84 between reading measures taken 5 to 6 years apart (first assessment at around 10 years) in a group of reading-impaired twin school students, with an average across a variety of reading measures of about .80, high stability indeed. Their analyses showed that 86 percent of this "phenotypic" stability is genetic in origin. The environment, especially the environment that twins share such as family and school, contributed very little to the developmental stability. These figures are in line with those obtained from other behaviour-genetic analyses of children comprising normal-range samples. For example, Harlaar, Dale, and Plomin (2007) report stability estimates for reading of around .6 across the three ages of 7, 9, and 10 in the Twins Early Development Study in the United Kingdom, with between 68 and 77 percent of this phenotypic stability being genetically mediated. Data from adopted and non-adopted children and their related and unrelated siblings are also genetically-informative. Wadsworth, Corley, Plomin, Hewitt, and DeFries (2006) report relatively high developmental stability for reading across an age-span of 9 years (7 to 16) in the Colorado Adoption Project, with values ranging between .58 and .71 across different ages within this span. Between 53 and 86 percent of the stability was mediated by genes.

It is important to note that the estimates of longitudinal stability we have discussed so far are all limited by measurement error. When the common variance across multiple measures of a skill is modelled as a latent trait, the latent trait is free from measurement error. The longitudinal stability for individual differences in a word-reading latent trait from age 10 to 16 years was estimated at .98 (Hulslander, Olson, Willcutt, & Wadsworth, 2010). This underlines the strength of stability over time in reading and reading disability.

Longitudinal research can also reveal the degree to which the same genes are affecting variation in reading as children advance through school. Most of this research is with unselected samples of twins (rather than twin pairs in which there is evidence of reading disability), but on the widely-accepted view that reading disability is determined by the same genes that influence full-range variation (Plomin & Kovas, 2005), this research is also informative about the developmental pattern for dyslexia. One important observation is that the genes that influence word decoding are also those that influence reading comprehension early in schooling (Byrne et al., 2006), in line with the companion observation that the correlation between word identification skills and comprehension are high in the first one or two school grades. However, by fourth grade there is more phenotypic separation between word identification and comprehension, and this is accompanied by greater genetic diversity. Keenan et al. (2006) showed that genes affecting listening comprehension combine with those affecting word identification to generate virtually all of the genetic variation in reading comprehension (as predicted by Hoover and Gough's [1990] "simple view"). The important point for developmental reading disability is that new sources of (genetically-driven) variation come into play as schooling progresses, meaning that disability for genetically-compromised children could emerge early or late, with detection depending on the judicious selection of assessments (the inclusion of reading and/or listening comprehension in the case of dyslexia).

Comorbidity

Behaviour-genetic analyses can illuminate the nature of comorbidity among developmental disabilities, and longitudinal designs can be even more informative. It is well known that reading impairment and attention deficit/hyperactivity disorder (ADHD) co-occur, with around 20–40 percent of children diagnosed with dyslexia also meeting criteria for ADHD (more strictly, the inattention component; Willcutt & Pennington, 2000). There is evidence that the two disorders are pleiotropic (arise in part from shared genes; Willcutt, Pennington, Olson, & DeFries, 2007).

In a longitudinal twin study over 3 years, kindergarten to Grade 2, Ebejer et al. (2010) showed that both reading and inattention became more genetically complex with development (new genes entering to influence scores with advancing grades), but that all of the shared genes were in evidence in the first (kindergarten) year. Comorbidity shows its hand early. From the results of another longitudinal study with twins spanning 5 years into adolescence, it is clear that comorbidity matters because children who are diagnosed with both disorders have less favourable long-term outcomes, academically and socially, than those with a single diagnosis (Willcutt, Betjemann et al., 2007). For example, word reading became worse in those diagnosed with both disorders over time, even though there were no differences in the severity of reading disability at the start of the study. Thus, intervention for both disorders is called for when both exist in the same child, and the intervention should start early because comorbidity starts early.

Longitudinal perspectives on intervention

Most intervention research is longitudinal in that it is common practice to assess children prior to and after the intervention, which generally takes time. However, we want to emphasize longer-term follow-up after the completion of the intervention, up to several years. There are probably hundreds of research studies of intervention with reading disability alone, many with long-term follow-up, and it is beyond the scope of this chapter to summarize this literature. Instead, we select examples to illustrate why a longitudinal perspective matters, and to present some findings that may be of special interest in this volume.

The primary value of a longer-term perspective is that short-term outcomes may not last, or may have apparently deleterious effects. Chapman, Tunmer, and Prochnow (2001), for example, showed that the commercial intervention program, Reading Recovery (Clay, 1993), generated actual *declines* in reading and general academic self-concept over the 3 years following its use with groups of reading disabled first-graders (as well as showing no short-term improvement in reading but some progress in phonological awareness).

Wise, Ring, and Olson (2000) instituted a training study for second- to fifth-grade reading-impaired children that contrasted phonologically-based training (phonological awareness, articulatory concepts, direct phonics instruction) with accurate reading-in-context, both within a computer-assisted program. Immediately following the interventions, the phonological group was ahead of the other group in phoneme deletion, an index of the success of the phonologically-based intervention, and in word and nonword reading. The advantage in phoneme deletion was maintained over the 2-year follow-up period, but that for reading dissipated over the same period (although both groups maintained gains).

Elbro and colleagues (Borstrom & Elbro, 1997; Elbro & Peterson, 2004) selected family-risk children for kindergarten intervention. In this Danish study, which included non-trained-risk children as controls, the focus was on teaching the children about individual phonemes in words, supported by letter instruction. Regular kindergarten teachers who had participated in lengthy training administered the teaching program on a whole-of-class basis, about half an hour each day for 17 weeks, with one or more risk children in each class. Comparison children, both at risk and not, were taught in classes that included some attention to phonological awareness but at a considerably less extensive and intensive level than the experimental training. In Grades 2 and 3, the instructed risk children outperformed the risk controls on each measure of reading administered, including silent and oral reading, real and nonword reading, and speed as well as accuracy. By Grade 7, the trained children were still ahead of the controls on only three of eight measures, including real word reading fluency, nonword reading and pseudohomophone detection. The nonadvantage on five of the tests contrasts with the situation in the earlier grades, when the trained group outperformed the risk controls on all measures. Further, the experimental training was not a panacea. At Grade 7, many more risk than non-risk children were below the 5th and 20th percentile cutoffs determined by the non-risk group. Averaged over the reading measures, approximately 16 percent of the trained-risk children were below the 5 percent cutoff and 42 percent below the 20 percent cutoff. The trained-risk children generally fared better than the non-trained ones (percentages of 25 and 47, respectively, compared with the 16 and 42 just reported), but this was only significant in 2 out of 16 cases (where case = the 5th or 20th percentile on a test, with eight tests in all). Thus the additional kindergarten focus on phonemic awareness and letters assisted the risk children to achieve higher than otherwise-expected levels of reading, especially in early school grades, but by Grade 7 at least some of the advantage over non-trained-risk children had evaporated.

The study by Hindson et al. (2005), mentioned earlier, was an intervention with family-at-risk (FAR) preschool children. It followed on from earlier work by Byrne and Fielding-Barnsley and colleagues in which a preschool intervention for phonemic awareness was created and subject to a randomized control trial for short-and long-term effectiveness (Byrne & Fielding-Barnsley, 1991, 1993, 1995; Byrne, Fielding-Barnsley, & Ashley, 2000), with children from a community sample. The key insight we taught was phoneme identity, i.e., that two words can begin, or end, with the same sound, as in *sail* and *sun*, or *drum* and *worm.* On the whole, the results were encouraging in that there were immediate improvements in phonemic awareness that transferred to reading over both short and long terms, with small to modest effects still visible after 6 years. The main point in the present context is that numbers of children from the experimental group were nevertheless poor readers in school, and that the best indicator of long-term prospects in reading was not the level of phonemic awareness (phoneme identity) that the children reached following the early intervention but how many lessons they required to first show that they understood the phoneme identity (Byrne et al., 2000), a learning *rate* rather than *attainment* measure.

In the light of this result, we designed the FAR intervention study to allow for quantification of (a) the learning rate for the core insight we were teaching, the idea of phoneme identity, and (b) the final level attained. We sought to teach the children to criterion across a sample of phonemes. If on a single instructional session, comprising a single phoneme such as beginning/s/, the child failed to reach a reasonably strict criterion of success, he or she repeated that lesson on the next teaching occasion. The total number of lessons required to complete the program, which consisted to 11 phoneme/position combinations, formed the measure of responsiveness. We also administered a post-instruction test of phoneme identity, using both taught and untaught phonemes, leaving us with two variables that we dubbed Progress (number of lessons required) and Outcome (post-test score).

Follow-up assessment at the end of kindergarten (first school year), on average 18 months after the intervention, showed, first, that the FAR children reached levels comparable with a "typical" control group from an earlier project, but that some appeared to be struggling readers nevertheless, a greater number than normally expected. The same pattern emerged in the following 2 years; scores on standardized tests indicative of grade-appropriate performance in decoding for the risk group as a whole, but a higher-than-normal number of children remaining in the impaired reader range (Byrne, Shankweiler, & Hine, 2008). The best predictor of kindergarten reading was the Progress measure – entered first into a regression model, it accounted for around 24 percent of variance in school decoding and spelling, with Outcome adding no more variance explained; entered in the other order, Progress added to variance explained on top of Outcome. In Grades 1 and 2, Progress and Outcome each made independent contributions to variance explained in a combined literacy measure, to totals of 35 percent in Grade 1 and 22 percent in Grade 2.

The pattern of results underlined for us the importance of learning rate in addition to learning attainment as a predictor of subsequent reading success. We have explored this variable in our own behaviour-genetic studies of literacy development. In particular, we have shown that learning the orthographic patterns of newly-encountered printed words is affected by genes (heritability around 43 percent of total variance), and, importantly, that the same genes also affect performance on decoding and spelling previously encountered words (Byrne, Olson et al., 2008). The genetic correlations among these variables approach 1.

The quantification of learning rate requires, by definition, a longitudinal perspective. And as with other predictors of future success, the longer-term effects of rate require sustained evaluation across several years, at least while the child is progressing through periods of normally rapid advance in achievement, as applies in the early school years for reading (McCoach, O'Connell, Reis, & Levitt, 2006). We are unaware of other studies that use rate of progress in learning in other developmental disabilities, such as dyscalculia, but we suggest that this variable may be a valuable addition to the research toolkit.

Combining correlational and experimental methods in longitudinal research

Quantitative research in psychology takes two main forms, correlational (what goes with what) and experimental (what affects what). These two approaches can be combined when, in an intervention study (basically, an experiment), attempts are made to identify factors that best predict outcomes (basically, a set of correlations). The predictors can be classified as mediators, intervening variables that are thought to account for the influence of the treatment on the outcome, and moderators, often categories such as race or gender, that influence the effectiveness of the intervention (Breitborde, Srihari, Pollard, Addington, & Woods, 2010). As usual, we contend that studying these factors in a longitudinal context will generate the most informative data. We have already given examples of this kind of amalgamation in the project described in Hindson et al. (2005) and Byrne, Shankweiler, and Hine (2008) – the rate of early progress in mastering a core component of literacy development, phoneme identity, proved to be a reasonable indicator of future reading prospects, suggesting that some basic learning process was at work in the intervention and in subsequent literacy growth – it was a mediator. Another example comes from Vellutino et al. (1996), who implemented an intensive, early intervention for the lowest-rated first graders in a New York school system and explored the characteristics of the children who were difficult versus easy to remediate. The follow-up assessment was conducted 1 year after the tutoring, and the researchers showed that difficult-to-remediate children already showed deficits in phonological, but not visual, syntactic or semantic, skills at the time the tutoring began. The results were interpreted as confirming a crucial role for phonological processes in the reading development – they too were mediators of the intervention.

An example of a moderator variable detected in an intervention study comes from van Otterloo, van der Leij, and Veldkamp (2006). These researchers were documenting the role of treatment integrity on the effectiveness of a home-based pre-reading intervention focused on phoneme awareness and letter knowledge for children at familial risk for dyslexia. Not surprisingly, they were able to show that treatment integrity, that is, the quantity and quality of the program administration, affected outcomes. But this relationship held strongly only for the children of the most highly educated mothers in the group. For children of low-educated mothers the relationship was non-existent for quantity and of lesser magnitude for quality. Interestingly, Friend, DeFries, and Olson (2008) have shown that for children who struggle with reading and who come from homes with higher levels of parental education reading ability appears to be more heritable than for struggling readers from less educated home environments. It may well be that the quality and quantity of intervention matters more in situations where genes also matter more.

In the case of our FAR study, we also investigated which earlier-assessed variables predicted the Progress metric itself, and found that vocabulary and verbal short-term memory did. It might be telling to trace the origins of all these variables further back still, perhaps even to the kinds of ERP measures of speech perception collected by Guttorm et al. (2005) in the child's first year of life. The prospects of a truly informative picture of the trajectories of developmental dyslexia, and developmental disabilities more broadly, might then be in prospect. The marriage of neuroscientific and cognitive methods can be seen to good effect in the work of Blomert and colleagues. They have shown that despite dyslexics often having full knowledge of letter–sound relations under standard testing arrangements ("knowing their letters"), more sophisticated measures using, for example, fMRI, can reveal that full integration of letters and their associated sounds has not occurred, even into adulthood (Blau et al., 2010; Blau, van Atteveldt, Ekkebus, Goebel, & Blomert, 2009). These observations also fit those of Lyytinen, Erskine et al. (2006)

mentioned earlier, that there is a group of dyslexics whose developmental trajectory starts with a rather specific difficulty in learning letters and progresses into a more general problem with written word identification. Here then is a good example of integration across neuroscientific, cognitive and longitudinal observations in the service of creating a more complete picture of developmental disabilities.

Summary and conclusion

Developmental disabilities all face issues of definition and proper characterization, such as how multi-factored the disability is, its (possibly changing) relations with other aspects of cognition and behaviour, and the status of subtypes. Some of these matters will yield to cross-sectional developmental research, but there are distinct advantages in being able to follow the same individuals over time, not least the elimination of between-individual differences as sources of uncertainty, as in the comparison of within- versus between-subject designs in psychological research in general.

Longitudinal research is the only means to track the emergence of developmental disabilities in cases where they cannot be diagnosed at birth (or earlier). For those with a substantial genetic load, such as reading impairment, family history of the disorder can be used to select children at risk, and there are several highly informative projects following the progress of these children prior to and during school instruction. An important conclusion from this research is that processes known to correlate with variation in reading ability already show their hand prior to the start of literacy instruction, evidence that variation in these processes is not simply a follow-on effect of reading skill. Other kinds of predictive studies, exemplified by prediction of progress of the disability from neural signals, show that longitudinal research can integrate with other designs to advance our understanding. For some disabilities, such as dyscalculia, some of these advantages are yet to be realized.

Genetically-sensitive research designs can tell us about the aetiology of developmental disabilities in the sense of identifying relative genetic and environmental influences on them, and they are additionally informative when conducted within a longitudinal framework. This combination can address questions about the degree to which genetic and environmental factors remain constant or change during development. Genetic factors are primarily responsible for the stability of reading disability over time, but that there can be new genetic sources coming "on stream" as children develop, an observation that may be especially useful for practitioners to explain how disabilities might emerge some way into a child's development. Longitudinal research can also track the entwined trajectories of comorbid disorders, important in practical terms for children burdened with dual diagnoses.

Intervention research with developmental disabilities also benefits from a longitudinal perspective. Outcomes can be short-lived, and long-term follow-up is required to discover whether they are sustained in comparison to some kind of control group. Finally, we outlined the merits of combining experimental and correlational methods in a longitudinal framework, an approach that may get us closer to a fuller picture of the complexities of developmental disabilities, especially when it is combined with insights from other methods such as those afforded by neuroscience.

References

American Psychiatric Association. (2000). *Diagnostic and statistical manual of mental disorders* (4th ed., text rev.). Washington, DC: Author.

American Psychiatric Association. (2012). *DSM-5 development: A13 Dyslexia* [Website]. Retrieved April 18th, 2012, from http://www.dsm5.org/ProposedRevision/Pages/proposedrevision.aspx?rid=84#

Anderson, R. C., & Nagy, W. E. (1992). The vocabulary conundrum. *The American Educator, 16*, 14–18, 44–47.

Andersson, U. (2010). Skill development in different components of arithmetic and basic cognitive functions: Findings from a 3-year longitudinal study of children with different types of learning disabilities. *Journal of Educational Psychology, 102*, 115–134.

Barkley, R. A., & Murphy, K. (1998). *Attention-deficit hyperactivity disorder: A clinical workbook* (2nd ed.). New York, NY: Guilford.

Blau, V., Reithler, J., van Atteveldt, N., Seitz, J., Gerretsen, P., Goebel, R., & Blomert, L. (2010). Deviant processing of letters and speech sounds as proximate cause of reading failure: A functional magnetic resonance imaging study of dyslexic children. *Brain, 133*, 868–879.

Blau, V., van Atteveldt, N., Ekkebus, M., Goebel, R., & Blomert, L. (2009). Reduced neural integration of letters and speech sounds links phonological and reading deficits in adult dyslexia. *Current Biology, 19*, 503–508.

Borstrom, I., & Elbro, C. (1997). Prevention of dyslexia in kindergarten: Effects of phoneme awareness training with children of dyslexic parents. In C. Hulme & M. Snowling (Eds.), *Dyslexia: Biology, cognition and intervention* (pp. 235–253). London, UK: Whurr.

Breitborde, N. J. K., Srihari, V. H., Pollard, J. M., Addington, D. N., & Woods, S. W. (2010). Mediators and moderators in early intervention research. *Early Intervention in Psychiatry, 4*, 143–152.

Bruck, M. (1992). Persistence of dyslexics' phonological awareness deficits. *Developmental Psychology, 28*, 874–886.

Butterworth, B., Varma, S., & Laurillard, D. (2011). Dyscalculia: From brain to education. *Science, 332*, 1049–1053.

Byrne, B. (1998). *The foundation of literacy: The child's discovery of the alphabetic principle.* Hove, UK: Psychology Press.

Byrne, B. (2005). Theories of learning to read. In M. J. Snowling & C. Hulme (Eds.), *The science of reading: A handbook* (pp. 104–119). Oxford, UK: Blackwell Publishing.

Byrne, B., Coventry, W. L., Olson, R. K., Samuelsson, S., Corley, R., Willcutt, E. G., . . . DeFries, J. C. (2009). Genetic and environmental influences on aspects of literacy and language in early childhood: Continuity and change from preschool to Grade 2. *Journal of Neurolinguistics, 22*, 219–236.

Byrne, B., & Fielding-Barnsley, R. (1991). Evaluation of a program to teach phonemic awareness to young children. *Journal of Educational Psychology, 83*, 451–455.

Byrne, B., & Fielding-Barnsley, R. (1993). Evaluation of a program to teach phonemic awareness to young children: A 1-year follow-up. *Journal of Educational Psychology, 85*, 104–111.

Byrne, B., & Fielding-Barnsley, R. (1995). Evaluation of a program to teach phonemic awareness to young children: A 2- and 3-year follow-up, and a new preschool trial. *Journal of Educational Psychology, 87*, 488–503.

Byrne, B., Fielding-Barnsley, R., & Ashley, L. (2000). Effects of preschool phoneme identity training after six years: Outcome level distinguished from rate of response. *Journal of Educational Psychology, 92*, 659–667.

Byrne, B., Khlentzos, D., Olson, R. K., & Samuelsson, S. (2010). Evolutionary and genetic perspectives on educational attainment. In K. Littleton, C. Wood, & J. K. Staarman (Eds.), *International handbook of psychology in education* (pp. 3–34). Bingley, UK: Emerald Press.

Byrne, B., Olson, R. K., Hulslander, J., Samuelsson, S., Wadsworth, S., DeFries, J. C., . . . Willcutt, E. G. (2008). A behavior-genetic analysis of orthographic learning, spelling, and decoding. *Journal of Research in Reading, 31*, 8–21.

Byrne, B., Olson, R. K., Samuelsson, S., Wadsworth, S., Corley, R., DeFries, J. C., & Willcutt, E. (2006). Genetic and environmental influences on early literacy skills: A review and update. *Journal of Research in Reading, 29*, 33–49.

Byrne, B., Shankweiler, D., & Hine, D. (2008). Reading development in children at risk for dyslexia. In M. Mody & E. Silliman (Eds.), *Brain, behavior, and learning in language and reading disorders* (pp. 240–270). New York, NY: Guilford Press.

Castles, A., & Coltheart, M. (1993). Varieties of developmental dyslexia. *Cognition, 47*, 149–180.

Castles, A., Datta, H., Gayan, J., & Olson, R. K. (1999). Varieties of developmental reading disorder: Genetic and environmental influences. *Journal of Experimental Child Psychology, 72*, 73–94.

Chapman, J. W., Tunmer, W. E., & Prochnow, J. E. (2001). Does success in the Reading Recovery program depend on developing proficiency in phonological-processing skills? A longitudinal study in a whole language instructional context. *Scientific Studies of Reading, 52*, 141–176.

Clay, M. M. (1993). *Reading recovery*. Auckland, New Zealand: Heinemann.

Coltheart, M. (2005). Modeling reading: The dual-route approach. In M. J. Snowling & C. Hulme (Eds.), *The science of reading: A handbook* (pp. 6–23). Oxford, UK: Blackwell Publishing.

DeFries, J. C., Singer, S. M., Foch, T. T., & Lewitter, F. I. (1978). Familial nature of reading disability. *British Journal of Psychiatry, 132*, 361–367.

Dowker, A. (2009). *What works for children with mathematical difficulties? The effectiveness of intervention schemes*. Department for Children, Schools and Families. Available from http://nationalstrategies.standards.dcsf.gov.uk/node/174504

Ebejer, J. L., Coventry, W. L., Byrne, B., Willcutt, E. G., Olson, R. K., Corley, R., & Samuelsson, S. (2010). Genetic and environmental influences on inattention, hyperactivity-impulsivity, and reading: Kindergarten to Grade 2. *Scientific Studies of Reading, 14*, 293–316.

Elbro, C., & Petersen, D. K. (2004). Long-term effects of phoneme awareness and letter sound training: An intervention study with children at risk for dyslexia. *Journal of Educational Psychology, 96*, 660–670.

Filipek, P. A., Accardo, P. J., Baranek, G. T., Cook, E. H. Jr., Dawson, G., Gordon, B., . . . Volkmar, F.R. (1999). The screening and diagnosis of autistic spectrum disorders. *Journal of Autism and Developmental Disorders*, *29*, 439–84.

Friend, A., DeFries, J. C., & Olson, R. K. (2008). Parental education moderates genetic influences on reading disability. *Psychological Science, 19*, 1124–1130.

Frost, S. J., Sandak, R., Mencl, W. E., Landi, N., Rueckl, J. G., Katz, L., & Pugh, K. R. (2009). Mapping the word reading circuitry in skilled and disabled readers. In P. McCardle & K. Pugh, (Eds.). *Helping children learn to read: Current issues and new directions in the integration of cognition, neurobiology and genetics of reading and dyslexia research and practice* (pp. 3–19). Mahwah, NJ: Psychology Press.

Gilger, J. W., Pennington, B. F., & DeFries, J. C. (1991). Risk for reading disability as a function of parental history in three family studies. *Reading and Writing: An Interdisciplinary Journal, 3,* 205–219.

Guttorm, T. K., Leppänen, P. H. T., Poikkeus, A.-M., Eklund, K. M., Lyytinen, P., & Lyytinen, H. (2005). Brain event-related potentials (ERPs) measured at birth predict later language development in children with and without familial risk for dyslexia. *Cortex, 41,* 291–303.

Harlaar, N., Dale, P. S., & Plomin, R. (2007). From learning to read to reading to learn: Substantial and stable genetic influence. *Child Development, 78,* 116–131.

Hallgren, B. (1950). Specific dyslexia (congenital word-blindness): A clinical and genetic study. *Acta Psychiatrica et Neurologica Supplement, 65,* 1–287.

Hindson, B. A., Byrne, B., Fielding-Barnsley, R., Newman, C., Hine, D., & Shankweiler, D. (2005). Assessment and early instruction of preschool children at risk for reading disability. *Journal of Educational Psychology, 94,* 687–704.

Hoeft, F., McCandliss, B. D., Black, J. M., Gantman, A., Zakerani, N., Hulme, C., . . . Gabrielli, J. D. E. (2011). Neural systems predicting long-term outcomes in dyslexia. *Proceeding of the National Academy of Sciences, 108,* 361–366.

Hoover, W. A., & Gough, P. B. (1990). The simple view of reading. *Reading and Writing: An Interdisciplinary Journal, 2,* 127–160.

Hulslander, J., Olson, R. K., Willcutt, E. G., & Wadsworth, S. J. (2010). Longitudinal stability of reading-related skills and their prediction of reading development. *Scientific Studies of Reading, 14,* 111–136.

Keenan, J. M., Betjemann, R. S., & Olson, R. K. (2008). Reading comprehension tests vary in the skills they assess: Differential dependence on decoding and oral comprehension. *Scientific Studies of Reading, 12,* 281–300.

Keenan, J.M., Betjemann, R., Wadsworth, S. J., DeFries, J. C., & Olson, R. K. (2006). Genetic and environmental influences on reading and listening comprehension. *Journal of Research in Reading, 29,* 75–91.

Klingberg, T., Hedehus, M., Temple, E., Salz, T., Gabrieli, J. D., Moseley, M. E., & Poldrack, R. A. (2000). Microstructure of temporoparietal white matter as a basis for reading ability: Evidence from diffusion tensor magnetic resonance imaging. *Neuron, 25,* 493–500.

Kovas, Y., Haworth, C. M. A., Dale, P. S., & Plomin, R. (2007). The genetic and environmental origins of learning abilities and disabilities in the early school years. *Monographs of the Society for Research in Child Development, 72*(3), 1–144.

Lovett, M. W. (1984). A developmental perspective on reading dysfunction: Accuracy and rate criteria in the subtyping of dyslexic children. *Brain and Language, 22,* 67–91.

Lyytinen, H., Aro, M., Holopainen, L., Leiwo, M., Lyytinen, P., & Tolvanen, A. (2006). Children's language development and reading acquisition in a highly transparent orthography. In R. M. Joshi & P. G. Aaron (Eds.), *Handbook of orthography and literacy* (pp. 47–62). Mahwah, NJ: Lawrence Erlbaum Associates.

Lyytinen, H., Erskine, J., Tolvanen, A., Torppa, M., Poikkeus, A.-M., & Lyytinen, P. (2006). Trajectories of reading development: A follow-up from birth to school age of children with and without risk for dyslexia. *Merrill-Palmer Quarterly, 52,* 514–546.

Lyytinen, H., Guttorm, T. K., Huttunen, T., Hämäläinen, J., Leppänen, P. H. T., & Vesterinen, M. (2005). Psychophysiology of developmental dyslexia: A review of findings including studies of children at risk for dyslexia. *Journal of Neurolinguistics, 18*, 167–195.

Maughan, B., Hagell, A., Rutter, M., & Yule, W. (1994). Poor readers in secondary school. *Reading and Writing: An Interdisciplinary Journal, 6*, 125–150.

McCoach, D. B., O'Connell, A. A., Reis, S. M., & Levitt, H. A. (2006). Growing readers: A hierarchical linear model of children's reading growth during the first 2 years of school. *Journal of Educational Psychology, 98*, 14–28.

Olson, R. K., Byrne, B., & Samuelsson, S. (2009). Reconciling strong genetic and strong environmental influences on individual differences and deficits in reading ability. In K. Pugh & P. McCardle (Eds.), *How children learn to read: Current issues and new directions in the integration of cognition, neurobiology and genetics of reading and dyslexia research and practice* (pp. 215–233). New York: Taylor & Francis.

Pennington, B. F., & Olson, R. K. (2005). Genetics of dyslexia. In M. J. Snowling & C. Hulme (Eds.), *The science of reading: A handbook* (pp. 453–472). Oxford, UK: Blackwell Publishing.

Plaut, D. C. (2005). Connectionist approaches to reading. In M. J. Snowling & C. Hulme (Eds.), *The science of reading: A handbook* (pp. 24–38). Oxford, UK: Blackwell Publishing.

Plomin, R., & Kovas, Y. (2005). Generalist genes and learning disabilities. *Psychological Bulletin, 131*, 592–617.

Rietveld, M. J. H., Hudziak, J. J., Bartels, M., van Beijsterveldt, C. E. M., & Boomsma, D. I. (2004). Heritability of attention problems in children: Longitudinal results from a study of twins, age 3 to 12. *Journal of Child Psychology and Psychiatry, 45*, 577–588.

Rodgers, B. (1983). The identification and prevalence of specific reading retardation. *British Journal of Educational Psychology, 53*, 369–373.

Samuelsson, S., Byrne, B., Quain, P., Wadsworth, S., Corley, R., DeFries, J. C., . . . Olson, R. K. (2005). Environmental and genetic influences on prereading skills in Australia, Scandinavia, and the United States, *Journal of Educational Psychology, 97*, 705–722.

Scarborough, H. S. (1989). Prediction of reading disability from familial and individual differences. *Journal of Educational Psychology, 81*, 101–108.

Shaywitz, S. E., Fletcher, J. M., Holahan, J. M., Shneider, A. E., Marchione, K. E, Stuebing, K. K., . . . Shaywitz, B. A. (1999). Persistence of dyslexia: The Connecticut Longitudinal Study at adolescence. *Pediatrics, 104*, 1351–1359.

Smith, B. H., Barkley, R. A., & Shapiro, C. J. (2006). Attention-deficit/hyperactivity disorder. In E. J. Mash & R. A. Barkley (Eds.), *Treatment of childhood disorders* (3rd ed., pp. 65–136). New York, NY: Guilford.

Snowling, M. J. (2000). *Dyslexia.* Oxford, UK: Blackwell.

Snowling, M. J., Gallagher, A., & Frith, U. (2003). Family risk of dyslexia is continuous: Individual differences in the precursors of reading skill. *Child Development, 74*, 358–373.

Stanovich, K. E. (1994). Annotation: Does dyslexia exist? *Journal of Child Psychology and Psychiatry, 35*, 579–595.

Stanovich, K. E. (2000). *Progress in understanding reading: Scientific foundations and new frontiers.* New York, NY: Guilford.

Stanovich, K. E, & Siegel, L. S. (1994). The phenotypic performance profile of reading-disabled children: A regression-based test of the phonological-core variable-difference model. *Journal of Educational Psychology, 89*, 114–127.

Thomas, C. J. (1905). Congenital word-blindness and its treatment. *Ophthalmoscope, 3*, 380–385.

Toll, S. W. M., Van der Ven, S., Kroesbergen, E., & Van Luit, J. (2011). Executive functions as predictors of math learning disabilities. *Journal of Learning Disabilities, 44*, 521–532.

van Otterloo, S. G., van der Leij, A., & Veldkamp, E. (2006). Treatment integrity in a home-based pre-reading intervention programme. *Dyslexia, 12*, 155–176.

Vellutino, F. R., & Fletcher, J. M. (2005). Developmental dyslexia. In M. J. Snowling & C. Hulme (Eds.), *The science of reading: A handbook* (pp. 362–378). Oxford, UK: Blackwell Publishing.

Vellutino, F. R., Scanlon, D. M., & Lyon, G. R. (2000). Differentiating between difficult-to-remediate and readily remediated poor readers: More evidence against the IQ-achievement discrepancy definition of reading disability. *Journal of Learning Disabilities, 33*, 223–238.

Vellutino, F. R., Scanlon, D. M., Sipay, E. R., Small, S. G., Pratt, A. . . . Denckla, M. B. (1996). Cognitive profiles of difficult-to-remediate and readily remediated poor readers: Early intervention as a vehicle for distinguishing between cognitive and experiential deficits as basic causes of specific reading disability. *Journal of Educational Psychology, 88*, 601–638.

Wadsworth, S. J., Corley, R. P., Plomin, R., Hewitt, J. K., & DeFries, J. C. (2006). Genetic and environmental influences on continuity and change in reading achievement in the Colorado Adoption Project. In A. Huston & M. Ripke (Eds.), *Developmental contexts of middle childhood: Bridges to adolescence and adulthood* (pp. 87–106). New York, NY: Cambridge University Press.

Wadsworth, S. J., DeFries, J. C., Olson, R. K., & Willcutt, E. G. (2007). Colorado longitudinal twin study of reading disability. *Annals of Dyslexia, 57*, 139–160.

Willcutt, E. G., Betjemann, R. S., Pennington, B. F., Olson, R. K., DeFries, J. C., & Wadsworth, S. J. (2007). Longitudinal study of reading disability and attention-deficit/hyperactivity disorder: Implications for education. *Mind, Brain, and Education, 4*, 181–192.

Willcutt, E. G., & Pennington, B. F. (2000). Psychiatric comorbidity in children and adolescents with reading disorder. *Journal of Child Psychology and Psychiatry, 41*, 1039–1048.

Willcutt, E. G. Pennington, B. F., Olson, R. K., & DeFries, J. C. (2007). Understanding comorbidity: A twin study of reading disability and attention-deficit/hyperactivity disorder. *American Journal of Medical Genetics Part B (Neuropsychiatric Genetics), 144B*, 709–714.

Wise, B., Ring, J., & Olson, R. K. (2000). Individual differences in gains from computer-assisted remedial reading with more emphasis on phonological analysis or accurate reading in context. *Journal of Experimental Child Psychology, 77*, 197–235.

Wolf, M., & Bowers, P. G. (1999). The double deficit hypothesis for the developmental dyslexias. *Journal of Educational Psychology, 91*, 415–438.

Zabell, C., & Everatt, J. (2002). Surface and phonological subtypes of adult developmental dyslexia. *Dyslexia, 8*, 160–177.

4 Modelling developmental disorders

Michael S. C. Thomas, Frank D. Baughman, Themis Karaminis, and Caspar J. M. Addyman

Introduction: why build models of developmental disorders?

A 6-year-old child is given a vocabulary test where he has to name pictures of objects. He scores poorly, and makes mistakes such as naming a picture of a guitar as a 'piano'. One explanation of the child's difficulty is that he has impoverished semantic (meaning) representations. Another child has problems reading words out loud, especially new words that she has not seen before. For example, she reads the novel word 'slear' as 'sear'. One explanation of her difficulty is that she has poorly specified phonological (speech sound) representations. What do these terms 'impoverished' and 'poorly specified' mean? How did the mental representations of meaning and speech sounds get this way? If a speech and language therapist or a specialist teacher wanted to intervene to remediate these problems, what intervention would be appropriate, and at what age? Should it be a different intervention if representations are impoverished versus poorly specified?

Computational models of developmental disorders represent one technique to improve our understanding of the nature of deficits, their origin, long-term outcomes and possible pathways for remediation. The majority of the models we consider in this chapter are developmental, in that they learn abilities by exposing a developmental system to a structured learning environment. The act of building a model – specifying the nature of the developmental system, its input and output systems, and the information present in the learning environment – forces a theory to be specified in much greater detail than would normally be the case in a verbal formulation. In the context of disorders, models allow detailed consideration of what could be affecting development: What is it that is different about the developmental system that is preventing strong learning? Is the information different in the learning environment? What exactly is different about meaning representations that are 'impoverished' or phonological representations that are 'poorly specified' and how does this lead to the kinds of error one sees in children with developmental impairments in productive vocabulary and reading, respectively?

The process of constructing a model, by its nature, involves simplification. The aim is to build a working system that embodies key constraints of the phenomenon under consideration, and simplifies aspects that are taken to be unimportant.

For the study of behaviour in children and adults with developmental disorders, empirical data from psychology form the most frequent constraints. For example, we might find that a child with a productive vocabulary deficit also has difficulty in providing definitions of words, indicating the type of information that is missing from the representations of meaning. Models then provide several benefits. As we have seen, the act of building a model forces greater clarity on existing explanations. In addition, a working model allows researchers to test the viability of certain theoretical claims. For example, a model of vocabulary development could test the claim that representations of meaning altered in a certain way indeed lead to naming errors of the type observed in the children. Models can serve to unify a range of empirical effects via a single working implementation. Models can sometimes produce emergent effects that are unexpected consequences of the theoretical assumptions. This is particularly the case where the model system has many components and complex interactions occur between them. Once the researcher has a working model, he or she can apply it to novel situations, to make predictions about behaviour that can then be tested empirically. With regard to development, the researcher can trace the behaviour of the model across time, for instance predicting the long-term outcome of early-observed deficits. And the researcher can carry out experiments on the model, for example, evaluating different forms of intervention to see which might best alleviate a developmental deficit.

In this chapter, we present examples of the use of computational modelling in the study of developmental disorders. In the next three sections, we illustrate three key ideas. The first section considers the use of models for testing the viability of theoretical proposals – in this case, to establish that certain kinds of deficits in the language system are sufficient to produce behavioural impairments across development, such as those found in Specific Language Impairment (SLI). This section focuses on the additional detail forced by implementation. The second section considers the role of the developmental process itself in producing the impairments, compared to building a static model and simulating deficits by breaking components of the model. This issue is considered in the context of models of reading development and dyslexia. The third section addresses the behaviour of complex cognitive architectures made up of many interacting components rather than individual systems, and explores the developmental consequences of initial limitations to individual components: Do deficits subsequently spread throughout the system, or can initially normal components serve to compensate for impaired ones, so alleviating deficits later in development? Once more, this example makes reference to dyslexia in reading. These three examples employ methods drawn from two approaches to computational modelling, artificial neural networks (sometimes called connectionism) and dynamical systems modelling. Reviews of these methods can be found in Spencer, Thomas, and McClelland (2009), Thomas and McClelland (2008), and Mareschal and Thomas (2007). Following these sections, we consider some of the latest models in the field, including those considering the effects of anomalies in reward-based learning and those modelling deficits at the population level rather than just the individual.

I. Models for evaluating the viability of theoretical proposals: examples from developmental language deficits

A number of studies have employed artificial neural network models to investigate the causes of developmental deficits in aspects of language. The studies shared a common methodology. They constructed a normal model intended to capture the profile of accuracy rates or error patterns in the target domain presented by typically developing children. A disorder model was then constructed by implementing manipulations of the parameter space of the default model in its initial untrained state. These involved altering the computational constraints or the quality of the input and output representations, or both. Examples of such manipulations are (1) the use of fewer units in the hidden layer of the network (e.g., Thomas & Redington, 2004) – these are the resources over which the system develops its own internal representations to learn the target domain; (2) the use of an activation function in the processing units that rendered them less sensitive to differences in the input that they received (e.g., Thomas, 2005); (3) the addition of noise to the activation levels of units throughout or in specific parts of the network architecture (e.g., Joanisse & Seidenberg, 1999; Joanisse, 2004); (4) the weakening of the strength with which certain types of input information were represented in the model (e.g., Hoeffner & McClelland, 1993); and, (5) the probabilistic pruning of weighted connections in the network (e.g., Joanisse & Seidenberg, 1999). When models with these altered constraints were exposed to the target language domain, they exhibited impaired developmental profiles, characterised by the errors shown by young children with language impairments.

The decision of which parameter to manipulate in the normal model was theoretically driven, i.e., linked to aetiological accounts of the language disorder addressed in each study (cf. Thomas & Karmiloff-Smith, 2003). For example, the model of Hoeffner and McClelland (1993) investigating the possible origin of deficits in children with SLI in inflectional morphology. Inflectional morphology is a domain of language that concerns how words change their form to indicate their grammatical status in a sentence (for instance, verbs may be in the present or past tense and nouns may be in the singular or plural). The model evaluated the effect of weakening phonological representations of words, in line with theoretical accounts positing that a low-level perceptual deficit results in the emergence of behavioural impairments at higher levels within the language system (e.g., Tallal & Piercy, 1973a, 1973b). By contrast, Thomas (2005) demonstrated that a similar deficit could be simulated in a learning system that had processing units with reduced sensitivity to variations in the incoming signal. This condition corresponds to theoretical views suggesting that SLI is caused by general processing limitations (e.g., Kail, 1994).

In the following examples drawn from the domain of inflectional morphology, the aim of connectionist studies of language disorders was to illustrate that when applied to normal models, certain computational constraints were sufficient to alter the acquisition of behaviour to capture the linguistic profile of the language disorders. The models thereby established the viability of the related theoretical account to explain the cognitive profile of the disorder in the target domain. Additionally, the implemented models offered more detailed mechanistic explanations for the application of the general principles of the theoretical proposals in the specific linguistic domains considered. We consider each study with respect to three factors, scope, implementation, and implications. The scope assesses the range of empirical phenomena the model simulated, the implementation addresses which computational conditions were used to simulate the deficit, and the implications consider the wider theoretical consequences for the field of psycholinguistics. The key emphasis throughout this section will be on how the models established the viability of theoretical accounts and added to their detail.

Hoeffner and McClelland (1993): verbal morphology in SLI

Hoeffner and McClelland (1993) addressed a wide range of deficits of children with SLI in verbal morphology, including those found in the production of base, third person singular, progressive, past tense, and past participle forms of verbs. The normal model was a connectionist attractor network, in which a phonological and a semantic layer were connected bi-directionally. This network was required to learn mappings between distributed phonological and semantic representations of base and inflected verb forms from an artificial language of monosyllabic verb stems design to parallel features of English. An important assumption of the model was that in normal development, certain speech sounds, including word-final stops and fricatives, whether morphemic (e.g., the -*d* in changed) or non-morphemic (e.g., the -*d* in need), are characterised by lower phonetic saliency for language learners. Therefore, less strong phonological representations were used to represent these phonemes. The reduction of the strength for these representations was implemented in the following manner. Phonemes were represented by activation of the articulatory features that described a given phoneme. For high-salience phonemes, a value of 1 was used for active features. For low-salience phonemes, a value of 0.3 was employed.

The impaired model of Hoeffner and McClelland (1993) evaluated a theoretical proposal that a perceptual deficit may be the root cause of SLI (Tallal & Piercy, 1973a, 1973b). To implement this deficit, the atypical model was given weaker phonological representations for *all phonemes*; for low-salience phonemes, this meant that they were weaker still: thus word-final stops and fricatives were now represented by activation values of 0.1.

With this manipulation present throughout training, the model of Hoeffner and McClelland (1993) successfully simulated a range of morphological deficits presented by children with SLI. Notably, these deficits had been considered strong evidence for an underlying failure of the rule-based system of language by other researchers (e.g., Gopnik, 1990; Gopnik & Crago, 1991). By contrast, the model employed associative learning and did not contain rule-based representations. The model captured the differential degrees of impairment observed in SLI across the different inflections – more pronounced in the third singular, the past tense and past participle, and less severe in the progressive and in verb stems with non-morphemic word-final stops and fricatives (cf. Leonard, 1999). Impaired performance was associated with an increased percentage of inflectional suffix omission errors, also observed in children with SLI (Rice, Wexler, & Cleave, 1995). Finally, within the semi-regular domain of English past tense, the model simulated a greater degree of impairment in regular than in irregular inflection reported by Gopnik (1990; see also Gopnik & Crago, 1991). It should be noted, however, that the subsequent literature has not confirmed this pattern as characteristic of SLI – rather, lower levels of performance are observed for both regular and irregular verbs, with a residual small advantage for regular verbs (e.g., van der Lely & Ullman, 2001; see Joanisse, 2004, for discussion). For Hoeffner and McClelland (1993), the model supported the viability of the claim that a general perceptual deficit within the learning system could reproduce a profile of a rule-based impairment, similar to that suggested by language-specific accounts of SLI.

Joanisse (2004): past tense in SLI

Joanisse (2004) implemented a model for the learning of past tense based on an attractor network architecture trained on mappings between distributed phonological and localist semantics (lexical semantics) representations of English verbs. In a similar fashion to Hoeffner and McClelland (1993), this model also considered an underlying phonological deficit for SLI (based on Leonard, 1999; Tallal, Miller, & Fitch, 1993). However, here the deficit was implemented by the addition of small amounts of random noise to the phonological representations.

The impaired model was weaker in learning both regular and irregular past-tense forms, while performance in generalising the 'past-tense rule' to novel verbs was very low. Joanisse (2004) argued that his model demonstrated that children's representation of phonology is important for all aspects of the acquisition of the past tense. Moreover, he suggested that SLI could not be solely a rule-learning deficit, since irregular inflection was also affected, both in the model and empirical data (e.g., van der Lely & Ullman, 2001).

Thomas and Karmiloff-Smith (2003): past tense in Williams Syndrome

Thomas and Karmiloff-Smith (2003) investigated the acquisition of past tense in Williams syndrome (WS), a rare genetic disorder in which language is a relative strength against a background of learning disability. The authors employed a three-layered feed forward connectionist network in which the input layer contained distributed representations of phonology and localist representations of semantics of base forms of verbs, while the output layer was required to produce the phonological form of the past tense of the verb. The training set was an artificial language with monosyllabic stems constructed so as to represent the domain of the English past tense. Thomas and Karmiloff-Smith (2003) considered a wide range of theoretically-driven manipulations of the parameter space of their normal model to contrast five hypotheses for the underlying mechanisms of atypical language development in WS. In particular, they considered atypical conditions that corresponded to (i) a delay, (ii) a hyper-phonological morphological system, (iii) atypically structured phonological representations, (iv) lexical-semantic anomalies, or (v) an integration deficit. Multiple possibilities of atypical conditions were examined for each hypothesis. These ranged from alterations in the number of hidden units or the sensitivity of the activation function to incoming activation, to changes in the architecture or the representational schemes for the different types of information in the model. Thomas and Karmiloff-Smith (2003) showed that different low-level constraints in the computational system could lead to different atypical developmental trajectories, comparable to behavioural data observed in WS (Thomas et al., 2001).

Thomas (2005): past tense in SLI

In the study of Thomas (2005), the normal architecture of the Thomas and Karmiloff-Smith (2003) model was used to evaluate a proposal of Ullman and Pierpont (2005) with respect to SLI. The Procedural Deficit Hypothesis argues that the language impairments in SLI stem from a deficit in the procedural memory system, in this case in the brain structures involved in the learning of rule-based aspects of language. Importantly, a compensation mechanism from the complementary declarative memory system, which supports lexicon-based inflections, was also proposed. This would explain why aspects of inflectional morphology in SLI sometimes indicate residual knowledge of rule-based inflection, such as over-regularisation errors in irregular verbs (e.g., 'thinked') or generalisation of the past-tense rule to novel forms (e.g., 'wugged') (Leonard, Bortolini, Caselli, McGregor, & Sabbadini, 1992). In Ullman and Pierpont's proposal, the residual knowledge stems from the operation of compensatory declarative mechanisms rather than the procedural system.

Simulations in Thomas (2005) showed that when processing units had activation functions of low sensitivity, so that the units were not good at discriminating small differences in input activations, the model exhibited a qualitative fit to the developmental profile of SLI in past-tense production. However, these impaired units were not part of a system dedicated to regular inflections, as postulated by the Procedural Deficit Hypothesis. Instead, the manipulation was to a low-level constraint in a general processing channel; the constraint happened to be more important for the learning of regular verbs than irregular verbs (that is, it was *domain-relevant*, cf. Karmiloff-Smith, 1998). Importantly, changing the computational properties of this shared processing channel also changed the balance between how the model used its two information sources: it came to rely more heavily on lexical semantic input, and less heavily on phonological input, to drive its residual behaviour. In this sense, the model reflected the compensatory character of Ullman and Pierpont's proposal. Overall, the study demonstrated the importance of implementation for specifying the nature of compensatory processes in atypical language development.

Karaminis and Thomas (2010): noun, verb, and adjective morphology in English and Modern Greek SLI

Models of language acquisition need to be general in two ways. They need to account for both typical and atypical language acquisition, and at the same time, they should be able to address language development across languages with different typological characteristics. Karaminis and Thomas (2010) addressed how SLI might emerge in two languages with such different characteristics: English and Modern Greek. Their normal model, called the Multiple Inflection Generator (MIG), combined elements of previous connectionist models of morphology (e.g., Hoeffner & McClelland, 1993; Joanisse & Seidenberg, 1999; Plunkett & Marchman, 1991; Plunkett & Juola, 1999). The architecture is shown in Figure 4.1. The MIG implemented a more general process of producing inflected forms that would encompass multiple grammatical classes and multiple inflections within a grammatical class. While this adds somewhat to the complexity of the learning in English morphology, for the much richer inflectional paradigms found in Modern Greek, it presents a formidable challenge. The architecture considered was a three-layered feed-forward neural network, which learned to integrate multiple cues presented in the input layer (input phonology, lexical semantics, grammatical class, and target inflection) to output the phonological form of a word that would be appropriate to the grammatical sentential context in which the word was to be produced.

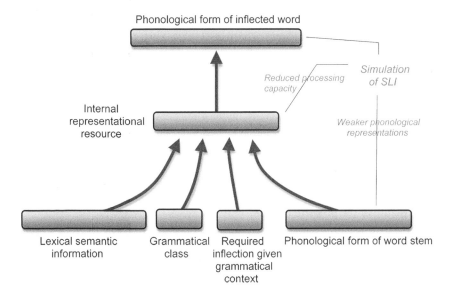

Figure 4.1 Architecture of the Multiple Inflection Generator (MIG), which integrates multiple cues to output the phonological form of content words appropriate to the sentential grammatical context (Karaminis & Thomas, 2010). The model has been applied to simulating the acquisition of inflectional morphology in English and in Greek, for both typically developing children and children with SLI (Karaminis, 2011). Blocks represent layers of simple processing units.

The same architecture was used to learn mappings from artificial languages incorporating characteristics of the inflectional systems of English and Modern Greek. In the latter case, the training corpus consisted of a notably greater number of mappings, reflecting the complexity and the fusional character of the Modern Greek system of inflectional morphology (Stephany, 1997). In both languages, the default version of the MIG simulated a wide range of empirical phenomena in morphological acquisition in typical development.

The impaired version of the MIG (Karaminis, 2011) combined the use of fewer hidden units in the hidden layer with an implementation of the weaker phonological representations utilised by Hoeffner and McClelland (1993). The same constraint was considered for the English and the Modern Greek version of the MIG. In both cases, the model simulated morphological deficits of children with SLI (e.g., English: van der Lely & Ullman, 2001; Modern Greek: Stavrakaki, Koutsandreas, & Clahsen, 2012). Importantly, English-speaking and Greek-speaking children with SLI show subtly different patterns of deficit, which the model was able to capture. For example, in past-tense elicitation tasks (e.g., van der Lely & Ullman, 2001), English-speaking children with SLI produced a greater proportion of forms that were not marked for tense than typically developing children. The formation of the perfective past tense of verbs in Modern Greek requires fusing the stem with morphological features marking the past tense and those marking the perfective aspect. Tense indicates the time when an event happened (past, present, future) while aspect indicates its state at that point in time (imperfective = ongoing, or perfective = a simple whole event). Stavrakaki, Koutsandreas, and Clahsen (2012), who considered a perfective past-tense production task, found that the deficits of Greek-speaking children with SLI were more pronounced in the marking of aspect (perfective) than in the marking of tense (past). For the English and Modern Greek versions of the MIG, the same atypical processing constraints produced the increase in unmarked forms in the English case, and the greater deficit in the marking of aspect than tense in the Greek case.

With regards to the aetiology of SLI, the model demonstrated the viability of the idea that weaker representations and processing limitations could provide a unified account of the impairment across different linguistic domains and across languages, with the manifestation of behavioural deficits in each domain and each language depending on an interaction between atypical processing constraints and the structure of the problem domain.

II. The importance of the developmental process as an explanation of developmental deficits: the example of reading and dyslexia

In this section we examine models of developmental dyslexia. We compare the two computational models of reading, the Dual Route Cascade (DRC) model of Coltheart and colleagues (Coltheart, Curtis, Atkins, & Haller, 1993; Coltheart, Rastle, Perry, Langdon, & Ziegler, 2001) and the triangle model of Seidenberg and McClelland (Plaut, McClelland, Seidenberg, & Patterson, 1996; Seidenberg &

McClelland, 1989). The models crucially differ with respect to the role of development. The former is an explicit, cognitive model, with hand-wired structures while the latter is a connectionist learning model. While both were implemented as models of skilled adult reading, here we consider how well they account for the varieties of developmental dyslexia.

Reading is a hard-won skill and some children find it much harder than others. Developmental dyslexia is a behaviourally defined disorder associated with poor reading. It is diagnosed when there are severe problems with reading against a background of otherwise normal sensory acuity and cognitive ability, and where the deficit could not be wholly attributable to inadequate instruction, opportunity or motivation to learn. Yet dyslexia is also a developmental disorder where early detection and intervention show remarkable remedial success (e.g., Kujala et al., 2001). Nevertheless, without a properly developmental and computational account it is hard to account for the success (and failure) of remedial programs.

From an evolutionary perspective, reading is a recent cultural invention where evolution is unlikely to have had any direct influence on its acquisition. Therefore it is a cognitive ability that requires a mechanistic account. This is not to say that biology is irrelevant. Learning to read recruits and reshapes pre-existing systems. In particular, it reorganises areas of the brain associated with visual object recognition and is constrained by the computational abilities of this area of the cortex (Dehaene, 2009). What is going wrong to cause dyslexia? Are there general deficits, which manifest themselves only in this particular cognitive domain? Or might dyslexia be attributable to specific deficits in particular brain regions or as a consequence of their connectivity? What does the developmental process itself contribute to poor reading?

There is one straightforward way in which dyslexia is developmental. Children with difficulties reading spend less time reading books. Gabrieli (2009) cites the surprising statistic that "outside of school in 5th grade, a good reader may read as many words in two days as a poor reader does in an entire year" (Gabrieli, 2009, p. 280). With this reduced input and less opportunity to practice, their ability will lag even further behind their peers. Likewise, interventions that increase a child's sensitivity to speech sounds (their 'phonological awareness') may have greatest effect if provided at critical early stages. (For a review of early intervention studies, see Torgesen, 2004.) Nevertheless, while environmental factors such as access to reading material and appropriate education can change the outcomes for poor readers, there is a strong genetic component to dyslexia. DeFries and Alarcón (1996) found a 68 percent concordance in identical (monozygotic) twins compared to 38 percent in fraternal (dizygotic) twins. This puts the heritability for dyslexia in the range 54–75 percent (Pennington, 1999). High heritability does not implicate a specific gene for dyslexia. It could be that multiple variants are present in the normal population each of which adds a small risk for reading deficits (see Newbury, this volume). Any genetic account, however, raises the question of how a specific deficit for reading can be heritable when reading is (in evolutionary terms) a recent cultural invention (Mareschal et al., 2007).

Two main types of developmental dyslexia have been described with respect to English (Castles & Coltheart, 1993). *Phonological* dyslexics have most difficulty with regular new words and pseudowords (i.e., word-like nonwords, like HEAN or STARN); *surface* dyslexics have difficulty reading irregular words (e.g., YACHT, HAVE); some children exhibit a mixed pattern with difficulty on both types of words. The dissociation between reading novel words and irregular words was instrumental in motivating models which posited two processing routes between print and speech, one based on a lexicon of whole words, the other based on links between particular letters/letter clusters and speech sounds.

Coltheart et al. (2001): the Dual Route Cascade model

The Dual Route Cascade model (Coltheart et al., 1993; Coltheart et al., 2001), shown in Figure 4.2(a), was a hand-coded computational model that fitted a wide range of data from laboratory tasks with skilled adult readers in English. The model was conceived as a comprehensive model of the fully formed adult reading system and conformed to a highly modular view of the reading system.

The Dual Route Cascade (DRC) model has two separate mechanisms for reading words out loud. It has a lexical route, which features an orthographic and a phonological node for each monosyllabic word in English, allowing for their recognition and pronunciation. It also maintains a set of grapheme-to-phoneme conversion rules that apply to all regular pronunciations in English. (A grapheme is a written letter or letter combination that corresponds to a single speech sound or phoneme.) When a word is encountered, it activates its representation in the lexical route and simultaneously it starts sequentially activating the conversion rules from left to right, grapheme by grapheme. The activation from both these pathways cascades through the network until a complete set of phonemes pass a pronunciation threshold. The model does not implement a further semantic route although this is thought to be important for discriminating between words that sound the same (homophones; e.g., HERE and HEAR).

The model provided a good fit to a wide range of adult behavioural data from non-word and pseudoword naming, capturing effects from frequency and regularity and neighbourhood size (that is, how many similar words there are to a given word in the lexicon). However, the parameters for the model were all hand-coded in order to fit the empirical data. The lexical route was trained to eliminate mistakes in its performance on tasks with non-word material. "Our odyssey through parameter space thus consisted of running exception word/nonword pairs" (Coltheart et al., 2001, p. 219). This is problematic because it means the focus of the fine-tuning of the model was based on non-word materials that would not normally be encountered by a child. Similarly the grapheme-to-phoneme conversion (GPC) rules were selected in advance to be optimal across all possible regular pronunciations in English.

Coltheart et al. (2001) were able to demonstrate that lesioning their model produced many of the characteristics of acquired dyslexia following brain damage. The model did not directly address developmental dyslexia but attributed surface

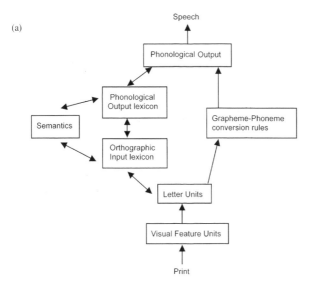

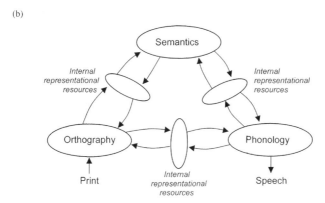

Figure 4.2 (a) The non-developmental Dual-Route Cascaded model of reading (Coltheart et al., 2001). (b) The 'triangle' model of reading development (Seidenberg & McClelland, 1989). Ellipses represent layers of simple processing units.

and phonological dyslexia, respectively, to a failure of the lexical route or GPC route to develop properly. Because the DRC architecture was not a learning model, it was unable to show how the developmental deficits could arise from the outcome of an atypical developmental process. Nevertheless, Coltheart et al. (2001) speculated on how the DRC model could inform these issues. They took a highly modular approach suggesting that "[a]n impairment in learning to read could [correspond to] an impairment in acquiring any one component of this architecture" (ibid, p. 246). A deficit in just the GPC route could lead to a specific difficulty in reading nonwords and could potentially account for phonological dyslexia. A deficit in some part of the lexical route would be manifested as a selective deficit with irregular words, as found in surface dyslexia. Coltheart, Dufty, and Bates (2000; cited in Coltheart et al., 2001) demonstrated that different post-hoc parameterisations of the DRC model could capture the performance of typically developing children and children with dyslexia between the ages of 7 to 15 years.

Despite its success in capturing a range of data, there are three limitations of the DRC model as applied to developmental dyslexia. First, research has demonstrated that the identical damage applied to the initial state of a developmental system can have a quite different effect to that applied to the end state. For instance, noise in processing is more damaging to a developing system than a trained system, while loss of resources is more damaging to a trained system than a developing system. Acquired and developmental deficits cannot be directly analogous (Thomas & Karmiloff-Smith, 2002). Second, the idea of developmental damage to one route of a multi-route system fails to consider the possibility of compensatory changes in initially undamaged routes (see next section). Third, the absence of a developmental process prevents the model from providing a means to investigate ways to intervene to improve a system that has begun to develop atypically. To the extent that the model captures patterns of developmental deficits, it may be doing so for the wrong reasons.

Seidenberg and McClelland (1989); Plaut et al. (1996): the Triangle model

The triangle model of reading was initially described by Seidenberg and McClelland (1989) and its architecture is shown in Figure 4.2(b). Here we focus on the version described in a later article (Plaut et al., 1996). The direct link between the written and spoken forms of words involves only a single route, a connectionist network which learns to associate a grapheme-encoded input with the appropriate phonemically-encoded outputs. The phonetic and orthographic representations also connect to an (unimplemented) semantic representation, and it is this three-way connectivity that gives the model its name. In Plaut et al. (1996), the inputs were 105 units encoding graphemes; these were fully connected to 100 hidden units which fed-forward to 61 fully connected phoneme units. In some simulations there were also recurrent connections in the output layer that served to clean up the selection. Activation passed through the network and training was performed by a standard backpropagation of error algorithm.

As with the DRC model, the triangle model focused on reading monosyllabic words and could produce a similarly high proportion of correct pronunciations. It also captured the influence of word frequency and regularity (and their interaction), as well as exhibiting similar performance to human pronunciation of nonwords with consistent or inconsistent neighbourhoods (Glushko, 1979). However, the triangle model did not *a priori* divide the reading problem into regular and irregular words. In an analysis of hidden units, Plaut et al. (1996) showed that units could not be partitioned according to which type of word they responded. The contribution to the solution was distributed across all hidden nodes in both cases.

Harm and Seidenberg (1999) adapted this model to look at the early development of reading and dyslexia. Children come to reading with an extensive knowledge of the phonology of their native language. So Harm and Seidenberg first had their model acquire phonological representations before learning to map visual word forms onto phonological output. They were then able to investigate how impaired phonological representations affected learning. Mild impairments only affected non-words while severe impairments produced a mixed deficit. Reducing the computational capacity of the network (by removing hidden units before training) produced a pattern similar to surface dyslexia. Harm, McCandliss, and Seidenberg (2003) extended this work utilising the model to demonstrate why giving poor readers remedial training in spelling–sound correspondences is more effective than phonological awareness training (McCandliss, Beck, Sandak, & Perfetti, 2003). In line with the literature, they showed in their model that improvements due to phonological awareness training are only effective in an early sensitive period. Importantly, by virtue of its developmental process, the model was able to shed light on the role of timing on intervention: the quality of phonological representations needs to be improved before links are learned to orthography. Links between orthography and poor phonological representations are hard to unlearn.

Of course, both models have limitations. As in the previous section, models of language processing need to be general not just across typical and atypical development, but also across languages. Both models remain at the cognitive level, with few established links to the neural substrates that may underlie successful and unsuccessful acquisition of reading skills. Lastly, neither model addresses why a heritable disorder should be specific to reading. The suspicion is that whatever properties are atypical in these reading models, they must be properties that are more general in the language or visual systems, but less easily detected when they are awry outside the realm of reading.

III. Deficit spread versus compensation across development in complex cognitive architectures

In this section we outline a form of computational modelling called *dynamical systems modelling*, which has recently been applied to the study of developmental disorders (see Spencer, Thomas, & McClelland, 2009, for a general introduction to the approach). We begin by offering a brief background to the approach and a description of some of its core aims. We then step through a more detailed example in order to demonstrate a key virtue often extolled of dynamical systems: *that complex behaviours of a system can emerge as a consequence of dynamic interactions during development between a number of relatively simple component processes*. We describe recent work in which dynamical systems models addressed the specificity of impairments in developmental disorders (Baughman & Thomas, 2008). Following on from the previous section, we use developmental dyslexia as our focus and examine key issues related to the degree of specificity in the reading disorder, and the neurocomputational conditions that may deliver the observed behavioural deficits.

Dynamical systems models are one of a number of mathematical modelling approaches that study change over time. These approaches are derived from *dynamical systems theory* (Thelen & Smith, 1994) and they include, for example, *dynamic field theory, growth modelling, catastrophe theory,* and *population dynamics*. The phenomena targeted by these approaches vary, as does the time course over which change is observed. For example, within the study of infant sensory and motor development, dynamic field theory has been used to explain changes over the millisecond and second range in children's ability to reach and control their movements for objects (Spencer, Perone, & Johnson, 2009; Thelen, Schöner, Scheier, & Smith, 2001). Within the study of the development of language, growth modelling has been used to study how children acquire vocabulary, over a period of days, weeks, months and years (van Geert, 1991). Catastrophe theory has been used to explore changes over hours, days and weeks, in children's ability to reason (van der Maas & Molenaar, 1992). Population dynamics has been used to study the effects of biological and environmental variables on changes to population numbers, over years, decades and centuries (Hofbauer & Sigmund, 1998).

Though these examples of dynamical systems are varied, a common purpose unifies them within the context of human learning and development – this is to understand the *mechanics* that underlie change in complex systems and that allow those systems to alter their behaviour (i.e., to learn and produce new behaviours). To illustrate what we mean by 'mechanics', let us briefly consider the example mentioned earlier, of van Geert's use of growth modelling. Van Geert (1991) was interested in identifying the key influences on language development. He began by simplifying the process of the development of vocabulary to a component process, defined by a single growth curve. The growth of this process was constrained by a number of variables, or parameters that related to: (1) a given, initial level of linguistic proficiency, (2) the rate of linguistic growth, (3) the level of resources in the environment, and (4) the level of environmental feedback. By testing the effects of small manipulations to these parameters, van Geert showed how in a single model (representing a single learner) the trajectory of development could be dramatically altered. Additionally, van Geert demonstrated how the interactions *between* two models (i.e., two learners) also had markedly different effects on the two models' developmental outcomes. In particular, he found that a combination of supportive and competitive interactions between models best simulated language growth. The mechanics underlying dynamical systems may thus simply be thought of as comprising two aspects, firstly the variables (both biological and environmental) that influence the development of component processes, and secondly the way that these processes are organised and interact (henceforth referred to as the system or network *architecture*).

Dynamical systems approaches offer an advantageous framework for researchers interested in studying cognitive development because at a behavioural level, models exhibit several features that closely resemble change observed in human development. Dynamical systems models can exhibit profiles of change that are non-linear, with the emergence of new abilities often being preceded by periods of marked instability. Around these times of instability, behaviour is influenced both by previously learned, latent knowledge and newer, active representations of knowledge. Additionally, significant changes in the performance of dynamical models often occur suddenly, giving the appearance of stage-like transitions. However, analysis reveals that increases in ability are due neither to the emergence of new, more advanced underlying processes, nor the restructuring of existing processes. Rather, they are the result of continuous change within the interactions of the underlying properties of the system.

Dynamical systems models applied to the study of developmental disorders

Dynamical systems models provide a useful framework for exploring how the process of development contributes to the emergence of abilities and disabilities by virtue of their distinction between the component processes of a system, the variables that influence their growth, and the nature of the interactions between those processes. To explore the possible source of developmental disorders such as developmental dyslexia, we must establish what these mechanics might be. To guide this search, we turn to the literature pertaining to cognitive theories of developmental disorders. Here, we find that one of the common assumptions is that by adulthood, cognition is organised largely in a *modular* manner. That is, the range of cognitive abilities that humans come to develop is the product of a number of functionally specialised cognitive components. While we described the DRC model in these terms, it was also true of the triangle model of reading, in its distinction between orthographic, semantic, and phonological representations of knowledge.

Evidence for claims of functional specialisation is often derived from studies of adult patients who, following brain damage or disease, have been shown to exhibit dissociations in their cognitive abilities. That such cases appear to show that the cognitive system may become 'fractionated' has been used as the basis for developing models of the normal adult cognitive architecture (Shallice, 1988). The use of modular architectures to explain the causes of developmental disorders is an issue of contention, inasmuch as they risk de-emphasising or even ignoring the developmental process, as we saw in the previous section (see Temple, 1997; Thomas & Karmiloff-Smith, 2002; Thomas, 2006). Within modular accounts of disorders, one finds that the root cause of a disorder is often explained in terms of either a 'delay' or, a 'deficit' to the functioning of a single cognitive module, or process (illustrated in the application of the DRC model to developmental dyslexia). Yet, such modular explanations rest on two assumptions: (1) that the cognitive system of the child is also modular, and (2) that during the process of development, module-specific deficits can persist without compensation by or spread to other causally linked cognitive processes. Both these assumptions have been challenged (e.g., Filippi & Karmiloff-Smith, this volume; Karmiloff-Smith, 1998). Whilst uneven profiles of cognitive abilities are often found during childhood, current debates concern precisely how deficits emerge and the true extent of specificity of a deficit in a developmental disorder.

The answers to these questions very much depend on the nature of the cognitive architecture present in children. For example, distributed theories (of the sort inspired by McClelland & Rumelhart, 1988) lead to doubts that any deficit, however domain specific to begin with, could remain so across development. In such theories, cognitive processes are graded and interactive, relying on the contribution of many different components. Evidence from the neurosciences supports the view that the brain is highly interactive and capable of compensation following some forms of early damage (Thomas & Karmiloff-Smith, 2002; Thomas, 2003). Between the extremes of fully modular and fully distributed theories lie various positions that propose more limited degrees of cognitive differentiation. For example, hemispheric specialisation may be important even if functions are interactive within each hemisphere, as evidenced by the emergence of laterality effects after unilateral brain damage in the domains of language (Bates & Roe, 2001) and spatial cognition (Stiles, 2001). Some accounts focus on the importance of a central executive (see e.g., Baddeley, 1996), while others emphasise hierarchical organisation in cognition (e.g., Anderson & Lebiere, 1998).

Computational modelling once more provides the opportunity to test the viability of different theoretical accounts. By taking a modelling approach, we can explicitly assess the consequences of assuming a given architecture for the development of an impairment. In the following illustrative example, we simplified the simulation of developmental processes at the level of individual components in order to focus on the implications of their interactivity in five large-scale architectures. The simplification involved assuming that the development of a cognitive process can be captured by a growth curve defined by a small number of parameters, including its onset, rate of growth, and final asymptotic value. Variations in these parameters were then used to depict heterogeneous underlying mechanisms and domains. By postulating different global architectures (fully distributed, hemispheric, central processor, hierarchical, and modular, shown in Figure 4.3), we then examined the consequences on development of damage that initially occurred to a single process – these are the conditions that modular theories propose to be responsible for apparently domain-specific developmental deficits like developmental dyslexia.

A dynamical systems model

The dynamical systems model we used was based upon a framework developed by van der Maas and colleagues. Van der Maas et al. (2006) proposed a dynamical model of the development of intelligence. It simulated cognitive development for a number of different components via non-linear growth curves in a fully connected system (depicted in Figure 4.4).

A fundamental feature of the model is that all of the processes within the system co-operate throughout development. Unique parameters help guide the development of individual processes, but development is also influenced dynamically by the performance of all other processes. These interactions result in mutually

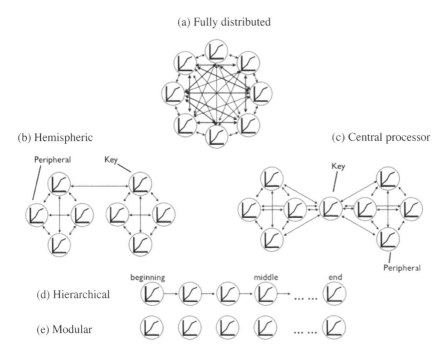

Figure 4.3 Candidate architectures for multi-component cognitive systems. A growth curve is depicted within each processing component.

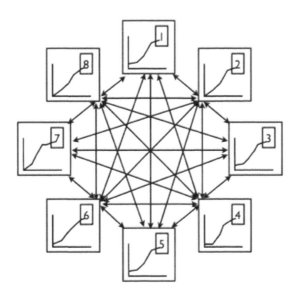

Figure 4.4 The mutualism model, applied to the study of disorders (Baughman & Thomas, 2008).

beneficial and positive influences over development. Hence, the model was referred to as the 'mutualism' model. The following coupled differential equation specifies the dynamics of the mutualism model.

$$\frac{dx_i}{dt} = a_i x_i \left(1 - x_i / K_i\right) + a_i \sum_{\substack{j=1 \\ j \neq i}}^{w} M_{ij} x_j x_i / K_i$$

The mutualism equation was derived from population dynamics and the *Lotka-Volterra* equation. The equation states that at each point in time (t) the change in the performance level x of a given process i (dx_i) is a product of the sum of the interaction weights of each process j with which it is functionally connected ($M_{ij} x_j x_i$), multiplied by the rate of growth of process i (a_i) times the current level of performance of process x_i, divided by the asymptote level for that process (K_i). For each process, changes in x_i at each time step are constrained by the performance (and thus the individual properties) of all other processes to which it is connected. Because the parameters that influence the model's behaviour are relatively few (i.e., a, K and x) and because the functional architecture can be explicitly specified via a matrix of functional connectivity (M), we considered the model to be a useful framework for investigating issues surrounding specific developmental impairments under various architectures.

Due to the fact that the model necessarily sits at a fairly high level of abstraction, one consequence is that it becomes more difficult to elucidate what each of the model parameters relates to, in terms of *specific* biological, or environmental factors. At this level of simplification, the model parameters reflect largely a blend of influences from both. For instance, the growth (a) of a given cognitive process may likely be influenced by both biological and environmental factors. On the other hand, the initial level (x) of a process (which may be initially constrained by growth) may be primarily dependent on environmental input. The capacity of a process (K) may be influenced both by environmental and biological factors, and the degree of interconnectivity (M) may initially be largely dependent on biological factors, but susceptible to effects in the environment.

Once a cognitive architecture has been specified, one must decide where it is appropriate to apply an initial deficit. Within each architecture, processes differ in their interconnectivity, and thus are likely to differ in the amount of influence they exert on the development of the system as a whole. To illustrate, take the following comparison between the fully distributed model and the central processor model, shown in Figure 4.3(a) and 4.3(c), respectively. In the fully distributed model one can see that all processes share the same degree of connectivity. Therefore, the effect of damage to one process should be equivalent to the effect of damage to any other. In contrast, in the central processor model, the degree of connectivity differs between processes. Whereas the central process has the greatest number of connections (it is connected to all processes), the connectivity of any other process is more limited (each process is connected only to the processes within the same cluster). Within each architecture, therefore, the consequences of an initial deficit should vary, depending on whether it is applied to a *peripheral* process (one with relatively fewer connections) versus a *key* process (one with a relatively greater number of connections). For each of the architectures given in Figure 4.3, we applied an initial focal deficit to a single component, either to its onset, growth rate, final asymptote, or combinations of these three. We then traced the effects of the deficit separately on both peripheral and key processes, over the full architecture as development proceeded. Deficits were applied to the start state of a population of simulated individuals, who had minor variations in the initial values of their onsets, growth rates, and asymptotes, but all of whom shared a common architecture.

An illustrative example of deficit spread versus compensation

With respect to developmental dyslexia, the most pertinent result concerns conditions where simulations produced lasting deficits for a single process (corresponding, say, to the GPC component in the DRC model). We found that a large impairment (e.g., a 75 percent reduction of the normal level) to just one parameter (the K parameter, asymptote level) was sufficient to produce this outcome across the range of models. We assessed two additional properties. *Compensation* was assessed based on whether the performance of the initially damaged process was reliably different to if it had developed in isolation, unconnected to any other process. *Deficit spread* was assessed based on whether the performances of the initially undamaged processes were reliably different to those same processes in the normal model. Figure 4.5 depicts the developmental profiles for each of the individual processes for each architecture. Black lines show the trajectories of each process in the normally developing models and grey lines show the trajectories of each process in developmentally disordered models. Horizontal dashed lines depict the level of performance that is predicted for the level of damage, were the process to develop in isolation, and against which the action of compensation was gauged.

Unsurprisingly, in the modular architecture, early selective damage to a single process resulted in a dramatic drop in the performance level for that process. Also of no surprise was the fact that in the modular model the initially unaffected processes developed normally. Due to the lack of interconnectivity, the modular network exhibited no spread of deficit and equally, offered no compensation to the damaged process. In this case, an early deficit would result in a truly specific impairment. The pattern was different in the other four architectures. As the process of development unfolded, the effects of early damage to a single process were not isolated. Figure 4.5 illustrates the extent of deficit spread for each of the architectures (shown via the lower-than-normal developmental trajectories for initially unaffected processes) and compensation (where performance for the damaged process was above the level predicted).

Notably, while the performance of the damaged component in the latter architectures was significantly lower than the normal model, there was no reliable difference in performance between the initially undamaged processes and their normally developing counterparts, *against the background of variability in the population*

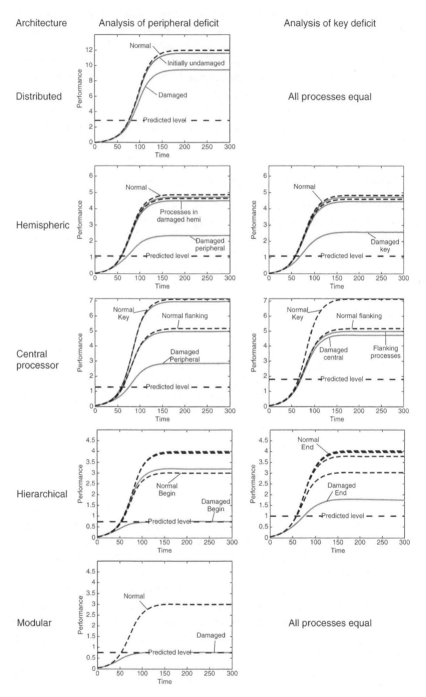

Figure 4.5 Developmental trajectories for each architecture, distinguishing between key and peripheral processes.

as a whole. That is, the spread of the deficit over development was masked by the fact that the performance was *within the normal range* for the population, even though it was below the level it would have been if the starting conditions in each system were normal (see Figure 4.6). Superficially, the behavioural profile suggests that specific impairments, of the sort reported in cases like developmental dyslexia, are possible under a variety of neurocomputational conditions, including those that did not specify a modular functional architecture; in fact, in non-modular, interactive cognitive architectures, the effects of the damage were never truly specific but instead were widespread and subtle, with the system's dynamics determining the degree of deficit spread and the amount of compensation following early forms of damage. The implication of these findings is that if the functional architecture of cognition in the child is not modular, then a range of other cognitive domains outside the primary deficit may show subtle deficits, even under conditions where the initial deficit began as more restricted (see also, Williams & Lind, this volume). Whether these subtle deficits can be detected depends in part on the range of variability that the wider population exhibits in the relevant domains.

Computational simulations of this kind have the potential to reconcile views of the apparently specific nature of behavioural impairments in disorders such as developmental dyslexia with those that posit the highly distributed nature of cognition. The task of narrowing down the range of candidate architectures requires the combined efforts of empirical (both behavioural and neurosciences) and computational approaches. For example, if it were the case that current assessment techniques do not detect the subtle developmental effects of a deficit in one domain on other cognitive domains, then a good starting point would be to utilise more sensitive behavioural measures of the apparently normally functioning

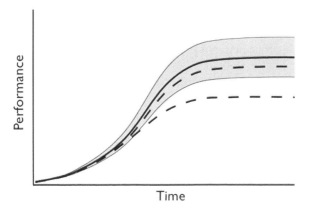

Figure 4.6 A simulated typical developmental trajectory with upper and lower bands depicting variability in the population, along with two examples of atypical trajectories (dashed). The upper dashed line represents an atypical trajectory that, while showing a deficit compared to the level that this individual could have achieved without initial damage, would not be detectable since it falls within the normal range for the population.

domains. Indeed, studies aimed at refining the methods for assessing children's cognitive abilities are underway (see e.g., Bornstein, 2011; Rezazadeh, Wilding, & Cornish, 2011). By more accurately profiling the abilities of children, it may be possible to eliminate some architectures from enquiry. Converging evidence from the neurosciences will be invaluable in this matter. For example, studies targeting whole-brain patterns of activity are beginning to identify the causal, functional relations between cognitive domains (see e.g., Bressler & Menon, 2010; Hu et al., 2011; Jolles, van Buchem, Crone, & Rombouts, 2011; Menon, 2010).

Indeed, some of this work has suggested that the functional architecture of cognition may be organised according to the properties of *small-world networks*. Small-world networks offer another example of a dynamical system in which a network consists of a number of component processes, between which are varying amounts of connectivity. While each process is causally related to each other process, their influence can be exerted via shorter or longer pathways. Interactions between any two processes can take place either via direct connections or via pathways employing variable numbers of intermediate nodes. In the case of a *regular* small-world network shown in Figure 4.7(a), where a regular relationship exists for all processes, connections are limited to processes that are near each other. Longer-range interactions will require many intermediate nodes. In other cases, shown in Figure 4.7(b) and 4.7(c), small-world networks exhibit additional *random* connections. The effect of these random connections is a shortening of paths, and thus more direct influence between processes from diverse areas of the system.

The dynamics of small-world networks have been studied in a variety of contexts (e.g., social networks and in the spread of disease in populations). However, their relevance here comes from the use of brain-imaging techniques, which have demonstrated that distributed patterns of activity resembling small-world networks underlie a range of cognitive activities (Boersma et al., 2011; Ferrarini et al., 2009; Fransson, Aden, Blennow, & Lagercrantz, 2011; van den Heuvel & Pol, 2010). In these cases, the view that is emerging is that cognition is comprised of regions of highly connected processes or 'cortical hubs' (Achard, Salvador, Whitcher, Suckling, & Bullmore, 2006) and regions where connectivity between processes is more diffuse. The functional differences in the properties of these

(a)   (b)   (c)

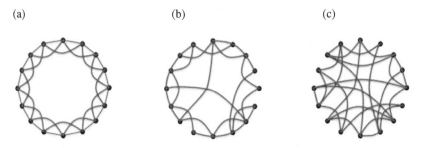

Figure 4.7 The connectivity of 'small world' architectures: (a) connections are limited to processes that are near each other; (b) and (c): small-world networks with additional random connections that shorten pathways.

networks have been examined in disorders such as Alzheimer's disease (Stam et al., 2009), schizophrenia (Liu et al., 2008) and attention deficit hyperactivity disorder (ADHD) (Wang et al., 2009). Our current simulation work is extending dynamical systems modelling of developmental deficits to small-world scenarios.

Despite these advances, the challenge of modelling at the level of cognitive architectures is to understand for a given disorder exactly how widespread the neurocomputational differences are in the atypically developing brain, and how the effects of these differences unfold through the intricacies of the developmental process (see also, Filippi & Karmiloff-Smith, this volume).

Forthcoming work in the modelling of developmental disorders

The previous models have captured developmental deficits in terms of neurocomputational limitations to the representations or processing within associative learning systems. However, there are other types of learning which provide alternative candidate pathways for developmental deficits. Reinforcement learning involves learning cognitive operations, actions, or sequences of actions that maximise rewards. It is possible that individuals with disorders find different aspects of their environments rewarding compared to typically developing children. This in turn may change the way children with disorders interact with and attend to their environments and indeed, the subjective nature of the environments to which they are exposed. One example comes from the domain of eye gaze behaviour. Typically developing infants learn to use the direction of their caregiver's gaze to predict where to find interesting objects in the immediate environment. Infants and children with autism tend to avoid looking at caregivers' eyes, leading to disruptions in the development of dyadic (two-person) interactions. By contrast, in WS, infants and children seem captivated by the faces of caregivers, yet they show deficits in triadic interaction, where there is failure to establish shared attention between child and adult on an object. Triesch, Teuscher, Deak, and Carlson (2006) constructed a computational model of the development of infant eye-gaze following based on reinforcement learning. In this model, the simulated infant learned that if she looked at her caregiver's direction of eye gaze, this might serve as a predictive cue of where in the environment interesting objects might be found, which the infant could then fixate. Through a sequence of exploratory behaviour in the simulated environment, the infant came to maximise the reward she gained from fixating her caregiver and from using the direction of her caregiver's gaze to look at rewarding objects around her. Triesch et al. then simulated two conditions of atypical development, building in constraints from autism, where faces are hypothesised to be intrinsically less rewarding, and WS, where faces are hypothesised to be more rewarding than normal. In both cases, the simulated infants showed developmental deficits in gaze following behaviour, where faces were either avoided, so attenuating caregiver eye gaze direction as a predictive cue, or fixated for longer than normal, so failing to move on to fixate objects in the environment. In both cases, the atypical reward conditions led to emergent deficits in the development of gaze following. Notably, these two atypical models for autism and WS, distinguished only by the reward value attached to faces, looked very similar in the early stages of development. However, the small difference in the start state led to a radical divergence between the systems across development, until they exhibited very different behaviour. (See Richardson & Thomas, 2006; Williams & Dayan, 2005, for related work modelling reward learning in ADHD.)

Kriete and Noelle (2011) recently postulated that problems in reward-based learning might contribute to deficits in executive functioning observed in adolescents and adults with autism. The authors used as their model of normal development the Cross-Task Generalisation (XT) model of pre-frontal cortex task control (Rougier, Noelle, Braver, Cohen, & O'Reilly, 2005). The objective was to capture two pieces of empirical evidence regarding executive dysfunction in older individuals with autism: perseverative errors on the Wisconsin Card Sort Task (WCST) and normal performance on the Stroop task. In the WCST, subjects must show cognitive flexibility in altering the dimensions over which they sort cards (e.g., by colour, by shape). In the Stroop task, subjects must respond to a single dimension of a stimulus and ignore another potentially more salient dimension. The original XT model combined both reinforcement learning and associative learning to simulate performance on the WCST and Stroop tasks, in adults and in individuals suffering acquired frontal brain damage.

Kriete and Noelle pursued the hypothesis that dopamine may be reduced in autism, thereby dysregulating the interaction of the mesocortical dopamine system with the prefrontal cortex (PFC). The dopaminergic neurotransmitter system implements reward-based learning in PFC. The postulated deficit in the reward signal in the XT model affected a gating mechanism that destabilised short-term PFC representations supporting task performance. Destabilisation was key for flexibility in behaviour, since it opened the PFC to change its task configuration. A change of task configuration is crucial in WCST but is not required in the Stroop task. As a result, the reduction in destabilisation in the autism condition led to perseverative behaviour in a simulation of WCST (i.e., continuing to sort the cards by a dimension that was no longer relevant) but did not alter performance on the Stroop task. In addition, Kriete and Noelle found that the WCST impairment was late emerging in the development of the autistic model, because the PFC component only adopted the role of supporting cognitive flexibility once associative mechanisms (modelling posterior cortex) had acquired relevant abilities. The model therefore provides a novel causal explanation of why behavioural deficits in executive function may be late emerging in autism, even though their primary cause (a reduction in dopamine) is in place throughout development.

As the Kriete and Noelle (2011) paper illustrates, one advantage of using computational models based on principles of neurocomputation is the opportunity to make links to evidence from neuroscience. Ultimately, the causal explanation of a disorder will span many levels of description. The known genetic basis of some disorders (such as the genetic mutations in disorders like Down syndrome and WS) and the high heritability observed in behaviourally-defined disorders (such as autism and dyslexia) implies that the lowest level of description will be genetic. Yet there are puzzles that arise from genetic accounts of disorders. One of these is that genetic mutations and gene variants are often only probabilistically associated with behavioural outcomes observed in disorders. There must be other risk and protective factors that modulate the relationship between a given genetic cause and the behavioural phenotype observed in a disorder. Moreover, some common gene variants have been associated with more than one disorder (e.g., developmental language impairment and autism; Vernes et al., 2008).

A new simulation approach based on population modelling has begun to investigate the probabilistic nature of the causes of developmental deficits. Population modelling involves simulating large numbers of individuals undergoing both typical and atypical development. Apart from the hypothesised cause of the disorder, the framework includes the possibility of population-wide variation in the neurocomputational properties of all children, as well as variations in the quality of the environment to which all children are exposed. One model utilising this approach, by Thomas, Knowland, and Karmiloff-Smith (2011), evaluated the hypothesis that autism may be caused by disruptions in connectivity occurring during synaptic pruning. During development, the brain initially produces exuberant connectivity, which is subsequently pruned back in childhood. This gives the brain greater plasticity in early development, to adapt to the environment in which it finds itself, while saving on metabolic resources later in development. However, if the pruning process is too aggressive, rather than just removing spare computational resources, it can compromise the neurocomputational properties of the system or even lead to regression in behaviour. Notably, Thomas et al. found that the cause of the disorder in their networks (over-aggressive synaptic pruning) interacted with other dimensions that varied in the general population, such as the amount of computational resources, the rate of learning, and the richness of the learning environment to which the individual was exposed. These risk and protective factors led to a probabilistic relationship between the (in the model, known) cause of the disorder and its manifestation in behavioural deficits. Moreover, the authors demonstrated how a direct cause of one disorder (e.g., slow development) could be a risk factor for another (e.g., slow development makes the effects of aggressive synaptic pruning worse). This would explain why there should be shared causal factors (such as gene variants) between different disorders: the shared factor indexes the cause of one disorder and the elevated risk (but not direct cause) or another. Bishop (2006) recently advocated that researchers move to an explanatory framework of developmental disorders based on risk and protective factors, rather than necessary and sufficient conditions. Population modelling is a new approach that is consonant with this shift to viewing causal factors as probabilistic against a background of variability.

Lastly, population-level models also permit a consideration of the effects of variations in the quality of the environment. Thomas, Ronald, and Forrester (2012) recently modelled the effects of socio-economic status (SES) on language development at the population level, evaluating the idea that one way that SES might operate on cognitive development is via a manipulation of the amount of information available to the child. This model generated the novel prediction that SES should be statistically associated with good developmental outcomes in children but not with bad developmental outcomes. Empirical data from the acquisition of inflectional morphology (Bishop, 2005) offered direct support for this novel prediction. Crucially, because the operation of the model was understood, it was possible to show that this asymmetric statistical relationship was misleading. Poor environment did indeed cause poor developmental outcomes in the model. However, because a range of other neurocomputational factors could also compromise developmental outcomes, the unique statistical predictive power of the environment was lost. By contrast, for a good developmental outcome, all factors must be good (i.e., a good learning system and a good environment). Presence or absence of good SES then becomes more uniquely predictive. In this way, the implemented mechanistic model offered a deeper understanding of causal relations than that available through simply identifying correlations between behaviour and factors in the environment.

Using models to investigate intervention

Implemented computational models of developmental deficits provide the foundation to explore possible interventions, and indeed allow for a much wider range of interventions to be considered than in human studies, where there are both practical and ethical limitations. Nevertheless, work on simulated interventions has been relatively limited so far, the greater focus having been on building accurate models of the disorders themselves. The model of dyslexia in reading offered one example of a simulated intervention. Harm, McCandliss, and Seidenberg (2003) demonstrated how improving the internal structure of poor phonological representations via training on component sounds of whole words was successful in improving the subsequent acquisition of mappings between print and sound. The model in addition demonstrated why such an intervention was more effective before the start of literacy training – once the system started to learn mappings between orthography and poorly structured phonology, these bad mappings were hard to unlearn.

A number of questions are brought to the fore in considering simulated interventions in a developmentally disordered system. First, where a cognitive system has an atypical processing property, can this be normalised by the intervention? Second, where there has been a history of development with the atypical property, can the consequences of this development be undone? In part, this relates to how the plasticity of the target cognitive system changes with age. Third, should the intervention target atypical processing properties directly, or should it operate through exposing the child to a differently structured learning environment? Fourth, if it is not possible to normalise the processing properties of the system by an intervention (so that the child cannot feasibly hope to master all aspects of a target domain), which subset of behaviours should be optimised?

These questions can be illustrated by some examples. In the model of dyslexia discussed above, it was possible to normalise the system by intervention – training to improve phonological awareness altered phonological representations sufficiently for normal mappings to be learned between orthography and phonology. However, the consequences of a history of atypical development were harder to undo – the intervention was less successful if literacy acquisition had already commenced. In the Thomas, Knowland, and Karmiloff-Smith (2011) model of autism, which simulated the disorder via over-aggressive pruning of connections in an artificial neural network, normalisation would not be possible – the connectivity was permanently lost. In this model, interventions could only aim to generate the best behavioural outcome that the altered connectivity pattern would allow. Direct interventions that target atypical processing properties might be possible in the future. Researchers working with animal models of Down syndrome have reported that a drug intervention that reduced (excess) neural inhibition in a mouse model led to improved learning on a novel object recognition task (Fernandez et al., 2007). Nevertheless, one might expect most interventions to operate via engaging the child with differently structured learning environments – perhaps those that exaggerate key dimensions of the task to be learned, or focus on prototypical behaviours.

One key challenge to be addressed is how such behavioural interventions can successfully generalise beyond the items used in the intervention itself. Given that generalisation is a much-studied dimension of computational learning systems, it is an ideal challenge to be addressed by computational models of developmental disorders. In short, the modelling approach holds great promise to study and predict effective interventions and work is indeed underway in a number of labs, but the approach has yet to deliver substantial results.

Conclusion

In this chapter, we outlined the advantages offered by computational modelling in advancing our understanding of the causes of developmental deficits. By implementation, models force greater specification on theoretical proposals, and test their viability. They generate novel testable predictions, and allow the model system to be evaluated in new conditions, for example to test possible interventions. We considered examples from language and reading development, and from disorders including SLI, dyslexia, autism, and WS. We considered individual cognitive systems, large-scale cognitive architectures, and interactions between reward-based learning and associative learning. We outlined the new approach of population modelling to investigate risk and protective factors modulating the relationship between disorder cause and behavioural outcome. Throughout, central to our argument has been that explanations of developmental deficits need to focus on the nature of the developmental processes itself (Karmiloff-Smith, 1998), and that computational modelling offers the means to do so.

Of course, a computational model can never demonstrate that a proffered explanation of a developmental deficit is the correct one. Models can only demonstrate that a given account is a viable one. And, as we pointed out earlier, by their nature, models will always contain simplifications, which can under some circumstances, compromise their applicability. Despite their merits, researchers should be cautious in evaluating models. For example, a number of questions might be asked of any computational model of a cognitive process: (1) How robust are the target data that are being simulated? (2) Does the model leave out any key psychological, neural, or environmental constraints? (3) Does the model include anything irrelevant or incorrect in its implementation that is instrumental in producing the target behaviour? And (4), does the model unify a range of empirical effects and/ or produce testable predictions?

Although they must be interpreted with caution, we believe, nevertheless, that computational models have great potential to complement behavioural and neuroscience methods in understanding the causes of disorders, and ultimately, in identifying the best interventions to remediate the negative consequences of these disorders on the developing child.

Acknowledgements

This research was supported by ESRC grants RES-062–23–2721 and RES-062–23–0819 and a Leverhulme Study Abroad Fellowship to Michael Thomas held at the University of Chicago. The studies of Themis Karaminis were funded by the Greek State Scholarship Foundation (IKY) and the Greek Ministry of Education. We would like to thank Marc Joanisse for his helpful comments on an earlier draft of this chapter.

References

Achard, S., Salvador, R., Whitcher, B., Suckling, J., & Bullmore, E. (2006). A resilient, low-frequency, small-world human brain functional network with highly connected association cortical hubs. *The Journal of Neuroscience, 26*, 63.

Anderson, J., & Lebiere, C. (1998). *The atomic components of thought.* Mahwah, NJ: Lawrence Erlbaum Associates, Inc.

Baddeley, A. (1996). Exploring the central executive. *The Quarterly Journal of Experimental Psychology, 49A*, 5–28.

Bates, E., & Roe, K. (2001). Language development in children with unilateral brain injury. In C. Nelson & M. Luciana (Eds.), *Handbook of developmental cognitive neuroscience* (pp. 281–307). Cambridge, MA: MIT Press.

Baughman, F. D., & Thomas, M. S. C. (2008). Specific impairments in cognitive development: A dynamical systems approach. In B. C. Love, K. McRae, & V. M. Sloutsky (Eds.), *Proceedings of the 30th Annual Conference of the Cognitive Science Society* (pp. 1819–1824). Austin, TX: Cognitive Science Society.

Bishop, D. V. M. (2005). DeFries-Fulker analysis of twin data with skewed distributions: Cautions and recommendations from a study of children's use of verb inflections. *Behavior Genetics, 35*, 479–490.

Bishop, D. V. M. (2006). Developmental cognitive genetics: How psychology can inform genetics and vice versa. *Quarterly Journal of Experimental Psychology, 59*, 1153–1168.

Boersma, M., Smit, D. J. A., de Bie, H. M. A., Van Baal, G. C. M., Boomsma, D. I., de Geus, E. J. C., . . . Stam, C. J. (2011). Network analysis of resting state EEG in the developing young brain: Structure comes with maturation. *Human Brain Mapping, 32*, 413–425.

Bornstein, R. F. (2011). Toward a process-focused model of test score validity: Improving psychological assessment in science and practice. *Psychological Assessment, 23*, 532–544.

Bressler, S. L., & Menon, V. (2010). Large-scale brain networks in cognition: Emerging methods and principles. *Trends in Cognitive Sciences, 14*, 277–290.

Castles, A., & Coltheart, M. (1993). Varieties of developmental dyslexia. *Cognition, 47,* 149–180.

Coltheart, M., Curtis, B., Atkins, P., & Haller, M. (1993). Models of reading aloud: Dual-route and parallel-distributed-processing approaches. *Psychological Review, 100,* 589–608.

Coltheart, M., Rastle, K., Perry, C., Langdon, R., & Ziegler, J. (2001). DRC: A Dual Route Cascaded model of visual word recognition and reading aloud. *Psychological Review, 108,* 204–256.

DeFries, J. C., & Alarcón, M. (1996). Genetics of specific reading disability. *Mental Retardation and Developmental Disabilities Research Reviews, 2,* 39–47.

Dehaene, S. (2009). *Reading in the brain: The science and evolution of a human invention.* New York, NY: Penguin Viking.

Fernandez, F., Morishita, W., Zuniga, E., Nguyen, J., Blank, M., Malenka, R. C., & Garner, C. C. (2007). Pharmacotherapy for cognitive impairment in a mouse model of Down syndrome. *Nature Neuroscience, 10,* 411–413.

Ferrarini, L., Veer, I. M., Baerends, E., van Tol, M. J., Renken, R. J., van der Wee, N. J. A., . . . Milles, J. (2009). Hierarchical functional modularity in the resting-state human brain. *Human Brain Mapping, 30,* 2220–2231.

Fransson, P., Aden, U., Blennow, M., & Lagercrantz, H. (2011). The functional architecture of the infant brain as revealed by resting-state FMRI. *Cerebral Cortex, 21,* 145–154.

Gabrieli, J. D. E. (2009). Dyslexia: A new synergy between education and cognitive neuroscience. *Science, 325,* 280–283.

Glushko, R. J. (1979). The organization and activation of orthographic knowledge in reading aloud. *Journal of Experimental Psychology: Human Perception and Performance, 5,* 674–691.

Gopnik, M. (1990). Feature blind grammar and dysphasia. *Nature, 344,* 715.

Gopnik, M., & Crago, M. (1991). Familial aggregation of the developmental language disorders. *Cognition, 39,* 1–50.

Harm, M. W., & Seidenberg, M.S. (1999). Phonology, reading acquisition, and dyslexia: Insights from connectionist models. *Psychological Review, 106,* 491–528.

Harm, M. W., McCandliss, B. D., & Seidenberg, M. S. (2003). Modeling the successes and failures of interventions for disabled readers. *Scientific Studies of Reading, 7,* 155–182.

Hoeffner, J. H., & McClelland, J. L. (1993). Can a perceptual processing deficit explain the impairment of inflectional morphology in developmental dysphasia? A computational investigation. In E. V. Clark (Ed.), *Proceedings of the 25th Child Language Research Forum* (pp. 38–49). Stanford, CA: CSLI Publications.

Hofbauer, J., & Sigmund, K. (1998). *Evolutionary games and population dynamics.* Cambridge, UK: Cambridge University Press.

Hu, X., Guo, L., Zhang, D., Li, K., Zhang, T., Lv, J., . . . Liu, T. (2011). Assessing the dynamics on functional brain networks using spectral graph theory. In *Biomedical imaging: From nano to macro, 2011 IEEE international symposium.* April, 2011, Chicago, IL, USA.

Joanisse, M. F. (2004). Specific language impairments in children: Phonology, semantics and the English past tense. *Current Directions in Psychological Science, 13,* 156–160.

Joanisse, M. F., & Seidenberg, M. S. (1999). Impairments in verb morphology after brain injury: A connectionist model. *Proceedings of the National Academy of Sciences, 96,* 7592–7597.

Jolles, D. D., van Buchem, M. A., Crone, E. A., & Rombouts, S. A. R. B. (2011). A comprehensive study of whole-brain functional connectivity in children and young adults. *Cerebral Cortex, 21,* 385.

Kail, R. (1994). A method for studying the generalized slowing hypothesis in children with specific language impairment. *Journal of Speech and Hearing Research, 37*, 418–421.

Karaminis, T. N. (2011). *Connectionist modelling of morphosyntax in typical and atypical development for English and Modern Greek.* Unpublished PhD Thesis, University of London.

Karaminis, T. N., & Thomas, M. S. C. (2010). A cross-linguistic model of the acquisition of inflectional morphology in English and Modern Greek. In S. Ohlsson & R. Catrambone (Eds.), *Proceedings of 32nd Annual Conference of the Cognitive Science Society.* Portland, OR, USA.

Karmiloff-Smith, A. (1998). Development itself is the key to understanding developmental disorders. *Trends in Cognitive Sciences, 2*, 389–398.

Kriete, T., & Noelle, D. C. (2011). *Dopamine and the development of executive dysfunction in autism spectrum disorders.* Manuscript submitted for publication.

Kujala, T., Karma, K., Ceponiene, R., Belitz, S. Turkkila, P. Tervaniemi, M., & Naatanen, R. (2001). Plastic neural changes and reading improvement caused by audiovisual training in reading-impaired children. *Proceedings of the National Academy of Sciences, 98*, 10509–10514.

Leonard, L. B. (1999). *Children with specific language impairment.* Cambridge, MA: The MIT Press.

Leonard, L. B., Bortolini, U., Caselli, M. C., McGregor, K. K., & Sabbadini, L. (1992). Morphological deficits in children with specific language impairment: The status of features in the underlying grammar. *Language Acquisition, 2*, 151–179.

Liu, Y., Liang, M., Zhou, Y., He, Y., Hao, Y., Song, M., . . . Jiang, T. (2008). Disrupted small-world networks in schizophrenia. *Brain: A Journal of Neurology, 131*, 945.

Mareschal, D., & Thomas M. S. C. (2007). Computational modeling in developmental psychology. [Special Issue on Autonomous Mental Development]. *IEEE Transactions on Evolutionary Computation, 11*, 137–150.

Mareschal, D., Johnson, M. H., Sirois, S., Spratling, M. W., Thomas, M. S. C., & Westermann, G. (2007). *Neuroconstructivism: How the brain constructs cognition* (Vol. 1). Oxford, UK: Oxford University Press.

McCandliss, B. D., Beck, I., Sandak, R., & Perfetti, C. (2003). Focusing attention on decoding for children with poor reading skills: Design and preliminary tests of the word building intervention. *Scientific Studies of Reading, 7*, 75–104.

McClelland, J. L., & Rumelhart, D. E. (1988). *Computational models of cognition and perception: Explorations in parallel distributed processing: A handbook of models, programs, and exercises.* Cambridge, MA: The MIT Press.

Menon, V. (2010). Large-scale brain networks in cognition: Emerging principles. In O. Sporns (Ed.), *Analysis and function of large-scale brain networks* (pp. 43–53). Washington, DC: Society for Neuroscience.

Pennington, B. F. (1999). Dyslexia as a neurodevelopmental disorder. In H. Tager-Flusberg (Ed.), *Neurodevelopmental disorders* (pp. 307–330). Cambridge, MA: MIT Press.

Plaut, D. C., McClelland, J. L., Seidenberg, M. S. & Patterson, K. (1996). Understanding normal and impaired word reading: Computational principles in quasi-regular domains. *Psychological Review, 103*, 56–115.

Plunkett, K., & Juola, P. (1999). A connectionist model of English past tense and plural morphology. *Cognitive Science, 23*, 463–490.

Plunkett, K., & Marchman, M. (1991). U-shaped learning and frequency effects in a multi-layered perceptron: Implications for child language acquisition. *Cognition, 38*, 43–102.

Rezazadeh, S. M., Wilding, J., & Cornish, K. (2011). The relationship between measures of cognitive attention and behavioral ratings of attention in typically developing children. *Child Neuropsychology*, *17*, 197–208.

Rice, M., Wexler, K., & Cleave, P. (1995). Specific Language Impairment as a period of extended optional infinitive. *Journal of Speech and Hearing Research*, *38*, 850–863.

Richardson, F., & Thomas, M. S. C. (2006). The benefits of computational modelling for the study of developmental disorders: extending the Triesch et al. model to ADHD. *Developmental Science*, *9*, 151–155.

Rougier, N. P., Noelle, D. C., Braver, T. S., Cohen, J. D., & O'Reilly, R. C. (2005). Prefrontal cortex and flexible cognitive control: Rules without symbols. *Proceedings of the National Academy of Sciences*, *102*, 7338–7343.

Seidenberg, M. S., & McClelland, J. L. (1989). A distributed, developmental model of word recognition and naming. *Psychological Review*, *96*, 523–568.

Shallice, T. (1988). *From neuropsychology to mental structure*. Cambridge, UK: Cambridge University Press.

Spencer, J. P., Perone, S., & Johnson, J. S. (2009). The dynamic field theory and embodied cognitive dynamics. In J. Spencer, M. S. C. Thomas, & J. L. McClelland (Eds.), *Toward a new unified theory of development: Connectionism and dynamical systems theory reconsidered* (pp. 146–202). Oxford, UK: Oxford University Press.

Spencer, J., Thomas, M. S. C., & McClelland, J. L. (2009). *Toward a new unified theory of development: Connectionism and dynamical systems theory re-considered*. Oxford, UK: Oxford University Press.

Stam, C. J., de Haan, W., Daffertshofer, A., Jones, B. F., Manshanden, I., van Cappellen van Walsum, A. M., . . . Scheltens, P. (2009). Graph theoretical analysis of magneto-encephalographic functional connectivity in Alzheimer's disease. *Brain: A Journal of Neurology*, *132*, 213–224.

Stavrakaki, S., Koutsandreas, K., & Clahsen, H. (2012). The perfective past tense in Greek children with specific language impairment. *Morphology, 22*, 143–171.

Stephany, U. (1997). The acquisition of Greek. In D. I. Slobin (Ed.), *The cross-linguistic study of language acquisition* (Vol. 4). Hillsdale, NJ: Erlbaum.

Stiles, J. (2001). Spatial cognitive development. In C. A. Nelson & M. Luciana (Eds.), *Handbook of developmental cognitive neuroscience* (pp. 399–414). Cambridge, MA: MIT Press.

Tallal, P., & Piercy, M. (1973a). Defects of non-verbal auditory perception in children with developmental aphasia. *Nature*, *241*, 468–469.

Tallal, P., & Piercy, M. (1973b). Developmental aphasia: Impaired rate of non-verbal processing as a function of sensory modality. *Neuropsychologia*, *11*, 389–398.

Tallal, P., Miller, S., & Fitch, R. (1993). Neurobiological basis of speech: A case for the pre-eminence of temporal processing. *Annals of the New York Academy of Sciences*, *682*, 27–47.

Temple, C. M. (1997). Cognitive neuropsychology and its application to children. *Journal of Child Psychology and Psychiatry*, *38*, 27–52.

Thelen, E., & Smith, L. B. (1994). *A dynamic systems approach to the development of cognition and action*. Cambridge, MA: MIT Press.

Thelen, E., Schöner, G., Scheier, C., & Smith, L. B. (2001). The dynamics of embodiment: A field theory of infant perseverative reaching. *Behavioral and Brain Sciences*, *24*, 1–34.

Thomas, M. S. C. (2003). Limits on plasticity. *Journal of Cognition and Development*, *4*, 95–121.

Thomas, M. S. C. (2005). Characterising compensation. *Cortex, 41*, 434–442.

Thomas, M. S. C. (2006). Williams syndrome: Fractionations all the way down? *Cortex, 42*, 1053–1057.

Thomas, M. S. C., Ronald, A., & Forrester, N. A. (2012). *Modelling socio-economic status effects on language development*. Manuscript submitted for publication.

Thomas, M. S. C., & Karmiloff-Smith, A. (2002). Are developmental disorders like cases of adult brain damage? Implications from connectionist modelling. *Behavioural and Brain Sciences, 25*, 772–780.

Thomas, M. S. C., & Karmiloff-Smith, A. (2003). Modeling language acquisition in atypical phenotypes. *Psychological Review, 110*, 647–682.

Thomas, M. S. C., & McClelland, J. L. (2008). Connectionist models of cognition. In R. Sun (Ed.), *Cambridge handbook of computational cognitive modelling* (pp. 23–58). Cambridge, UK: Cambridge University Press.

Thomas, M. S. C., & Redington, M. (2004). Modelling atypical syntax processing. In W. G. Sakas (Ed.), *COLING 2004: Psycho-Computational Models of Human Language Acquisition* (p. 87–94). Geneva, Switzerland: COLING.

Thomas, M. S. C., Grant, J., Barham, Z., Gsodl, M., Laing, E., Lakusta, L., . . . Karmiloff-Smith, A. (2001). Past tense formation in Williams syndrome. *Language and Cognitive Processes, 16*, 143–176.

Thomas, M. S. C., Knowland, V. C. P., & Karmiloff-Smith, A. (2011). Mechanisms of developmental regression in autism and the broader phenotype: A neural network modeling approach. *Psychological Review, 118*, 637–654.

Torgesen, J. K. (2004). Preventing early reading failure. *American Educator, 28*, 6–9.

Triesch, J., Teuscher, C., Deak, G., & Carlson, E. (2006). Gaze following: Why (not) learn it? *Developmental Science, 9*, 125–147.

Ullman, M., & Pierpont, E. (2005). Specific Language Impairment is not specific to language: The Procedural Deficit hypothesis. *Cortex, 41*, 399–433.

van den Heuvel, M. P., & Pol, H. E. H. (2010). Exploring the brain network: A review on resting-state fMRI functional connectivity. *European Neuropsychopharmacology, 20*, 519–534.

van der Lely, H. K. J., & Ullman, M. (2001). Past tense morphology in specifically language impaired children and normally developing children. *Language and Cognitive Processes, 16*, 177–217.

Van Der Maas, H. L. J., Dolan, C. V., Grasman, R. P., Wicherts, J. M., Huizenga, H. M., & Raijmakers, M. E. J. (2006). A dynamical model of general intelligence. *Psychological Review, 113*, 842–861.

van der Maas, H. L. J., & Molenaar, P. C. (1992). Stage-wise cognitive development: An application of catastrophe theory. *Psychological Review, 99*, 395–417.

van Geert, P. (1991). A dynamic systems model of cognitive and language growth. *Psychological Review, 98*, 3–53.

Vernes, S. C., Newbury, D. F., Abrahams, B. S., Winchester, L, Nicod, J., Groszer, M., . . . Fisher, S. E. (2008). A functional genetic link between distinct developmental language disorders. *New England Journal of Medicine, 359*, 2337–2345.

Wang, L., Zhu, C., He, Y., Zang, Y., Cao, Q. J., Zhang, H., . . . Wang, Y. (2009). Altered small-world brain functional networks in children with attention-deficit/hyperactivity disorder. *Human Brain Mapping, 30*, 638–649.

Williams, J. O. H., & Dayan, P. (2005). Dopamine, learning, and impulsivity: A biological account of ADHD. *Journal of Child and Adolescent Psychopharmacology, 15*, 160–179.

5 Teasing apart disadvantage from disorder

The case of poor language

Penny Roy and Shula Chiat

When children's development is out-of-step with expectations (for example, if they lack social or language skills appropriate for their age), this may reflect factors internal to the child, external factors, or, indeed, a combination of these. While the genetic basis for autism and ADHD is clear (see Newbury, this volume) approximately half the children that Rutter and colleagues studied who were adopted from Romanian orphanages following 6 months or more of institutional care had autistic-like features, cognitive delay, inattention/hyperactivity, and disinhibited attachment (Kreppner et al., 2007). This is a much higher proportion than would be expected to demonstrate these traits in the general population who have not suffered such horrific early deprivation. Similar observations can be made about language impairment: while genetic sources for developmental language deficits have been demonstrated (see again Newbury, this volume), as many as 50 percent of children from socially disadvantaged backgrounds do not have language skills appropriate to their age (Locke, Ginsborg, & Peers, 2002). Again, this greatly exceeds expected rates of impairment arising from child-internal factors. We would obviously expect some of those Romanian orphans to have had autism or ADHD, and some children with low SES to have language impairment; we might also expect that effects of external factors will be intertwined with internal factors (see Thomas, Baughman, Karaminis, & Addyman, this volume). But if children have impaired language skills, does it matter what lies behind these?

Teasing apart the contribution of external and internal factors, we argue, is important if we are to understand the developmental pathways that lead to poorer-than-expected performance, and if we are to offer appropriate intervention. Addressing the distinction between poor language due to disadvantage and intrinsic language disorder is therefore important in theory and practice.

In this chapter, we review studies of speech and language in preschool children and primary school aged children from low socioeconomic backgrounds. We will draw on evidence from the UK, US and our own studies of preschoolers. We begin by considering what factors comprise SES classifications, discuss the nonlinear relationship between language performance and SES, and evaluate the extent to which SES-related differences are due to differences in care-giving. This is followed by a more detailed discussion of what is meant by language impairment and the nature of SES-related poor language performance, including the knotty issue of whether and how, theoretically and empirically, we can tease apart language delay due to 'disadvantage' as opposed to 'disorder', and the kind of measures that are required to do this. We highlight social and cultural biases of standard measures used to assess children's language, and make a case for measures proposed to be less affected by differences in environment and experience, drawing on evidence from others' studies. We then present unexpected findings from our own studies using these measures, and discuss the implications for language delay in children from low SES backgrounds, including the role of attention, executive function, and self-regulation. The conclusions we draw have implications for the types of intervention needed to promote language skills in children in socially disadvantaged communities.

Classification of SES

'Socioeconomic disadvantage' and 'low SES' are relative, not absolute, terms that vary according to which reference factors and cut-offs are adopted. Classifications are derived from single or combined measures (Hollingshead, 1975) of factors thought to relate to families' 'living conditions', including occupational, educational and income levels of main carers (see Hernandez & Blazer, 2006, Chapter 2, for a full discussion of these social environmental variables and their relation to health). Primary and secondary caregivers, either singly or combined, may be targeted, and information gained either directly or through self-completed questionnaires. SES levels may refer to individual factors (e.g., occupational status [Hart & Risley, 1995] or parental education level [Fenson et al., 2000]). Separate SES measures are significantly interrelated (Hart & Risley, 1995; Roy & Chiat, 2012). Broader classifications of SES are often adopted (e.g., low, middle, and high) based on either composite measures or single factors. Although income has been found to be more predictive of cognitive development and vocabulary (Duncan, Brooks-Gunn, & Klebanov, 1994; Marulis & Neuman, 2010), education level has probably been more widely used in research on early language acquisition. Parents are often more willing to provide education and occupation data than income data (Noble, McCandliss, & Farah, 2007). Measures may extend beyond individual families to the wider community, and such measures have been adopted in studies of SES and early language development (e.g., free school meals [Locke et al., 2002]; ACORN [A Classification of Residential Neighbourhood; Dodd, Holm, Zhu, & Crosbie, 2003]; the Index of Multiple Deprivation [Roy, Chiat, & Dodd, 2010]). Whatever measures are adopted, SES indices influence outcomes through the quality of the physical and psychological environments that children experience. Significant factors associated with SES and poverty in the pre-, peri- and post-natal periods include, for example, exposure to toxins and psychological stress, nutritional levels, parenting styles, cognitive stimulation and educational experiences.

Differences in reported language outcomes across studies are likely to be a function of the nature and heterogeneity of the sample, the range in SES variables and the stringency of cut-offs for defining low SES groups (Arriaga, Fenson,

Cronan, & Pethick, 1998). There is increasing evidence that the relation between SES and language outcomes is nonlinear: poorest outcomes are disproportionately associated with the most socially and economically disadvantaged groups (Duncan, Yeung, Brooks-Gunn, & Smith, 1998; Hart & Risley, 1995; Roy, Kersley, & Law, 2004; Washbrook & Waldfogel, 2010). For example, in their nationally representative sample of 12,644 British 5-year-olds in the UK Millennium Cohort Survey, Washbrook and Waldfogel found that their poorest income group had vocabulary scores nearly a year below the middle income group, more than twice the gap between middle and high earners, although the income gap between middle and high earners was twice that between middle and bottom earners. Further, SES measures (such as education) that are highly discriminating for language outcomes in large, representative samples may not be discriminating in samples where the range in key SES variables is more limited (Hurtado, Marchman, & Fernald, 2008; Roy et al., 2010). Contrary to previous studies, we found that parent educational level within a low SES group was not significant for preschoolers' language outcomes (see section 'The Barking and Dagenham study' below for full description of the study). In contrast, maternal occupation, favouring the employed, was significant. It is likely that the unemployed mothers were not only worse off financially, but were also more socially isolated than those at work. Social isolation is related to individuals' well-being, which in turn is likely to impact on the quality of interaction with their children. Broad measures of SES, although useful in identifying gaps in performance at a group level, tell us little about individual children's language experiences and how these impact on their developing language.

Low SES, language delay and associated problems

Across the last two decades, there has been increasing evidence of poor language performance in young children from socioeconomically disadvantaged backgrounds. Their performance on a range of language measures has been found to be significantly lower than that of their more advantaged peers (Fish & Pinkerman, 2003; Hart & Risley, 1995; King et al., 2005; Locke et al., 2002; Locke & Ginsborg, 2003; Nelson, Welsh, Vance Trup, & Greenberg, 2011; Qi, Kaiser, Milan, Yzquierdo, & Hancock, 2003; and see Ginsborg, 2006). Average scores of children from low SES groups are reported to be three-quarters to one standard deviation (*SD*) below average scores for the general population. According to some studies, as many as 50 percent have scores in the low range (1 *SD* or more below average) and about 10 percent have very low scores (2 *SD*s or more below average) which is about four times the proportion in the general population. Furthermore, the distribution of standard scores is skewed towards the low end: not only do a disproportionate number of children have below average scores, but relatively few perform in the above average range.

Most of these studies used standardised language measures. An exception is Hart and Risley's study of 42 US families from three SES groups ('professional, working class, and welfare'). Their measures of parents' language and children's vocabulary were based on direct observations and transcriptions of audio record-ing, starting when the children were 10 months old and finishing when they were 3 years old. Arguably, these measures are less subject to the inherent SES bias found in standard assessments that we discuss in more detail later. Yet marked discrepancies in children's vocabulary use and growth were evident by the age of 3, with SES accounting for 40 percent of the variance in scores.

Although our main focus is on language delay, this may not be the only problem that children from low SES backgrounds face. They are also known to be at risk of literacy problems (Flus et al., 2009), poor academic achievement (Snow, Porsche, Tabors, & Ross Harris, 2007) and socioemotional problems (Washbrook, 2010), but we know less about the nature of the relationships between these co-occurring problems and SES-related language delay. Nelson et al. (2011) addressed these questions in a large sample of socioeconomically disadvantaged 4-year-old US preschoolers attending Head Start programmes. A high proportion of children had language problems and there was a step-wise relationship between language delay and the measures of academic and socioemotional skills. Children with Strong Language Delay (2/3 language variables at least 1 *SD* below norms and one vari-able at least 1.5 below norms) had the poorest outcomes and those with High Language status (at least average scores) the best. It is not known to what extent reported associations between language delay and co-occurring problems in the general population are carried by the more socioeconomically deprived children.

Likewise, we know there are negative long-term implications of early speech and language problems on educational achievement, social inclusion and employ-ment opportunities (Johnson et al., 1999; Johnson, Beitchman, & Brownlie, 2010; Law, Rush, Schoon, & Parsons, 2009; Schoon, Parsons, Rush, & Law, 2010; Snow et al., 2007; Snowling, Bishop, Stothard, & Kaplan, 2006; Stothard, Snowl-ing, Bishop, Chipchase, & Kaplan, 1998). Once again we do not know if low SES groups are at greater risk of negative outcomes, nor if the developmental trajectories for children with early language delay differ across SES groups. A key question we address in this chapter is the extent to which early language delays are comparable across SES groups. Apparently similar speech and language profiles may be underpinned by different mechanisms and have different histories that may have implications for their long term sequelae.

Caregiving variables and language

Although it is parents' status that decides children's SES membership, for young children it is their first-hand, day-to-day experience of parenting and care that shapes their worlds. Beyond the individual, research at group level has shown there are systematic SES-related differences in the ways parents communicate with their infants that impact on early language development.

Hart and Risley (1995) found a huge disparity between their SES groups in the quantity of words the children were exposed to. One- to two-year-olds in their 'welfare' group experienced about a quarter of the number of words heard by the children from professional families, an estimated difference of about 153,000 words per week. These 'meaningful differences' in early language exposure were related to later language development. The Matthew principle operated at many levels. How much parents talked to their children as infants was strongly related to the amount they talked to them at 3 years. Moreover, there was a close association between quantity and quality. The more words the children heard, the greater the richness and diversity of the language the children were exposed to and the lower the proportion of imperatives and prohibitions they received. The preschoolers' language mirrored that of their parents not only in terms of the size and make-up of their vocabulary, but also in interaction styles, which reflected the amount of positive and negative feedback they had received as infants. Although, as noted above, SES was highly predictive of children's vocabulary use and growth at 3 and language at 9, proximal measures of parenting language and style (based on analyses of their language output) did better, accounting for an additional fifth of the variance in children's scores. There was a huge disparity between their two extreme SES groups, the welfare group and the professional group, with little or no overlap of scores on any parenting variables or any of the children's outcome measures. However, there was much more variability and spread of scores in a middle 'working class' group comprised of low and middle class families. SES measures of this group were not predictive of language and cognitive scores at 3 and 9, but proximal parenting variables were.

Subsequent research has consistently shown that the quantity, diversity and complexity of parents' child-directed speech in daily interactions with their children affects the nature and speed of early language acquisition. Children from middle to high SES backgrounds compared with those from low SES families are more likely to experience opportunities such as shared book reading which is known to elicit more complex and lexically rich language in parents' conversations with their children. However, as Washbrook and Waldfogel (2010) showed, although parenting style may account for a significant amount of variance, it is far from the whole story. Amongst other factors they found that material deprivation and child-related health factors accounted for nearly a third of the income-related vocabulary gap. Other studies have found that the association with SES holds even after controlling for parenting style and how talkative the children are themselves (Hoff, 2003; Huttenlocher, Waterfall, Vasilyeva, Vevea, & Hedges, 2010).

The older the child gets the more the SES-related vocabulary exposure gap widens (Hart & Risley, 2003) and by school entry, the vocabularies of the most disadvantaged children are substantially smaller than their more advantaged peers. They continue to build their vocabularies at a slower rate, so the gap widens year-on-year (Anderson & Nagy, 1992). As Marulis and Neuman (2010) point out, 'interventions will have to accelerate – not simply improve – children's vocabulary to narrow the achievement gap' (p. 301). Their careful meta-analysis of the effects of preschool interventions to enhance vocabulary cast doubt on how feasible this is to achieve in practice. Indeed, their findings suggested that intervention may even exacerbate the income gap in performance, in that middle- and upper-income children were much more likely to benefit from vocabulary intervention than children from low-income backgrounds.

Likewise, in a follow-up study of clinically referred preschoolers (Roy & Chiat, 2012), we found that the children from middle- and high-income groups showed significantly greater gains in expressive and receptive language than those from the low-income group. Even at this very young age, interventions known otherwise to be effective are not sufficiently powerful to reduce, never mind close, the income gap.

A series of studies with low SES and high SES children by Hurtado, Marchman, and Fernald (2008) shed some light on the possible underlying mechanisms. In a longitudinal study they established links between infants' early language input, the speed and efficiency of their online speech processing skills and word comprehension, and their capacity to acquire and expand their vocabularies. Fernald (2010, p. 9) concluded that 'child-directed talk not only enables faster learning of new vocabulary – it also sharpens the processing skills used in real-time interpretation of familiar words in unfamiliar contexts, with cascading advantages for subsequent learning'. In our own studies of preschoolers (Roy et al., 2010; Roy & Chiat, 2012), we found evidence that low SES heightened the risk of having less efficient lexical processing skills, poorer speech and language abilities and reduced capacity to respond positively to intervention.

An alternative interpretation of these findings is that the poor language outcomes of socioeconomically disadvantaged children are due to heritable rather than environmental factors. There has been a body of evidence and arguments against this view (see e.g., Hoff, 2003, 2006; Huttenlocher, Vasilyeva, Cymerman, & Levine, 2002). A full discussion of gene × environment interaction is beyond the scope of this chapter (but see Hernandez & Blazer, 2006; Rutter, 2008). However, it is noteworthy that the receptive subscale that most discriminated the language performance of the low and mid–high SES groups in our Barking and Dagenham study was very similar to a task known to be largely environmentally determined (see below). In this context, recent findings from the the Bucharest Early Intervention Project (BEIP), a randomised control study, are of interest (Windsor et al., 2011). That paper reported on the language outcomes at 30 and 42 months of a sample of institutionalised children who had either been randomly assigned to foster care (FC) or remained in institutional care (IC). Overall the FC group had substantially better expressive and receptive language outcomes than the IC group, but timing of placement was crucial. The language skills of children placed early (under 15 months) did not differ from a community sample from intact families. In contrast, those placed after 2 years had severe language delays, comparable to children in the IC group. In other words, for the randomly placed FC children who shared the same genetic risks as the IC group, very early enriched verbal input and responsive parenting were effective in preventing a language delay associated with early, albeit severe, deprivation. Interestingly though, both groups made few grammatical errors and did not differ in this respect. The more impoverished linguistic input of the IC group had not affected their syntactic development, at least not at this age. The authors concluded that the language deficits seemed to be due to severe delay rather than disorder, and their language skills were aligned with their broader cognitive abilities.

Likewise, a longitudinal study of syntactic skills found no differences between SES groups in mastery of basic syntactic rules of simple sentences (Vasilyeva, Waterfall, & Huttenlocher, 2008). By 2;6, however, clear SES-related differences emerged in the production of more complex multi-clausal sentences, favouring those children whose mothers' educational qualifications exceeded the level of high school diploma. The authors suggested that task-related differences in performance may reflect different mechanisms involved in their production, with simple syntax relying on mechanisms that are available to all typically developing individuals. On the other hand, the amount and the nature of verbal input may be critical for the acquisition of complex structures.

Low SES and language impairment

The higher rates of low language performance found in children from low SES backgrounds are in line with the disproportionately high rates of specific language impairment (SLI) found in disadvantaged groups within the general population. Tomblin, Records, Buckwalter, Zhang, and Smith's (1997) landmark investigation of the prevalence of SLI in the US reported an overall prevalence figure of 7 percent. This was based on a large sample of kindergarten children attending public schools, stratified according to urban, suburban and rural residential settings, but not by SES background. The overall prevalence figure collapses across residential and SES strata, masking the possible occurrence and extent of differences in prevalence for different socioeconomic groups.

This becomes apparent in the more detailed breakdown of results which reveals variations in the prevalence rate observed in different ethnic groups, with higher rates in Native American and Afro-American children, followed by Hispanic children, then White children, and not one case of SLI amongst the Asian participants. Pointing out that 'these data are not adjusted for the socioeconomic background of the children participating', the authors comment that 'The confounding of race/ethnicity with the socioeconomic variables of parental education and income within the U.S. society is widely documented. . . . Thus, the fact that SLI occurred at a greater rate among African Americans, Native Americans, and Hispanics than among Whites was very likely due, at least in part, to the lower levels of parental education and income within these groups' (Tomblin et al., 1997, p. 1258).

At face value, the results of this prevalence study as well as results from studies of low SES groups lead to the conclusion that language impairment is relatively frequent in low SES groups and relatively rare in high SES groups. However, this conclusion begs questions about what is meant by language impairment, and whether all children who perform in the low range on tests of language are properly diagnosed as having a language impairment.

According to Tomblin et al.'s study, all children meeting their criteria for SLI have an impairment by dint of their language performance, whatever their social background and whatever the reasons for their poor performance. But if we take SLI to refer to poor language performance that cannot be explained by limitations in a child's language experience, reflecting an intrinsic difficulty in acquiring language (Bishop, 1997; Leonard, 1998), the picture is less clear. As pointed out above, children living in disadvantaged communities are at particular risk of reduced input and experience, and this may account in part or in full for limited language in at least some of these children. In the case of vocabulary acquisition, this is more than plausible: since each lexical item in a language is an arbitrary connection between a phonological form and a meaning, we can only acquire vocabulary items to which we are exposed. Given SES differences in children's vocabulary input, it is unsurprising that children from different socioeconomic backgrounds attain low levels of vocabulary.

What about other aspects of language? Diagnosis of SLI typically relies on omnibus measures of receptive and expressive language such as the Preschool Language Scales (PLS; Boucher & Lewis, 1997), the Test of Language Development (TOLD; Newcomer & Hammill, 1988) and the Clinical Evaluation of Language Fundamentals (CELF; Semel, Wiig, & Secord, 2006a). For example, in Tomblin et al.'s study of prevalence, children were assessed on five subtests of the TOLD-2:P (Newcomer & Hammill, 1988) and a narrative comprehension and production task (Culatta, Page, & Ellis, 1983). The TOLD subtests were Picture Vocabulary, Oral Vocabulary, Grammatic Understanding, Sentence Imitation, and Grammatic Completion. To be diagnosed with language impairment, children had to score at least 1.25 *SD* below the mean for their age on two out of five composite scores derived from these tests (Comprehension, Expression, Vocabulary, Grammar, Narrative). For diagnosis with SLI, their Performance IQ score had to exceed 85. These criteria invite several observations. First, performance below -1.25 *SD* on vocabulary and narrative would be sufficient for diagnosis of language impairment. As pointed out above, vocabulary knowledge is indisputably influenced by exposure. The role of exposure in the development of narrative is less clear-cut. Nevertheless, it is highly likely that experience of story-telling and books, as well as rich and varied social discourse, will influence children's understanding and production of narrative. As pointed out above, input to children from low SES backgrounds is relatively limited in all these respects (Tough, 1977, 2000; Tizard & Hughes, 1984). On these criteria, it is unsurprising that children from less advantaged backgrounds are disproportionately represented in the SLI group.

While the case is most obvious with vocabulary and narrative, closer consideration of the clinical instruments used to assess receptive and expressive language demonstrates that they too go beyond the basic language skills entailed in spontaneous language production, requiring skills that are better nurtured and developed in more socially advantaged groups. To appreciate why children from socially disadvantaged backgrounds may be at greater risk of poor performance on language tests even if they do not have a language impairment, we need to compare the demands of receptive and expressive language tests with the demands of everyday language comprehension and production.

To understand a sentence, children must recognise the constituent word forms and their order (in English, where meanings are encoded by word order), and must map these onto word meanings and meaning relations to arrive at a mental representation of the situation conveyed by the sentence (Chiat, 2001). Consider now what is entailed in tests of sentence comprehension. Most typically, such tests employ a picture selection or picture pointing task. In the TOLD, for example, the child is presented with three pictures, including the target and related distractors. To select the correct picture (at above chance level), the successful mapping of sound onto meaning is necessary. But this is not sufficient. The child must also scan and interpret the pictures, must not be deflected by partial overlaps between distractor pictures and word/relation meanings in the sentence, and must select the picture that matches the sentence in *all* key respects (i.e., consistent with words and their syntactic relations). This requires sustained and selective attention to verbal and visual input, comparison between these, and inhibition of partial interpretations. Where targets encode more complex meanings, correct interpretation relies on inferences about relations in pictures based on previous experience as well as verbal comprehension, and matching between information from these two modalities (see Silveira, 2010, for detailed argumentation and examples).

The 'Concepts and Directions' subtest of the Preschool CELF (Semel, Wiig, & Secord, 2006b) poses similar challenges. For example, presented with a picture showing big and small dogs, fish and monkeys, and the instruction 'Point to the big dog then point to the little monkey', the child must pay attention to and retain the two adjective-noun combinations in the verbal input in the face of a 'loaded' picture that includes the reverse as well as the target combinations. These demands go well beyond everyday comprehension, where the child hears utterances in contexts that rarely focus on decontextualised conceptual contrasts (e.g., in size, spatial order, temporal order) and rarely present minimal pairs, and where some aspects of the meaning may be predictable from situational experience, reducing the need to attend to *every* aspect of the input to form a full and correct mental representation of the meaning.

Exposing these wider demands of receptive language tasks does not invalidate them as measures of language comprehension, which clearly includes the ability to understand the full linguistically encoded meaning without contextual support, and the ability to extend interpretation through integration of linguistic meaning with context. Indeed, understanding language in school relies on these abilities and increasingly so through the school years. Performance on receptive language tasks is therefore informative about the range of verbal comprehension essential for take-up of school input. Our point is that such abilities go beyond basic language comprehension and that poor performance on these tasks may reflect limited experience of task demands such as cross-modal matching, interpretation of pictures and/or situations depicted in these, inferencing and sustained attention. Higher order cognitive functions such as the selection, shifting and sustaining of attention, the maintenance of information in working memory and inhibitory control involved in the regulation of goal directed behaviour are referred to collectively as executive function (EF) or executive control (Rueda, Posner, & Rothbart, 2005; Wiebe, Sheffield, Mize Nelson, Clark, & Espy, 2011). As will be seen, there is increasing evidence of EF deficits in children from socioeconomically disadvantaged backgrounds.

The same points can be made about expressive language. Basic language production entails the mapping of the child's own meaning intentions onto words and word combinations in conformity with the requirements of the language, i.e., with words in the appropriate order for intended meaning, and obligatory function words and inflections included. Expressive language tasks vary in the extent to which they exceed these basic demands. Being asked to produce a sentence to describe a picture using a given word, as on the CELF, is clearly different from expressing a self-generated meaning intention: the child must not only know the target word/structure, but must also focus on relevant aspects of the picture and adopt the intended semantic target before mapping this onto the appropriate word(s)/structure. In a task eliciting a grammatical marker such as past tense, the child must know the target morpheme (e.g., regular/irregular past tense), but must also recognise the requirement of the task to produce the verb presented in the input and mark this with the simple past tense rather than another auxiliary modifier even if this would be syntactically acceptable. Again, the wider demands of expressive language tests do not invalidate these as measures of children's verbal abilities. Schooling relies on and contributes to the development of the type of verbal skills they elicit: through the school years, children are increasingly required to adopt new perspectives and new meanings and to encode these in precise forms of language. Expressive language tests are therefore informative about children's readiness to meet the oral language demands of the classroom.

The higher-level language abilities measured by standard language tests are therefore essential for children's participation in and benefit from academic life, and indicate risk of academic struggle and failure, as follow-up studies of children confirm (see above). The basic language skills we have identified, on the other hand, are essential for children's everyday life. When children have difficulty understanding utterances in everyday contexts, and frequently 'get the wrong end of the stick', and when they have problems storing and accessing words, mispronounce words, struggle to convey familiar events using the usual range of verbs and verb structures, mix up temporal references and omit or substitute grammatical markers (required even if they make little difference to meaning), their difficulties affect more fundamental aspects of their lives: their social interaction and relations with family, peers, and the wider community. Such difficulties are hallmarks of SLI (Chiat, 2001; Leonard, 1998). But they are not necessarily problems for children who perform poorly on standard tests of receptive and expressive language, since these are liable to be influenced by input and experience in ways that basic language skills are not.

This claim finds support in evidence of SES effects on standard language measures where this is available. While standardised test manuals include information about the socioeconomic distribution of the standardisation sample, it is relatively rare for manuals to include a breakdown of scores according to socioeconomic grouping. Interestingly, though, Peers, Lloyd, and Foster (2000) included such analysis as part of the standardisation of the Clinical Evaluation of Language Fundamentals – Preschool[UK] (CELF-P), and found that moderate or severe language delay was more than five times as likely in children from low SES backgrounds.

However, Locke et al. (2002) suggested that the low performance of socially disadvantaged children does not arise from inherently lower language-learning abilities, but is more likely attributable to their early experience when 'it is likely that most of them have the potential for normal language development [but] they have lacked the input and opportunities to acquire vital linguistic skills' (p. 13). In Campbell, Dollaghan, Needleman, and Janosky's (1997, p. 519) words, 'poor performance may actually reflect the child's relative lack of experience with the test's format or stimuli, rather than indicating a more fundamental deficit'. Tomblin et al. (1997, p. 1258) make similar points about the findings of their prevalence study: 'The results showing a greater rate of SLI among most children of minority backgrounds were not surprising, given the cultural and linguistic bias of the clinical instruments employed'. These findings on test performance and language experience have important implications. If children attain low scores due to SES bias of the tests, they will require intervention to enhance their language knowledge and skills, thereby equipping them better to access and benefit from education. However, they will not require the clinical intervention targeting basic linguistic skills appropriate for children who have intrinsic difficulties in language acquisition.

Given the different possible causes of low language performance, associated with different repercussions and needs, we argue that a distinction should be made between deficits in basic language skills necessary for everyday interactions, and deficits in higher-level language skills particularly necessary for schooling and for participation in a highly literate culture, and propose that the term SLI or language disorder should be reserved for children who have deficits in everyday language. This accords with Vasilyeva et al.'s (2008) distinction between production of basic syntax, which was not affected by SES, in contrast to production of complex syntactic structures, which they took to be more affected by the nature of verbal input.

But if standard tests of language elicit poor performance in both cases, how can language disorder and language disadvantage be distinguished? Tomblin et al. (1997, p. 1248) suggest this may be 'a challenging if not intractable problem because epidemiologic research calls for highly standardized methods that are inherently insensitive to cultural differences'. Taking a different approach, Campbell et al. (1997, p. 519) observe that 'proposals for alternative or unconventional tests that are free of bias have been in short supply'. Nevertheless, they and others have identified measures that test language skills in ways that are minimally dependent on experience and established knowledge, and are relatively independent of SES, and that may therefore distinguish between language disorder and language disadvantage. The proposed measures are often designated as 'processing-dependent' as opposed to 'knowledge-dependent' (Campbell et al., 1997), since they minimise demands on children's language and cultural knowledge. In addition, some require minimal attention, no metalinguistic skills, and no inferencing, and they are less open to influence from everyday exercising or testing of language skills. Impairment on these tasks is known to relate to language disorder, and we refer to them as 'core language measures'.

Core language measures

Key amongst the proposed measures of core language are verbal repetition tasks. Word/nonword repetition and sentence repetition are known to probe important language skills: they relate to many other measures of language in mixed SES groups, and distinguish children with typical and atypical language development (Conti-Ramsden, Botting, & Faragher, 2001; Gathercole, 2006; Graf Estes, Evans, & Else-Quest, 2007; Seeff-Gabriel, Chiat, & Dodd, 2010). Both have been proposed as clinical markers for SLI (Bishop, North, & Donlan, 1996; Conti-Ramsden et al., 2001). Furthermore, word and nonword repetition have been found to predict later morphosyntactic skills as measured by sentence repetition and grammar score on the Renfrew Action Picture Test (Chiat & Roy, 2008; Roy & Chiat, 2008). At the same time, these tasks appear to be relatively unaffected by SES. No differences in nonword repetition performance were found between UK children from upper middle class and working class backgrounds (Burt, Holm, & Dodd, 1999). Similarly, Engel, Santos, and Gathercole (2008) found no differences between 6 to 7-year-old Brazilian children from high and low income families on nonword repetition, despite significant differences in vocabulary; Campbell et al. (1997) found no differences between 'minority' and 'majority' participants, aged 11–14 years, on a nonword repetition test, but significant differences on a broad-based measure of oral language. In our standardisation of the Early Repetition Battery (Seeff-Gabriel, Chiat, & Roy, 2008), we found that parental education level affected scores for whole sentence repetition, and to a lesser extent, word/nonword repetition, with children of parents who had no qualifications accounting for those effects that were observed. Interestingly, though, no SES effects were found for number of content words (all of which were early-acquired familiar items) and number of function words repeated correctly. The function word score, in particular, is taken to be a measure of basic morphosyntax; according to our findings, then, mastery of basic morphosyntactic skills is robust in the face of environmental differences.

The capacity to learn new words has also been proposed as a processing task that does not rely on prior knowledge. Vocabulary acquisition is a crucial aspect of language acquisition, and is known to be impaired in children with SLI. These children perform less well than typically developing children on tasks requiring fast mapping between novel word forms and their referents and retention of novel words for subsequent recognition and naming (Alt & Plante, 2006; Leonard, 1998; Oetting, 1999; Rice, Oetting, Marquis, Bode, & Pae, 1994). Horton-Ikard and Ellis Weismer (2007) investigated fast mapping skills in groups of African American children from low and middle SES backgrounds at age 30–40 months and found no significant difference between SES groups on this task, in contrast to the significant difference found on standard tests of receptive and expressive vocabulary.

The identification of processing tasks showing reduced if any effects of SES provided the motivation for our hypothesis that these tasks would help to distinguish language disorder from language disadvantage in preschool children living in a socially disadvantaged community. We investigated this hypothesis in a study of children living in a socially disadvantaged area of Greater London.

Standard and core language performance in a low SES sample: the Barking and Dagenham study

Participants in our study were 219 children with English as a first language who attended nurseries or reception classes in schools in Barking and Dagenham, a local authority ranked in the bottom 3–6 percent (out of 354) in England according to the Index of Multiple Deprivation (2007). The children were aged between 3;6–5;0, with an equal distribution across three 6-month age bands. Standard tests were administered to assess receptive and expressive language (CELF-Preschool-2; Semel et al., 2006b) and receptive vocabulary (BPVS-3; Dunn, Dunn, & Styles, 2009). To investigate core language, we identified four assessments that make minimal demands on knowledge and experience, and that test speech production, phonological processing and memory, and morphosyntax:

- The Diagnostic Evaluation of Articulation and Phonology (DEAP; Dodd, Crosbie, Zhu, Holm, & Ozanne, 2002), which identifies children with speech delay and disorder
- The two tests in our Early Repetition Battery (Seeff-Gabriel, Chiat, & Roy, 2008):
  - the Preschool Repetition Test (PSRep), which assesses children's repetition of real words and nonwords
  - the Sentence Imitation Test (SIT) which assesses children's repetition of content words and function words within sentences
- A novel word learning task.

The BAS-II (Elliott, Smith, & McCulloch, 1996) was used to measure nonverbal abilities. With the exception of the novel word learning task, all standard and core language measures were standardised assessments.

As well as comparing their performance with norms on standard and core measures, we made comparisons with performance of a mid–high SES sample of 168 age matched children drawn from socioeconomically more advantaged areas across London. The two samples differed significantly on all our key indices of SES (education, occupational levels and employment status of primary and secondary caregivers).

As expected, the distribution of language scores in our low SES group was consistently low, and significantly below the scores of the mid–high SES comparison sample. In contrast, performance below the average range was vanishingly rare in the mid–high sample. The nonverbal measure yielded similarly skewed performance in the two groups (see Figure 5.1 for mean scores of each group on each measure).

Broadly, then, our findings on standard language measures replicated the outcomes of previous studies of socially disadvantaged preschoolers (Fish & Pinkerton, 2003; King et al., 2005; Locke et al., 2002; Locke & Ginsborg, 2003; Qi

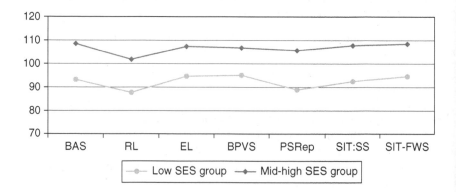

Figure 5.1 Distribution of the mean standard and core language scores and nonverbal scores for the low and mid–high SES groups (all tests with a mean of 100 and *SD* of 15).

Notes: BAS = British Ability Scales II; RL = Receptive CELF Preschool 2; EL = Expressive CELF Preschool 2; BPVS = British Picture Vocabulary Scale 3rd edition; PSRep = Preschool Repetition Test; SIT:SS = Sentence Imitation Test sentence score; SIT-FWS = Sentence Imitation Test function word score.

et al., 2003). However, profiles of performance across measures and across age contrasted with previous findings in some respects. While performance on receptive language was poor in our sample and the proportion below average similar to previous findings, expressive performance was relatively higher, and higher than previously reported for disadvantaged groups where expressive and receptive scores were found to be equally depressed. Many more children were identified with receptive-only problems or combined problems than expressive-only problems (contrasting not only with previous findings on low SES groups but with profiles observed in clinic samples: see Roy & Chiat, 2012). Whilst nonverbal performance did not account for the between-SES group differences in standard and 'core' language scores, a substantially higher proportion of the low SES group had below average nonverbal scores compared with the mid–high SES sample (27.4 percent vs. 4.8 percent). In both groups, children with below average nonverbal IQ were much more likely to have co-occurring LI than those with nonverbal scores in the average range.

While this profile of language performance was consistent across the three age groups in our study, the rate of poor performance was not equally distributed across the three 6–month age groups. Many more nursery children (3;6–3;11) were low scorers compared with the two older age groups (4;0–4;5 and 4;6–4;11) in reception class whose language skills were broadly comparable. Although receptive scores overall were lower than expressive, the age-related differences were more marked in receptive performance. In contrast, Locke et al. (2003), in their study of UK pre-schoolers (median 3;5), found little or no evidence of improvement with age, and the proportion of children with severe problems at follow-up (median 5;4) increased.

The nonlinear age differences in standard scores that we observed suggest that school, at least initially, had a positive impact on language performance. Evidence of a significant association between rate of school attendance and language performance, particularly in the youngest age group, supports this conclusion. Studies of low SES groups inevitably differ in details of sampling and methods, and while Locke et al.'s study is similar to ours in both respects, it is still possible that differences in sampling characteristics or in early years programmes may be responsible for different findings. However, conclusions from our study must remain tentative as the data are cross-sectional and may reflect cohort effects rather than true age-related changes. To test this out, we are in the process of running a small follow-up study of the youngest age group.

Whatever our eventual findings on 'catch-up' through school experience, the proportion of our low SES group with language impairment was disturbingly high, with nearly a third scoring in the impaired range according to knowledge-based standard language measures. But how did they perform on measures of core language previously found to be less affected by SES?

Results on these core language measures were not as we expected. Contrary to theoretical predictions and findings from previous studies (Campbell et al., 1997; Engel et al., 2008; Law, McBean, & Rush, 2011), the 'core' language performance of the low SES group was as depressed as their standard language performance (see Figure 5.1). Significantly more children in the low SES group failed the speech screen of the DEAP (17.8 percent, compared with 8.9 percent in the mid–high SES group). Full assessment of these children found more false positives in the low SES group, and while more children in this group than in the mid–high SES group were classified as having speech disorders (13.7 percent vs. 8.3 percent), this difference fell short of significance. However, speech problems classified as 'delayed' were disproportionately high in the low SES group: about four times greater than the rate found in the mid–high SES. Moreover, the therapists assessing the children reported that the spontaneous productions of some children in the low SES group were much less intelligible than their responses to the individual targeted DEAP items. In other words, the clinical measure might overestimate the children's intelligibility in everyday discourse and underestimate the speech problems in our low SES group. It seems that even basic speech processing is at increased risk of delay in these children. The distribution of performance on basic phonological and morphosyntactic skills (as measured by the Early Repetition Battery: Seeff-Gabriel et al., 2008) were again below the level expected in the general population. Poor performance was more marked on the word/nonword repetition of the PSRep, than the function words of the SIT, which nevertheless showed a gap of 1 *SD* between the SES groups. Moreover, speech disorders did not explain the unexpectedly poor PSRep performance in the low SES group. Our novel word learning task, reflecting children's fast mapping skills and phonological retrieval skills, was exceptional in eliciting equal scores for *comprehension* of the new words, but when it came to *production*, the significant disparity favouring the high SES group recurred.

As with the standard measures, the distribution of performance on core measures improved across age, and for function word scores, the distribution 'normalised'. In this case, as with sentence scores, improvement was linear across the three age groups, suggesting that maturation and/or increased input over time was more important than the specific input provided by school for the development of basic morphosyntactic skills.

Our findings at a group level are clearly at odds with our hypothesis: contrary to our predictions, performance on core language measures, presumed to rely less on experience and knowledge, was for the most part as affected by SES as performance on standard measures. At an individual level, on the other hand, there was some evidence of children with our hypothesised profile of language disadvantage: poor performance on standard language measures in the face of sound core language skills. On average, about a third of the children with poor standard language scores were in the normal range on core language measures. This nevertheless leaves a substantial proportion of children scoring poorly on core as well as standard measures, a profile we took to indicate impairment rather than disadvantage.

This unexpected outcome raises a number of questions and issues. First, why did we find depressed performance on measures previously found to be free of SES effects? This is most striking in the case of our word/nonword repetition test, which relies *least* on prior experience and knowledge (particularly in the case of nonwords since these are new to all children) yet showed markedly low performance across our age range. Previous studies of nonword repetition in low SES groups have involved children of 6 years and above (see section on 'Core language measures'). Our own study found that the rate of performance in the impaired range reduced across the age range. It is possible, then, that thresholds of experience required for 'normal' nonword repetition are reached later in socially disadvantaged groups, and that this 'core' measure would be more effective in differentiating disadvantage from disorder in school-age children. Comparing our findings on novel word learning with those of Horton-Ikard and Ellis Weismer (2007), who found no differences between their low and middle SES groups, it is striking that their sample size was small ($n = 15$ in each group), and as in our study, variability in scores was high. Therefore, as acknowledged by the authors, their study lacked power. Furthermore, their data show a difference in production of novel words favouring the middle SES group, but this difference was not analysed.

Taking into account findings of other studies, it seems that at least in the early years some experiences of social disadvantage are associated with poor core language performance as well as poor performance on standard tests of receptive and expressive language. Further research is needed to identify the indices of social disadvantage that are associated with poor performance on core as well as standard language measures. Whatever the outcome of such research, the findings in our Barking and Dagenham study bring us back to the issues we set out to address: whether poor performance in the low SES group can be differentiated from intrinsic language impairment in the wider population, and/or whether it reflects a considerably higher rate of intrinsic language impairment found in the wider population. Further reflection on our findings may throw some light on the sources of the disproportionately poor performance observed in our low SES group, even on core measures. First, our finding that CELF receptive language, and particularly the Concepts and Following Directions subtest, was most affected and changed most with school experience *is* in line with our argument and expectations: this task is most reliant on attention and inferencing skills that go beyond the processing skills needed for basic language comprehension (see above). Interestingly, the demands of this task are strikingly similar to the BAS Picture Comprehension task which Kovas et al. (2005) found had zero heritability estimates at the extreme low end of ability in their UK study of 787 pairs of 4- to 5-year-old twins. They put forward the argument that genetic influences in language development are much more evident in expressive than receptive skills where the genetic role is negligible, as mentioned above.

In the case of core language measures, while previous evidence suggested that these rely minimally on experience, it is clear that they rely on *some* experience: after all, children acquire the phonology and morphosyntax of the language to which they are exposed. Furthermore, even the least knowledge-based task of nonword repetition is now recognised to be affected by knowledge and experience since children are better able to repeat items if they are more like real words and contain more typical phonotactic sequences (Gathercole, 2006). The nonlinear effects of SES suggest that input and experience across the mid–high socioeconomic spectrum reach the threshold needed to consolidate core language skills. This does not rule out the possibility that input and experience of children in some low SES groups do not reach this threshold, so that more input is required to master even core language skills. Our finding that rates of speech delay, but not speech disorders, were disproportionately high in our low SES group is in line with this possibility. So is our finding that children's standard scores for repetition of sentences and more specifically function words show catch-up. Finally, there is some indication that prior exposure and item familiarity played some role in our findings on word/nonword repetition. For both SES groups, words were repeated better than nonwords, but there was a significant age group × SES group interaction with real words, due to significantly poorer real word repetition in the youngest age group in the low SES sample.

Rates of referral according to SES factors

Given the substantially higher rate of poor performance in the low SES group on core as well as standard measures, we might expect rates of clinical referral to be substantially higher. Contrary to this expectation, though in line with previous evidence (Zhang & Tomblin, 2000), SES factors were unrelated to SLT referrals. Just over 10 percent of *both* SES groups had experienced some contact with SLT services, with 6.4 percent of the low SES group and 7.1 percent of the mid–high SES group currently known to the services. Nor were there group differences in the number of SLT sessions the children had experienced, with the exception of one extreme outlier in the mid–high SES group who was reported to have had 100 sessions. A full three-quarters of the low SES group who had problems on our language and/or speech measures had no contact, either current or past, with SLT services, as was the case for half the mid–high SES group (but given the low rate of poor performance in this group, the actual number was small). Why are such a high proportion of children apparently being overlooked by services? Is this due to sheer weight of numbers in the low SES group? Or does it reflect the nature of the referral process, different thresholds for clinical referral in different SES groups (Roy & Chiat, 2012) and the type of problems that are noticed and lead to referral?

The profiles of children referred from low and mid–high SES groups are informative. The majority of the mid–high SES group in current contact with the services (60 percent) had no identifiable problems according to the measures and cut-offs we used, and the remainder had speech-only problems. Thus, no child referred in the mid–high group scored poorly on language measures in our study. In contrast, about a third of the referred children in the low SES group had language-only problems, and the remaining two-thirds had speech problems (with or without language). Our findings on rates of referral together with the profiles of referred children are in keeping with previous findings that speech has a stronger effect on receipt of intervention than language, and that receptive language problems, particularly characteristic of our low SES group, are likely to be overlooked (Zhang & Tomblin, 2000). Further, recent evidence has shown that children of low SES with language problems were less likely to have contact with SLT services (Bishop & McDonald, 2009) and referred children with adequate language development were more likely to be of higher SES (Keegstra, Knuff, Post, & Goorhuis-Brouwer, 2007).

Executive functions, low SES and language delay

Our argument that non-linguistic functions such as selective and sustained attention and working memory may be implicated in the weak receptive performance of our low SES group is in tune with recent research investigating associations between childhood poverty and neurocognitive development. These studies aimed to identify more fine grained functions that underpin the well established SES disparities in cognitive performance and school achievement in order to develop more effective interventions targeted at deficits in these functions. In addition to language, SES disparities in executive functions, working memory and attention have been found.

SES differences in EF have been identified from early infancy through the school years to young adulthood (Lipina, Martelli, Vuelta, & Colombo, 2005; Mezzacappa, 2004; Farah et al., 2006; Noble, Norman, & Farah, 2005; Noble et al., 2007). A US study of socioeconomically diverse first graders found SES was related to performance on language and a number of executive function tasks using composite scores (Noble et al., 2007). In terms of our findings and discussion of skills involved in receptive language performance, it is interesting to note that two individual tasks with high SES loadings and the highest intercorrelations amongst the adopted tests were the Peabody Picture Vocabulary Test language measure, and an auditory attention task, a measure of executive cognitive control. It is beyond the scope of this chapter to consider these studies in depth, but there have been a number of useful recent reviews in the area (see for example Hackman & Farah, 2009; Raizada & Kishiyama, 2010; Tomalski & Johnson, 2010). A series of three neurocognitive studies of young children at risk of language problems using event related potential (ERP) measures conducted by Stevens et al. (Stevens, Sanders, & Neville, 2006; Stevens, Fanning, Coch, Sanders, & Neville, 2008; Stevens, Lauinger, & Neville, 2009) are of particular relevance and will be discussed in more detail.

ERPs have been described as providing 'a biological window onto processes required for successful language learning' (Barry, Hardman, & Bishop, 2009). Two studies by Stevens et al. (2006, 2009) revealed that children with SLI and those from lower SES backgrounds (as measured by maternal education) had selective attentional auditory deficits compared with typically developing children or children whose mothers had higher levels of education. For both groups attention problems occurred in the early stages of perceptual processing. However, ERPs revealed between-group differences in the underlying neural mechanisms. Attentional deficits in the low SES group were due to reduced ability to filter out irrelevant auditory information, whereas the SLI group had reduced signal enhancement in the attended channel. The authors argued that both deficits are likely to have cascading consequences on the development of language and reading. Such deficits could underpin and differentiate the poor word/nonword repetition performance we found in our low SES sample, and may also be significant in their difficulties in learning novel words. To the best of our knowledge there are no ERP studies of children's nonword repetition skills, but a recent ERP study of adults with good and poor repetition skills concluded that deficits were due to an 'inability of encoding mechanisms to keep pace with incoming input' (Barry et al., 2009).

The third study by Stevens et al. (2008) was an intervention study. A detailed discussion of interventions is outside the scope of this chapter, but this study raises a number of crucial issues that need to be borne in mind, not least in understanding the complex nature of children's language difficulties. The study evaluated the effectiveness of Fast for Word-Language program (FFW: Tallal, 2004), an intensive computerised language training program (6 weeks, 100 mins/day) with a small sample of 6- to 8-year-olds with SLI and typically developing children. Although visual attention was not measured, the authors cited evidence that attention deficits in children with language disorders are domain general, and found in both linguistic and non-linguistic contexts. The program produced significant receptive language gains (as measured by CELF 3) in the SLI group and improved scores in neural measures of selective auditory attention, with changes localised to signal enhancement. The receptive gains were substantial, nearly a standard deviation, but contrary to predictions the gains in expressive skills were less marked. Previous evidence has been mixed (see Stevens et al., 2008, for a summary of evidence). It has been argued that language gains, when they occur, are non-specific and may work by training attention skills. If this is the case, the effect of training on expressive skills may be less immediate than the effect on receptive skills and gains may not be realised until much later. Stevens et al. argued that 'prior training in attention might help children with language deficits benefit more from targeted instruction in an academic domain' (2008, p. 63). In similar vein it has been suggested that enhancement of executive function skills and self-regulation may underpin the longer-term gains in academic achievement found in children who attended Head Start programmes from a young age despite the disappointing short-term fade out in cognitive skills found in their early years (see Raizada & Kishiyama, 2010, for fuller argument and evidence).

However, other factors in addition to training related changes in selective auditory attention may have been responsible for the receptive language gains, for example the large amount of attention that participants received from adults may have been significant. The coach–student ratio was excellent and the children were provided with lots of incentives for staying on task and engaged in the program. Informal observations of children's reactions to the assessment process in our community sample suggest that the effect of such interpersonal factors may be non-uniform across SES groups. Overall the children in the low SES group in our community sample relished the individual attention the assessments afforded, and stickers and praise were highly reinforcing and effective. In contrast, the children in the mid–high SES group were reported to be much less bothered about either adult attention or stickers. Although less extreme, there are some similarities between the desire for adult attention found in the low SES group and the social disinhibition observed in some children who have experienced early institutional care. Interestingly, this social disinhibition and lack of social selectivity was found to be highly correlated with observed and rated inattention/overactivity (Roy, Rutter & Pickles, 2004). Rueda, Purificación, and Rothbart (2010) have argued that individual differences in attentional control and self-regulation play an important role in school readiness, socioemotional development and academic success.

Conclusion

It is clear that the distinction between language disorder and disadvantage is by no means clear-cut: as might be expected, evidence points to compounding of social and intrinsic risk factors. Nevertheless, we have argued that a proportion of children from low SES backgrounds who perform poorly on standard measures of language have intact language potential. Hypothetically, if they had grown up in a more advantaged environment, they would perform in the normal range. For these children enhanced input is needed to realise their language potential. If home and community environments remain unchanged, they will continue to lag behind peers. The rationale for early group-based interventions for preschoolers such as Sure Start in the UK and Head Start in the US is that enriched input can compensate for the effects of earlier disadvantage. However, whilst such programmes might enhance their language skills they are not enough to close the SES gap in language performance, and this is not due in any simple way to the enormous differences in vocabulary exposure between children from the least and more advantaged backgrounds by the time they reach school.

We have seen that the effect of multiple factors associated with low SES on children's development is not restricted to language skills; executive functions and self-regulation are compromised too. Limitations in the development of EF skills may impact on both top-down and bottom-up processing skills involved in the understanding and use of language. Impairments in attention, inhibition and working memory can affect children's capacity to process and respond appropriately to the kind of decontextualised language and multiclausal instructions they face in academic settings. In addition, the deficits in selective auditory attention found in young children from low SES backgrounds may be implicated in the higher than expected speech delay, poor word/nonword repetition and novel word learning skills we found in our sample of preschoolers. The extent to which computerised training programmes designed to enhance attention can improve language skills in children from low SES backgrounds is not currently known. However, even if shown to be helpful, it is unlikely that such programmes will be sufficient to address fully the social emotional problems and academic difficulties known to co-occur with language delay in disadvantaged children and affect their life chances in the longer term (Snow et al., 2007). To stand a chance of keeping up, many such children will need continued enhanced input throughout the school years (Joffe, 2008, 2011).

Furthermore, where children have deficits in basic language skills, indicative of SLI in our terms, enhanced input is unlikely to suffice. We have argued that children with core deficits experience difficulties in everyday life not shared by their peers, calling for specialist intervention to develop their language skills, along with wider support for their social needs and for their families.

Acknowledgement

The Barking and Dagenham study was funded by the Nuffield Foundation, an endowed charitable trust that aims to improve social well-being in the widest sense. The Foundation funds research and innovation in education and social policy and also works to build capacity in education, science and social science research. The views expressed are those of the authors and not necessarily those of the Foundation. More information is available at www.nuffieldfoundation.org

References

Alt, M., & Plante, E. (2006). Factors that influence lexical and semantic fast mapping of young children with specific language impairment. *Journal of Speech, Language, and Hearing Research, 49*, 941–954.

Anderson, R. C., & Nagy, W. E. (1992). The vocabulary conundrum. *American Educator, 16*, 14–18, 44–47.

Arriaga, R. I., Fenson, L., Cronan, T., & Pethick, S. J. (1998). Scores on the MacArthur Communicative Development Inventory of children from low and middle-income families. *Applied Psycholinguistics, 19*, 209–223.

Barry, J. G., Hardiman, M. J., & Bishop, D. V. M. (2009). Mismatch response to polysyllabic nonwords: A neurophysiological signature of language learning capacity. *PLoS ONE 4*: e6270.

Bishop, D. V. M. (1997). *Uncommon understanding*. Hove, UK: Psychology Press.

Bishop, D. V. M., & McDonald, D. (2009). Identifying language impairment in children: Combining language test score with parental report. *International Journal of Language and Communication Disorders, 44*, 600–615.

Bishop, D. V. M., North, T., & Donlan, C. (1996). Nonword repetition as a behavioural marker for inherited language impairment: Evidence from a twin study. *Journal of Child Psychology and Psychiatry, 37*, 391–403.

Boucher, J., & Lewis, V. (1997). *Pre-school Language Scale-3 (UK Adaptation)*. London, UK: Harcourt Brace & Company Books.

Burt, L., Holm, A., & Dodd, B. (1999). Phonological awareness skills of 4-year-old British children: An assessment and developmental data. *International Journal of Language and Communication Disorders, 34*, 311–335.

Campbell, T., Dollaghan, C., Needleman, H., & Janosky, J. (1997). Reducing bias in language assessment: Processing-dependent measures. *Journal of Speech, Language, and Hearing Research, 40*, 519–525.

Chiat, S. (2001). Mapping theories of developmental language impairment: Premises, predictions and evidence. *Language and Cognitive Processes, 16*, 113–142.

Chiat, S., & Roy, P. (2008). Early phonological and sociocognitive skills as predictors of later language and social communication outcomes. *Journal of Child Psychology and Psychiatry, 49*, 635–645.

Conti-Ramsden, G., Botting, N., & Faragher, B. (2001). Psycholinguistic markers for specific language impairment (SLI). *Journal of Child Psychology and Psychiatry, 42*, 741–748.

Culatta, B., Page, J., & Ellis, J. (1983). Story retelling as a communicative performance screening tool. *Language, Speech, and Hearing Services in Schools, 14*, 66–74.

Dodd, B., Crosbie, S., Zhu., H., Holm, A., & Ozanne, A. (2002). *The Diagnostic Evaluation of Articulation and Phonology*. London, UK: Psychological Corporation.

Dodd, B., Holm, A., Zhu, H., & Crosbie, S. (2003). Phonological development: A normative study of British English-speaking children. *Clinical Linguistics & Phonetics, 17*, 617–643.

Duncan, G. J., Brooks-Gunn, J., & Klebanov, P. K. (1994). Economic deprivation and early childhood development. *Child Development, 65*, 296–318.

Duncan, G. J., Yeung, J., Brooks-Gunn, J., & Smith, J. R. (1998). How much does childhood poverty affect the life chances of children? *American Sociological Review, 63*, 406–423.

Dunn, L. M., Dunn, D. M., & Styles, B. (2009). *British Picture Vocabulary Scale* (3rd ed.). London, UK: GL Assessment.

Elliott C. D., Smith, P., & McCulloch K. (1996). *British Ability Scales II: Administration and scoring manual*. Windsor, UK: NFER-Nelson Publishing Company Ltd.

Engel, P. M. J., Santos, F. H., & Gathercole, S. E. (2008). Are working memory measures free of socioeconomic influence? *Journal of Speech, Language and Hearing Research, 51*, 1580–1587.

Farah, M. J., Shera, D. M., Savage, J. H., Betancourt, L., Giannetta, J. M., Brodsky, N. L., . . . Hurt, H. (2006). Childhood poverty: Specific associations with neurocognitive development. *Brain Research, 1110*, 166–174.

Fenson, L., Pethick, S., Renda, C., Cox, J. L., Dale, P. S., & Reznick, J. S. (2000). Short-form versions of the MacArthur Communicative Development Inventories. *Applied Psycholinguistics, 21*, 95–116.

Fernald, A. (2010). Getting beyond the "convenience sample" in research on early cognitive development. *Behavioral and Brain Sciences, 33*, 91–92.

Fish, M., & Pinkerman, B. (2003). Language skills in low-SES rural Appalachian children: Normative development and individual differences, infancy to preschool. *Applied Developmental Psychology, 23*, 539–565.

Flus, J., Ziegler, J. C., Warszawski, J., Ducot, B., Richard, G., & Billard, C. (2009). Poor reading in French elementary school: The interplay of cognitive, behavioural, and socioeconomic factors. *Journal of Developmental & Behavioral Pediatrics, 36*, 206–216.

Gathercole, S. E. (2006). Nonword repetition and word learning: The nature of the relationship. *Applied Psycholinguistics, 27*, 513–543.

Ginsborg, J. (2006). The effects of socio-economic status on children's language acquisition and use. In J. Clegg & J. Ginsborg (Eds.), *Language and social disadvantage: Theory into practice* (pp. 9–27). Chichester, UK: John Wiley & Sons Limited.

Graf Estes, K., Evans, J. L., & Else-Quest, N. M. (2007). Differences in the nonword repetition performance of children with and without Specific Language Impairment: A meta-analysis. *Journal of Speech, Language, and Hearing Research, 50*, 177–195.

Hackman, D. A., & Farah, M. J. (2009). Socioeconomic status and the developing brain. *Trends in Cognitive Sciences, 13*, 65–73.

Hart, B., & Risley, T. (1995). *Meaningful differences in the everyday experience of young American children.* Baltimore, MD: Brookes.

Hart, B., & Risley, T. (2003). The early catastrophe: The 30 million word gap. *American Educator, 27*, 4–9.

Hernandez, L. M., & Blazer, D. G. (2006). *Genes, behaviour, and the social environment: Moving beyond the nature-nurture debate.* Washington DC: National Academies Press (see http://iom.edu for downloadable copy).

Hoff, E. (2003). The specificity of environmental influence: Socioeconomic status affects early vocabulary development via maternal speech. *Child Development, 74*, 1368–1378.

Hoff, E. (2006). How social contexts support and shape language development. *Developmental Review, 26*, 55–88.

Hollingshead, A. B. (1975). *Four factor index of social status.* Unpublished manuscript, Yale University, New Haven, CT.

Horton-Ikard, R., & Ellis Weismer, S. (2007). A preliminary examination of vocabulary and word learning in African American toddlers from middle and low socioeconomic status homes. *American Journal of Speech-Language Pathology, 16*, 381–392.

Hurtado, N., Marchman, V. A., & Fernald, A. (2008). Does input influence uptake? Links between maternal talk, processing speed and vocabulary size in Spanish-learning children. *Developmental Science, 11*, F31–F39.

Huttenlocher, J., Vasilyeva, M., Cymerman, E., & Levine, S. (2002). Language input and child syntax. *Cognitive Psychology, 45*, 337–374.

Huttenlocher, J., Waterfall, H., Vasilyeva, M., Vevea, J., & Hedges, L. V. (2010). Sources of variability in children's language growth. *Cognitive Psychology, 61*, 343–365.

Joffe, V. L. (2008). Minding the gap in research and practice in developmental language disorders. In V. L. Joffe, M. Cruice, & S. Chiat (Eds.), *Language disorders in children and adults: New issues in research and practice* (pp. 68–97). Oxford, UK: Wiley-Blackwell.

Joffe, V. L. (2011). Secondary school is not too late to support and enhance language and communication. *Afasic Newsletter* (Winter Edition). London, UK: Afasic.

Johnson, C. J., Beitchman, J. H., & Brownlie, E. B. (2010). Twenty-year follow-up of children with and without speech-language impairments: Family, educational, occupational, and quality of life outcomes. *American Journal of Speech-Language Pathology, 19*, 51–65.

Johnson, C. J., Beitchman, J. H., Young, A., Escobar, M., Atkinson, L., Wilson, B., & Lam, I. (1999). Fourteen-year follow-up of children with and without speech/language impairments: Speech/language stability and outcomes. *Journal of Speech, Language, and Hearing Research, 42*, 744–760.

Keegstra, A. L., Knuff, W. A., Post, W. J., & Goorhuis-Brouwer, S. M. (2007). Children with language problems in a speech and hearing clinic: Background variables and extent of language problems. *International Journal of Pediatric Otorhinolaryngology, 71*, 815–821.

King, T. M., Rosenberg, L. A., Fuddy, L., McFarlane, E., Calvin, S., & Duggan, A. K. (2005). Prevalence and early identification of language delays among at-risk three year olds. *Developmental and Behavioral Pediatrics, 26*, 293–303.

Kovas, Y., Hayiou-Thomas, M. E., Oliver, B., Dale, P. S., Bishop, D. V. M., & Plomin, R. (2005). Genetic influences in different aspects of language development: The etiology of language skills in 4–5-year-old twins. *Child Development, 76*, 632–651.

Kreppner, J. M., Rutter, M., Beckett, C., Castle, J., Colvert, E., Groothues, C., . . . O'Connor, T. (2007). Normality and impairment following profound early institutional deprivation: A longitudinal follow-up into early adolescence. *Developmental Psychology, 43*, 931–946.

Law, J., McBean, K., & Rush, R. (2011). Communication skills in a population of primary school-aged children raised in an area of pronounced social disadvantage. *International Journal of Language and Communication Disorders, 46*, 657–664.

Law, J., Rush, R., Schoon, I., & Parsons, S. (2009). Modeling developmental language difficulties from school entry into adulthood: Literacy, mental health, and employment outcomes. *Journal of Speech, Language and Hearing Research, 52*, 1401–1416.

Leonard, L. B. (1998). *Children with specific language impairment*. Cambridge, MA: MIT Press.

Lipina, S., Martelli, M., Vuelta, B., & Colombo, J. (2005). Performance on the A-not-B task of Argentinian infants from unsatisfied and satisfied homes. *InterAmerican Journal of Psychology, 39*, 49–60.

Locke, A., Ginsborg, J., & Peers, I. (2002). Development and disadvantage: Implications for the early years and beyond. *International Journal of Language and Communication Disorders, 37*, 3–15.

Locke, A., & Ginsborg, J. (2003). Spoken language in the early years: The cognitive and linguistic development of three- to five-year-old children from socio-economically deprived background. *Educational and Child Psychology, 20*, 68–79.

Marulis, L. M., & Neuman, S. B. (2010). The effects of vocabulary intervention on young children's word learning: A meta-analysis. *Review of Educational Research, 80*, 300–335.

Mezzacappa, E. (2004). Alerting, orienting and executive attention: Developmental properties and sociodemographic correlates in an epidemiological sample of young urban children. *Child Development, 75*, 1373–1386.

Nelson, K. E., Welsh, J. A., Vance Trup, E. M., & Greenberg, M. (2011). Language delays of impoverished preschool children in relation to early academic and emotion recognition skills. *First Language, 31*, 164–194.

Newcomer, P., & Hammill, D. (1988). *Test of Language Development-2 Primary*. Austin, TX: Pro-Ed.

Noble, K. G., McCandliss, B. D., & Farah, M. J. (2007). Socioeconomic gradients predict individual differences in neurocognitive abilities. *Developmental Science, 10*, 464–480.

Noble, K. G., Norman, M. F., & Farah, M. J. (2005). Neurocognitive correlates of socio-economic status in kindergarten children. *Developmental Science, 8*, 74–87.

Oetting, J. B. (1999). Children with SLI use argument structure to cue verbs. *Journal of Speech, Language, and Hearing Research, 42*, 1261–1274.

Qi, C. H., Kaiser, A. P., Milan, S. E., Yzquierdo, Z., & Hancock, T. B. (2003). The performance of low-income African American children on the Preschool Language Scale-3. *Journal of Speech, Language and Hearing Research, 46*, 576–590.

Peers, I. P., Lloyd, P., & Foster, C. (2000). *Clinical Evaluation of Language Fundamentals – Preschool UK*. London, UK: Psychological Corporation.

Raizada, R. D. S., & Kishiyama, M. M. (2010). Effects of socioeconomic status on brain development, and how cognitive neuroscience may contribute to levelling the playing field. *Frontiers in Human Neuroscience, 4*, 1–11.

Rice, M., Oetting, J., Marquis, J., Bode, J., & Pae, S. (1994). Frequency of input effects on word comprehension of children with specific language impairment. *Journal of Speech and Hearing Research, 37*, 106–22.

Roy, P., & Chiat, S. (2008). Beyond outcomes: The importance of developmental pathways. In V. Joffe, M. Cruice, & S. Chiat (Eds.), *Language disorders in children and adults: Key issues in research and practice*. Chichester, UK: John Wiley.

Roy, P., & Chiat, S. (2012). *The impact of SES on language performance of young clinically referred children*. Manuscript submitted for publication.

Roy, P., Chiat, S., & Dodd, B. (2010). *Is language as poor as it looks? Assessment of language potential in socioeconomically disadvantaged preschoolers*. [End of award report for Nuffield Foundation grant EDU/36505].

Roy, P., Kersley, H., & Law, J. (2004). *The Sure Start Measure Standardisation Study*. Retrieved from http://www.surestart.gov.uk/doc/P0001797.pdf.

Roy, P., Rutter, M., & Pickles, A. (2004). Institutional care: Associations between over-activity and lack of selectivity in social relationships. *Journal of Child Psychology and Psychiatry, 45*, 866–873.

Rueda, M. R., Posner, M. I., & Rothbart, M. K. (2005). The development of executive attention: Contributions to the emergence of self-regulation. *Developmental Neuropsychology, 28*, 573–594.

Rueda, M. R., Purificación, C., & Rothbart, M. K. (2010). Contributions of attentional control to socioemotional and academic development. *Early Education & Development, 21*, 744–764.

Ruttter, M. (2008). Biological implications of gene-environment interaction. *Journal of Abnormal Child Psychology, 36*, 969–975.

Schoon, I., Parsons, S., Rush, R., & Law, J. (2010). Childhood language skills and adult literacy: A 29-year follow-up study. *Pediatrics, 125*, e459–e466.

Seeff-Gabriel, B., Chiat, S., & Dodd, B. (2010). Sentence imitation as a tool in identifying expressive morphosyntactic difficulties in children with severe speech difficulties. *International Journal of Language & Communication Disorders, 45*, 691–702.

Seeff-Gabriel, B., Chiat, S., & Roy, P. (2008). *Early Repetition Battery (ERB)*. London, UK: Pearson Assessment.

Semel, E., Wiig, E., & Secord, W. (2006a). *Clinical Evaluation of Language Fundamentals – 4[UK]*. London, UK: Harcourt Assessment.

Semel, E., Wiig, E., & Secord, W. (2006b). *Clinical Evaluation of Language Fundamentals – Preschool 2[UK]*. London, UK: Harcourt Assessment.

Silveira, M. (2010). *Specific Language Impairment (SLI) revisited: Evidence from a psycholinguistic investigation of grammatical gender abilities in Brazilian Portuguese-speaking children.* Unpublished PhD thesis, University College London, UK.

Snow, C. E., Porche, M. E., Tabors, P. O., & Ross Harris, S. (2007). *Is literacy enough? Pathways to academic success for adolescents.* Baltimore, MD: Paul H. Brookes Publishing.

Snowling, M. J., Bishop, D. V. M., Stothard, S. E., & Kaplan, C. (2006). Psychosocial outcomes at 15 years of children with a preschool history of speech-language impairment. *Journal of Child Psychology and Psychiatry, 47,* 759–765.

Stevens, C., Sanders, L., & Neville, H. (2006). Neurophysiological evidence for selective auditory attention deficits in children with specific language impairment, *Brain Research, 1111,* 143–152.

Stevens, C., Fanning, J., Coch, D., Sanders, L., & Neville, H. (2008). Neural Electrophysiological evidence from language-impaired and typically developing children, *Brain Research, 1205,* 55–69.

Stevens, C., Lauinger, B., & Neville, H. (2009). Differences in the neural mechanisms of selective attention in children from different socioeconomic backgrounds: An event-related brain potential study. *Developmental Science, 12,* 634–646.

Stothard, S. E., Snowling, M. J., Bishop, D. V. M., Chipchase, B. B., & Kaplan, C. A. (1998). Language impaired preschoolers: A follow-up into adolescence. *Journal of Speech, Language, and Hearing Research, 41,* 407–418.

Tallal, P. (2004). Improving language and literacy is a matter of time. *Nature Reviews Neuroscience, 5,* 721–728.

Tizard, B., & Hughes, M. (1984). *Young children learning: Talking and thinking at home and at school.* London, UK: Fontana.

Tomalski, P., & Johnson, M. H. (2010). The effects of early adversity on the adult and developing brain. *Current Opinion in Psychiatry, 23,* 233–238.

Tomblin, B. Records, N., Buckwalter, P., Zhang, X., & Smith, E. (1997). Prevalence of Specific Language Impairment in kindergarten children. *Journal of Speech, Language, and Hearing Research, 40,* 1245–1260.

Tough, J. (1977). *The development of meaning.* London, UK: George Allen & Unwin Limited.

Tough, J. (2000). Memorandum (EY 61). *Appendix to the Minutes of Evidence presented to the Select Committee on Education and Employment, the United Kingdom Parliament.* Retrieved from http://www.publications.parliament.uk/pa/cm200001/cmselect/smeduemp/33/33ap34.htm

Vasilyeva, M., Waterfall, H., & Huttenlocher, J. (2008). Emergence of syntax: Commonalities and differences across children. *Developmental Science, 11,* 84–97.

Washbrook, E. (2010). *A cross-cohort comparison of childhood behaviour problems.* Summary of preliminary findings from a project for the Sutton Trust.

Washbrook, E., & Waldfogel, J. (2010). *Cognitive gaps in the early years.* The Sutton Trust.

Wiebe, S. A., Sheffield, T., Mize Nelson, J., Clark, C. A. C., & A. Espy, K. (2011). The structure of executive function in 3-year-olds. *Journal of Experimental Child Psychology, 108,* 436–452.

Windsor, J., Benigno, J. P., Wing, C. A., Carroll, P. J., Koga, S. F., Nelson, C. A., . . . Zeanah, C. H. (2011). Effect of foster care on young children's language learning. *Child Development, 82,* 1035–1349.

Zhang, X., & Tomblin, J. B. (2000). The association of intervention receipt with speech-language profiles and social-demographic variables. *American Journal of Speech-Language Pathology, 9,* 345–357.

6 Issues of culture and language in developmental disorders

The case of dyslexia in Chinese learners

Simpson W. L. Wong, Moon X. Y. Xiao, and Kevin K. H. Chung

Introduction

Although developmental dyslexia affects an estimated 4 percent to 11 percent of the school-age population around the world (e.g., Chan, Ho, Tsang, Lee, & Chung, 2007; Salter & Smythe, 1997), it is not clear that it is the same phenomenon across different languages (Ziegler & Goswami, 2005). The majority of research into typical and atypical reading development has focused on English, resulting in an Anglocentric research agenda with arguably "limited relevance for a universal science of reading" (Share, 2008, p. 584). In this chapter we consider the growing body of research into the cognitive characteristics of dyslexia in a non-European language with a non-alphabetic orthography, namely Chinese (e.g., Chung & Ho, 2010; Chung, Ho, Chan, Tsang, & Lee, 2010; Chung, McBride-Chang, Wong, Cheung, Penney, & Ho, 2008; Wong & Ho, 2010). Not only does Chinese offer an important contrast to alphabetic orthographies, but there are important differences in how children from different Chinese societies are taught to read. Dyslexia in Chinese readers therefore provides a useful starting point for exploring issues related to culture and language in developmental disorders.

We start by introducing the languages and scripts of various Chinese societies, and the ways in which children are taught to read, as a background to subsequently exploring how these linguistic, orthographic and instructional factors affect the cognitive profiles of Chinese children with dyslexia. We also briefly review various subtypes of dyslexia in Chinese children, and recent evidence about the comorbidity between dyslexia, SLI and ADHD, before concluding with suggestions for future research.

Understanding dyslexia

Dyslexia is characterized by severe and often pervasive difficulty in learning to read and spell despite normal intelligence, and in the absence of sensory and neurological impairment or environmental deprivation (Lyon, Shaywitz, & Shaywitz, 2003; Rose, 2009). Dyslexia has been extensively investigated in languages with alphabetic orthographies, especially English, Dutch and Finnish. In these orthographies it is well established that a phonological processing deficit underlies the failure to acquire adequate word recognition and spelling (see Snowling, 2000; Spafford & Grosser, 2005). Because of the close connection between script and sound in alphabets, phonological sensitivity is particularly important in learning to read, and in turn makes it the key indicator of reading difficulties. Also important, and perhaps a separate cognitive skill issue, is deficient speeded naming, measured by a rapid automatized naming (RAN) procedure (Bowers & Wolf, 1993; Wolf & Bowers, 1999). This deficit in rapid naming which may signify the disruption of the automatic processes involved in extracting orthographic patterns, could represent a second core deficit in dyslexia (see Bowers & Wolf, 1993; McBride-Chang & Manis, 1996; Wolf & Bowers, 1999). This lack of fluency is more often observed in dyslexic children who learn to read a shallow orthography that has regular letter-to-sound correspondences (e.g., Finnish, German and Spanish). For example, German-speaking dyslexic children were found to have intact phonological decoding abilities but slow reading speed (Landerl & Wimmer, 2000). Alongside these deficits, dyslexic readers have additional difficulties in visual-orthographic processing (Corcos & Willows, 1993), and morphological awareness (Carlisle, 1995; Leong, 1999). These difficulties affect readers' ability to encode printed words, to manipulate word structures, and to analyze the meaning of morphologically complex words.

These findings raise the question of what underlies dyslexia in languages with non-alphabetic orthographies, such as Chinese. Do phonological deficits play as critical a role, or are other impairments (e.g., in rapid naming, visual-orthographic processing, morphological awareness) more important? Before discussing dyslexia in readers of Chinese, we present the main characteristics of the Chinese orthography.

Chinese orthography and literacy acquisition

Chinese orthography is sometimes described as a morpho-syllabic writing system, as each basic graphic unit of Chinese is a character that is linked to a morpheme (meaning unit) and syllable (DeFrancis, 1989; Mattingly, 1984). Unlike in alphabetic languages such as in English, where mappings between orthography and phonology are relatively transparent, a Chinese character represents both a morpheme and a syllable. Although a Chinese character represents a morpheme, there are no morphemic inflections for grammatical functions in Chinese as there are in English. In contrast, word formation in Chinese is via lexical compounding, and hence morphological compounding rules are more common and important in Chinese than in English. The basic graphic unit in Chinese is a character made up of different strokes. Strokes are combined to form stroke-patterns, also called radicals, which act as the basic orthographic units. Thus, unlike English where word length is a visual cue for recognition, individual strokes within a square-shape character are the primary visual information for word recognition.

Approximately 4,600–4,900 characters are commonly used in the traditional Chinese script (Cheung & Bauer, 2002). In Chinese, all characters are monosyllabic and there are no sub-syllabic segments related to meaning. A distinctive feature of Chinese compared to English is that there are tonal differences of a same syllable, i.e., one character representing a specific meaning corresponds to one syllable with a designated tone. There are four tones in Putonghua (the common speech used in mainland China). According to Cheng's (1982) study, there are 401 syllables in a corpus of over one million characters. Taking tonal variation into consideration, permutation of the four tones and the 401 syllables in Putonghua will theoretically result in around one thousand pronunciations, which correspond to around one million characters, and hence homophones abound. The existence of abundant homophones poses a challenge for Chinese disabled readers to differentiate meanings.

Although there is no script-sound relation in Chinese at the sub-lexical level, phonetic cues are encoded in some characters. Most characters comprise a combination of a semantic and a phonetic radical. An example is the character 清 /cing1/ "clean", which is composed of the semantic radical 氵, which gives a cue to the meaning of the character (i.e., water), and the phonetic 青, which itself is a character and is the phonetic radical providing a cue to the pronunciation of the character (Shu, Chen, Anderson, Wu, & Xuan, 2003). There are roughly 200 semantic and 800 phonetic radicals that have a certain positional regularity for a given character. Most semantic radicals occupy the left or top position within left-right (烤 /haau2/, "bake") or top-bottom (露 /lou6/, "dew") structure. Feldman and Siok (1997) estimated that approximately 75 percent of these radicals are on the left of a character. Even though most characters contain a phonetic radical, the information therein often provides an unreliable cue to pronunciation. Compared to the phonetic radicals, the semantic radicals provide more reliable cues (Shu, Chen et al., 2003). However, the association between radicals and the sound or the meaning of the whole character is neither entirely transparent nor completely reliable since different degrees of semantic and phonological regularity are found in characters (Shu & Anderson, 1997; Shu, Anderson, & Wu, 2000). This makes intuitive sense given that for the majority of characters the relationship between orthography and phonology is rather arbitrary and visual-orthographic processing is important for processing characters.

The majority of Chinese words are multisyllabic, with about two-thirds being bisyllabic (Taylor & Taylor, 1995). Most words are built and compounded from two or more morphemes. Many words sharing the same morpheme such as 餐桌 /faan6 zoek3/ "dining table", 電腦桌 /din6 nou5 zoek3/ "computer table", 木桌 /muk6 zoek3/ "wooden table" with the morpheme 桌 /zoek3/ "table", are semantically related because the semantic radical of a Chinese character often provides some indication of its meaning. There are also a relatively large number of syllables that share the same sounds or homophones, due to the limited number of syllables. Many syllables may have five or more homophones, which provide different meaning (Packard, 2000; Zhou, Zhuang, & Yu, 2002). For example, 東 /dung1/ "east", 冬 /dung1/ "winter". Given the characteristics of homophones and word compounding in Chinese, awareness of morphemes is of great importance in learning to read Chinese.

Chinese also differs from English and many other languages in that it lacks explicit grammatical rules such as tenses, subject–verbal agreement, gender, plurals or prepositions. Chinese relies primarily on morphosyntax, i.e., semantic-based word compounding, to fulfill various syntactic functions. For example, in order to express plural form of nouns, nouns which can be used in either singular or plural form like 書 "book", 床 "bed", 人 "person" may be combined with quantifiers like 很多 "many", 一些 "some", 很少 "a few" to indicate their plurality. Similarly, to indicate different tenses of verbs, function verbs could be added after the main verbs together to show an action status. For example, 着 (function verb to denote continuous action) is used to be combined with 看 "look", (i.e., 看着), expressing the action of "looking". The semantic-driven nature of Chinese may partly determine a rather loose word order system in Chinese compared with English. Although the canonical word order for Chinese sentences is Subject-Verb-Object (SVO), in many situations, if the topic of a conversation happens to be the object of a sentence, Object-Subject-Verb (OSV) order is also allowed, in order to emphasize the object. For instance, the SVO sentence 我打破了花瓶 "I hit break PERF (perfective aspect) vase" can be converted to an OSV sentence 花瓶被我打破了 "Vase bèi I hit break PERF (perfective aspect)". By using the preposition 'bèi', the subject 我 (I) was placed after the object 花瓶 (vase). Form-class classifications for many Chinese words are unclear. Because of the lack of inflections and word boundaries in Chinese, readers have to monitor the semantic relations of character sequence in a sentence. Morphosyntax and word ordering therefore become important aspects of syntax in Chinese, and need to be mastered for successful sentence reading at discourse level.

Apart from the characteristics of Chinese orthography introduced above, Chinese is spoken and taught quite differently across different Chinese societies. For example, in mainland China, over 70 percent of the population speaks the national language Putonghua (the common speech) (Grimes, 2002), while Cantonese (one dialect of Chinese) is spoken primarily in the regions of Guangdong (south part of mainland China), Hong Kong and Macau. Putonghua is also spoken in Taiwan and Singapore. Another difference across Chinese societies is the existence of auxiliary phonological coding system in some societies. In mainland China, a system of phonetic symbols, i.e., Hanyu Pinyin, was developed to notate the sounds of Putonghua and characters. The Hanyu Pinyin system uses consonants and vowels as well as tone to represent the sound of a character. It should be emphasized that the Hanyu Pinyin system was devised for annotation of the pronunciation of characters, and is not an independent alphabetic system such as English. The Pinyin system is used in mainland China and Singapore to teach Chinese. For example, children in mainland China are introduced to Pinyin at the first term of grade one before formal literacy instruction. Teachers put much emphasis on Pinyin when teaching characters. They usually present a new character with its Pinyin symbol on it as a cue to strengthen the association of pronunciation and orthography in the character. Most importantly, characters in textbooks are presented alongside Pinyin to prompt children's reading. By repeated practice, children eventually become very familiar with Pinyin and use it to remember the sounds of characters. A similar situation occurs in Taiwan, where Zhuyin fuhao was created to facilitate Chinese acquisition. On the other hand, no phonological coding system is used to teach character recognition in Hong Kong.

Another regional difference relevant to Chinese instruction is the use of two different scripts in different Chinese societies. The traditional script is used in Hong Kong and Taiwan, whereas a simplified script is used in mainland China and Singapore. The simplified characters originated from the traditional characters after the foundation of the People's Republic of China (PRC). The character simplification project launched by the PRC government in the 1950s eventually yielded 2,000 or so characters simplified either by incorporation of simplified components or by analogy with traditional characters (Rohsenow, 2004). The remaining characters share the same written forms across these two scripts. The simplified Chinese characters have reduced much of the memory burden for beginning readers, but at the same time this simplification may ignore visual information important for character recognition. In mainland China, several important skills or strategies are explicitly taught to children, including recognition of basic strokes, radicals, and structures of characters, conversion of a character and its Pinyin, discrimination of homophones, and orthographically or phonetically similar characters, and dictionary usage based on Pinyin and orthographic knowledge. The scenario in Hong Kong is quite different from that in mainland China. Lacking a phonological system such as Pinyin, the approach to teaching Chinese in primary schools relies heavily on rote memorization of the association between the sound and the orthography of a character – in other words the look-and-say method. Characters are often taught as a whole unit and no strategy of orthographic decomposition is applied systematically in reading instruction.

Cognitive profiles of Chinese dyslexic readers

Given the differences in the relationships between the spoken language and written script, and in the instructional methods used in different Chinese societies, Chinese dyslexia may present a different profile of cognitive-linguistic deficits from that in alphabetic languages. Chinese individuals with dyslexia show poor performance in several cognitive-linguistic areas that are critical for explaining their reading difficulties. As suggested by Yin and Weekes (2003), dyslexia in Chinese could be caused by psycholinguistic impairments at any of the levels of orthography, semantics (morphology), and phonology. Recent studies in Hong Kong showed that children with dyslexia could have a variety of multiple cognitive deficits, the most dominant being speed processing (or rapid naming), and visual-orthographic processing compared to phonological processing (Chan et al., 2007). Apart from these difficulties, morphological awareness, syntactic awareness, and verbal memory were also found to be core deficits in dyslexia for Chinese individuals (e.g., Chik et al., 2012; Chung et al., 2010; Shu, McBride-Chang, Wu, & Liu, 2006). We now discuss each of these deficits in turn.

Phonological awareness

Phonological awareness is consistently shown to be predictive of reading ability in English (Torgesen & Mathes, 2000; Wagner & Torgesen, 1987) and Chinese (Ho & Bryant, 1997; McBride-Chang & Kail, 2002; Shu, Peng, & McBride-Chang, 2008). Phonological awareness, which is the ability to reflect on, analyze and manipulate the sounds of language, is essential for learning to read as it facilitates awareness of the relationship between the sound and the printed word (e.g., Wagner, Torgesen, & Rashotte, 1994; Wagner & Torgesen, 1987). It has been considered as the main cause of reading deficit in dyslexic English readers. Similarly, several studies have demonstrated that Chinese dyslexic children have lower phonological awareness particularly in the measures of onset and rime awareness compared to normally achieving children (Chan et al., 2007; Ho, Chan, Tsang, & Lee, 2002; Ho, Chan, Lee, Tsang, & Luan, 2004). Conventionally, Chinese syllables are divided into onsets (initial sound) and rimes (final sound), thus studies of Chinese tend to focus on awareness of three sound units: syllables, onsets, and rimes. The majority of Chinese dyslexic children were found to have deficits in syllable awareness (Chow, McBride-Chang, & Burgess, 2005), onset-rime detection (Ho, Law, & Ng, 2000), and to use fewer phonetic cues in learning characters (Ho & Ma, 1999; Ho et al., 2000). However, phonological awareness deficit has been reported to be less frequent than other cognitive-linguistic deficits in Hong Kong dyslexic children (Ho et al., 2004). The low incidence of phonological deficit could be explained by the way Hong Kong Chinese children learn to read with a look-and-say method rather than through the use of Pinyin. Indeed, phonological awareness deficit has been more commonly found among dyslexic readers in Beijing than in Hong Kong populations, probably because Pinyin is used as the aid to reading instruction (see further discussion in the next section).

Visual-orthographic knowledge

In addition to phonological awareness, visual-orthographic knowledge has been found to be important for learning to read (Cassar & Treiman, 1997) and orthographic deficits contribute significantly to reading failure (e.g., Chung et al., 2010; Hultquist, 1997; Wolf, 1999). Visual-orthographic knowledge refers the processing of orthographic information (e.g., frequency of letter sequences) that alters the unit of perception by enabling the reader to move from processing individual letters to letter sequences. In Chinese, visual-orthographic knowledge refers to individual's awareness of conventional rules in structuring Chinese characters and their ability to identify or distinguish real Chinese characters from a pool of pseudocharacters, noncharacters, and visual symbols. Research findings have generally reported that orthographic deficits are the major cognitive-linguistic deficits in Chinese dyslexia (Ho et al., 2002, 2004). An orthographic deficit in Chinese dyslexic children may be a problem in developing a relationship between the orthographic and phonological processor and in forming a strong orthographic representation of words in their mind, thus contributing to failures in reading. Given the prominence of the complex orthographic rules and the lack of reliable grapheme-phoneme correspondence in Chinese characters, orthographic deficit has been considered as one of the prominent problems faced by Chinese dyslexic readers; indeed, it may be the crux of the problem in Chinese dyslexia (Ho et al., 2004).

Rapid automatized naming

Rapid automatized naming (RAN) has also been shown to be associated with reading in English and Chinese (e.g., Ho & Lai, 1999; Wimmer, Mayringer, & Landerl, 2000). Generally, RAN refers to an automatic process that retrieves verbal representations from orthographic patterns in the mental lexicon and maps arbitrary symbols to spoken language (Manis, Seidenberg, & Doi, 1999; Wolf & Katzir-Cohen, 2001). A substantial body of evidence has established that RAN is related to reading acquisition (e.g., Ho & Lai, 1999; Manis, Doi, & Bhadha, 2000; Parrila, Kirby, & McQuarrie, 2004) and reading impairment (e.g., Chung et al., 2010; Ho & Lai, 1999; Shu, Meng, & Lai, 2003). Because the orthography-to-phonology mapping is more arbitrary in Chinese than it is in English, RAN has been shown to be strongly correlated with reading performance in Chinese. Studies of the relationship between RAN and Chinese reading have indicated that Chinese dyslexic readers tend to respond more slowly than their typically developing peers in naming digits, colors, pictures, and Chinese characters, suggesting that slow rapid naming may be an indicator of difficulty in learning arbitrary associations and slowness in the speed of lexical access (Chung et al., 2010; Ho & Lai, 1999). Such slow rapid naming is likely to reflect slowness in developing stable and strong orthographic and multi-morphemic representations. Apart from orthographic deficits, a RAN deficit has been suggested as another core cognitive-linguistic deficit in Chinese dyslexia (Chan et al., 2007; Ho et al., 2002, 2004).

Morphological awareness

Morphological awareness is another skill that has been found to be important for reading acquisition and impairment in English and Chinese (e.g., Casalis & Louis-Alexandre, 2000; McBride-Chang, Wagner, Muse, Chow, & Shu, 2005; Shu, McBride-Chang, Wu, & Liu, 2006). Morphological awareness is defined as the ability to reflect upon and manipulate morphemes, and use word formation rules in understanding and creating new complex words (Kuo & Anderson, 2006). In Chinese, morphological awareness is defined as the ability to distinguish meanings among morpheme homophones or as the ability to manipulate and access morphemes in words with two or more morphemes. Given a large number of homophones and compound words in Chinese, morphological awareness is important for learning to read (e.g., McBride-Chang et al., 2005) and has been found to be impaired in Chinese dyslexic readers (e.g., McBride-Chang et al., 2008; Shu et al., 2006). A series of research studies have shown that dyslexic readers have poorer morphological awareness skills than typically developing readers (e.g., Chung et al., 2010; Shu et al., 2006). Shu et al. (2006) also found that among a number of cognitive-linguistic measures, morphological awareness is one of the most distinguishable skills to differentiate dyslexic children from average readers. In an attempt to identify cognitive-linguistic skills that might distinguish Chinese kindergarteners at risk of dyslexia, morphological awareness was one of the skills that differentiated children in the familial risk group (defined as having a sibling diagnosed with dyslexia) from the children with no familial risk or language delay (McBride-Chang et al., 2008; McBride-Chang et al., 2011). Weakened morphological awareness appears to be a significant contributor to the deficits in reading characteristic of dyslexic readers.

Syntactic awareness

Converging research has also shown a strong link between syntactic awareness and word-level and text-level reading in English (Bryant, MacLean, & Bradley, 1990; Muter, Hulme, Snowling, & Stevenson, 2004; Nation & Snowling, 2000; Plaza & Cohen, 2003; Tunmer & Bowey, 1984) and Chinese (Chik et al., 2011; So & Siegel, 1997). Research that includes a variety of measures of syntactic awareness from oral cloze, word order, and morphosyntax (e.g., judgment/error correction) tasks, has demonstrated that syntactic awareness is highly correlated with reading acquisition (e.g., Chiappe, Siegel, & Wade-Woolley, 2002; Muter et al., 2004) and reading failure in English (e.g., Wimmer et al., 2000; Wolf et al., 2002). There is increasing evidence for the importance of syntactic awareness in reading acquisition and for its causal role in reading impairment in Chinese (e.g., Chik et al., 2011; So & Siegel, 1997). For instance, Chik et al. (2011) reported that Chinese dyslexic children perform significantly less well than age controls in word order and morphosyntax measures. Their syntactic awareness skills also lagged behind those of their peers. Xiao and Ho (2011) also found a weak relation between word order and reading performance in Chinese dyslexic children. Taken together, the findings of these studies are thought to be strong evidence that syntactic awareness is another significant contributor to reading difficulties.

Verbal memory deficits

Finally, verbal memory has been found to be another important skill for reading acquisition in both alphabetic and Chinese languages (e.g., Kormos & Sáfár, 2008; Savage & Frederickson, 2006; Seigneuric & Ehrlich, 2005). It taps into an individual's ability to hold onto an ordered sequence of verbal information for a short duration of time. Such associations are particularly marked when children with and without reading difficulties are compared. Zhang, Zhang, Chang, and Zhou (1998) and Chung et al. (2010) found that Chinese readers with reading problems performed worse than did typically developing readers in verbal memory tasks such as repetition of digits, letters, words, and nonwords. From these findings, Chinese dyslexic readers appear to have difficulties in storing speech sounds and processing verbal information in their short-term memory, adversely affecting their development of stable graphic-sound associations and their acquisition of visual-orthographic knowledge. The converging evidence thus points to the existence of verbal memory deficits in Chinese dyslexia.

Cognitive profiles of dyslexic readers in different Chinese societies

Even though the sets of cognitive-linguistic deficits described above are correlated with reading difficulties in Chinese orthography, their associations may vary across different Chinese populations. Despite the large differences in spoken Chinese dialects, they all share the same writing system, and Putonghua and Cantonese are widely spoken in China. Luan (2005) examined the cognitive profiles of Chinese dyslexic children in Beijing, and Hong Kong. The most prevalent deficit in Beijing dyslexic children is morphological awareness deficit (29.6 percent), followed by phonological awareness deficit (27.6 percent), and rapid naming deficit (27.6 percent), while the three dominant deficits in Hong Kong dyslexic children are rapid naming deficit (52 percent), morphological awareness deficit (26.5 percent), and visual-orthographic deficit (24 percent). The most notable difference in cognitive profile of dyslexic children from Beijing as compared with that from Hong Kong lies in the proportion of deficits in phonological awareness (27.6 percent vs. 12 percent) and rapid naming (27.6 percent vs. 52 percent).

These findings may be a result of differences in the instruction method used for teaching recognition of Chinese character and nature of the script across these two communities. In Beijing, children read the simplified Chinese script and are taught to learn Chinese characters with the assistance of Pinyin when they enter primary school. The Pinyin system is alphabet-based, which highlights grapheme-phoneme conversions. Weakness in phonological awareness would undoubtedly impede Beijing dyslexic children using Pinyin in learning to read Chinese characters. However, in Hong Kong, traditional Chinese script is used and Chinese characters are usually taught with the look-and-say method that mainly stresses learning characters holistically with rapid retrieval of the name of characters. Successful reading acquisition may depend on the ability to pair printed words with print and sound for Hong Kong dyslexic readers. As such, paired associate learning which underpins the success in rapid retrieval of information and automatic processes involved in the extraction and induction of orthographic patterns is thought to be importantly related to Hong Kong dyslexic children. Difficulty with paired associate learning and slow naming speed in Hong Kong dyslexic children may be a marker of the acquisition of visual-verbal correspondences and the disruption of the automatic processes involved in the extraction and induction of orthographic patterns. Using different instructional methods and scripts may affect the reading process within Chinese language thereby producing different cognitive profiles of dyslexia across different Chinese societies.

Subtypes of Chinese dyslexia

Given that not all readers with dyslexia suffer from the same level of cognitive deficits (see also Byrne, Olson, & Samuelsson, this volume), unraveling different subtypes of dyslexia that have specific and distinguishable cognitive-linguistic deficits is essential for developing appropriate training and intervention methods.

Two major frames of reference have been used for classifying English speakers of dyslexia into subgroups, the dual-route model and the cluster-analytic approach, which looks at a variety of cognitive functions.

The dual-route model focuses mainly on two varieties of dyslexia: phonological dyslexia (or deep dyslexia) and surface dyslexia subtypes (Castles & Coltheart, 1993; see also Thomas, Baughman, Karaminis, & Addyman, this volume). According to this, reading a word or a letter string involves a direct route and a phonological route. Familiarity with a word or a letter string plays an important role in which route is activated. When a reader encounters a familiar word, the direct route is activated and the reader can access its semantic representation via its phonological representation. However, unfamiliar words do not have a lexical entry and so are unlikely to be read accurately by this route. When a reader encounters an unfamiliar word, it has to be decoded through the grapheme-phoneme correspondence by the phonological route. This route is very useful for reading unknown words and nonwords such as "brane", but may produce incorrect pronunciation of irregular words, for instance, [heIv] (rhyming with "cave" and "rave") for "have". Based on this model, readers can have differential performance on reading irregular words and nonwords, and so two types of dyslexia, namely surface dyslexia and phonological dyslexia, could be identified by using irregular word and nonword reading performance. Children whose irregular word reading is impaired but nonword reading is not especially impaired have a faulty direct route and are classified as having surface dyslexia, whereas those who have relatively intact irregular word reading but poor nonword reading have an impaired indirect route and are identified as phonological dyslexia (Castles & Coltheart, 1993). In studies of different subtyping in English speakers using the dual-route model, phonological dyslexia has dominated (e.g., Manis, Seidenberg, Doi, McBride-Chang, & Petersen, 1996; Stanovich, Siegel, & Gottardo, 1997). Given the very distinctive linguistic features between English and Chinese, differential impairments in Chinese subtypes may be found according to the dual-route model.

In a follow up subtyping study of Chinese dyslexia, surface and phonological (or deep) dyslexia could be classified according to children's performance on the reading of exception characters and pseudocharacters (Ho, Chan, Chung, Lee, & Tsang, 2007). Exception characters are real characters within which the phonetic radicals do not hint at the pronunciation of the whole character. For example, both 秋 /cau1/ and 狄 /dik6/ are exception words because they contain the phonetic radical 火 /fo2/ but are pronounced differently from their phonetic radical. Because of the phonological irregularity and inconsistency, exception characters cannot be read via the phonological route. Successful oral reading of exception characters is then thought to rely on the lexical route in the dual-route model. Pseudocharacters, or made-up words, consist of a semantic radical and a phonetic radical in their legal positions but carry no meaning. To make a correct prediction of the pronunciation of this kind of pseudocharacter, one can make analogy to other characters that contain the same phonetic radical. As such, the performance of pseudocharacter reading reflects the ability to utilize the sublexical route. Using a dual-route model, 18 out of 29 Chinese dyslexic children were classified as surface dyslexics while none of them was phonological dyslexic (Ho et al., 2004). The absence of phonological dyslexia in this Chinese sample suggested that dyslexic children were able to acquire and apply the orthographic-phonology correspondence rules. This is consistent with the results of a novel word learning experiment showing that Chinese surface dyslexics were more impaired in learning irregular than regular and pseudocharacters (Ho, Chan, Tsang, Lee, & Chung, 2006). The impaired exception word reading may be attributed to poor phonological working memory or paired-associate learning skills (Li, Shu, McBride-Chang, Liu, & Xue, 2009), which are supportive of the retention of lexical information and formation of the mapping between orthography and phonology. Nevertheless, these findings suggest that surface dyslexia seems to be dominant in Chinese dyslexia, a pattern less commonly found in English-speaking dyslexic populations (e.g., Manis et al., 1996).

Another frame of reference considers subgroups of dyslexia as a manifestation of a complex disorder that involves multiple dimensions of cognitive and related processing. Using a cluster-analytic approach to identify dyslexia subtypes based on the individual's differential deficits in different cognitive domains, Morris et al. (1998) identified seven clusters of dyslexia that consisted of two subtypes showing global deficiency in language skills, four displaying weakness in phonological awareness with variations in verbal memory and rapid naming, and the last subtype was deficient in processing rate. Similar findings obtained for Chinese were reported by Ho et al. (2004), whose dyslexic readers had seven subtypes: global deficit, orthographic deficit, phonological memory deficit, mild difficulty, and three other subtypes with rapid naming-related deficits. Taken together, these studies using the cluster-analytic approach provide good insights into different subgroups of dyslexia with specific and distinguishable cognitive-linguistic functions. Future studies may employ the cluster-analytic approach to take in additional cognitive-linguistic functions such as morphological and syntactic awareness. Differentiating among dyslexia types may create a taxonomic foundation for future research into the physiological correlates and genetic contributions of different subtypes in Chinese dyslexia.

Cognitive profile of Chinese children with comorbid dyslexia, specific language impairment (SLI) and attention-deficit/hyperactivity disorder (ADHD)

Dyslexia commonly co-occurs with specific language impairment (SLI) and attention-deficit/hyperactivity disorder (ADHD). Estimates of co-occurrence of dyslexia, SLI and ADHD vary widely from 17 percent to 75 percent (e.g., Gross-Tsur, Manor, & Shalev, 1996; McArthur, Hogben, Edwards, Heath, & Mengler, 2000; Shaywitz, Escobar, Shaywitz, Fletcher, & Makuch, 1992). Comorbidity of these three difficulties has been shown to be significantly more frequent than would be expected if they had independent aetiology. Despite the relatively high rates of co-occurrence between dyslexia, SLI and ADHD, the underlying mechanisms for the overlap are still unknown, particularly in Chinese communities. The comorbidity between dyslexia, SLI and ADHD may therefore be affected differently by the characteristics of the spoken language and orthography in Chinese.

Dyslexia and SLI are two of the most common difficulties in alphabetic readers. The overlap between dyslexia and SLI is estimated at between 25 percent and 75 percent (McArthur et al., 2000). Little is known about such comorbidity in languages with non-alphabetic orthographies. Three possible hypotheses have been proposed to explain the basis of the comorbidity of SLI and dyslexia (Catts & Kamhi, 2005). The Severity hypothesis suggests that SLI and dyslexia share a common manifestation, with SLI being affected more severely than dyslexia (Kamhi & Catts, 1986; Snowling, Bishop, & Stothard, 2000), whereas the Distinct hypothesis proposes that SLI and dyslexia have different manifestations with different underlying cognitive deficits (Catts, Adlof, Hogan, & Weismer, 2005). The Dyslexia-plus hypothesis posits that both SLI and dyslexia share a similar level of manifestation in phonological processing deficit, but SLI may have extra cognitive deficits (Bishop & Snowling, 2004).

To examine these hypotheses further in Chinese communities, a recent study conducted by Wong, Kidd, Ho, and Au (2010) attempted to investigate the overlap between dyslexia and SLI in a sample of Hong Kong Chinese children. The SLI-only group displayed the same weakness in a broad range of cognitive-linguistic skills such as phonological retrieval, phonological memory and awareness, and morphological awareness as was shown by the comorbid diagnosis of dyslexia group (SLI-D). The SLI-only group also performed less well in the grammar knowledge but better on the visual-orthographic knowledge than the SLI-D group. These findings appeared to show preliminary support to the Dyslexia-plus hypothesis. Nonetheless, it is worth noting that the sample size of the different groups was relatively small and a group of children with a singular diagnosis of dyslexia was not included.

In addition to the co-occurrence of dyslexia and SLI, the overlap between dyslexia and ADHD is estimated at about 40 percent to 50 percent (Shaywitz et al., 1992). For children with ADHD, executive function deficits that may include the components of response inhibition, planning, rule abstraction/set shifting and working memory are central to the disability (Sergeant, Geurts, & Oosterlaan, 2002; Willcutt, Doyle, Nigg, Faraone, & Pennington, 2005). When examining the comorbidity of dyslexia and ADHD, Purvis and Tannock (2000) found that children with both dyslexia and ADHD and those with dyslexia only were identifiable with deficits in phonological processing and rapid naming, but those with ADHD only were not. These results were consistent with the phenomimicry hypothesis (Pennington, Groisser, & Welsh, 1993), suggesting that dyslexia could produce just the behavioral characteristics of ADHD, or vice versa, without producing the cognitive deficits characteristic of ADHD having executive function deficits. However, Bental and Tirosh (2007) and Willcutt et al. (2005) reported that the ADHD and dyslexia group shared the impairments in attention and executive function with the pure ADHD group and in rapid naming, phonological processing and reading-related cognitive functions with the dyslexia only group. The comorbidity group exhibited similar levels of impairment in executive function, phonological processing and processing speed as in dyslexia only and ADHD only, suggesting that these cognitive deficits could share common cognitive risk factors. These findings support the common etiology hypothesis (Willcutt et al., 2003).

Two studies of Chinese (Chan, Hung, Liu, & Lee, 2008; Ho, Chan, Leung, Lee, & Tsang, 2005) found that the dyslexia and ADHD group displayed similar cognitive profile with significant deficits in rapid naming and visual-orthographic knowledge to those of pure dyslexia. However, neither a control group of typically developing individuals nor measures of executive function were included. Thus, it remains to be seen whether general deficits in rapid naming, executive functions of response inhibition and working memory and other specific deficits in visual-orthographic and phonological processing could possibly be shared cognitive risk factors in dyslexia and ADHD in Chinese children (see also the discussion by Williams & Lind, this volume).

The cognitive profile of Hong Kong Chinese children with comorbid dyslexia, SLI and ADHD discussed above may display evidence of cognitive-linguistic weakness, yet the extent to which the overlap between these difficulties may differ in the degree of severity in different cognitive-linguistic skills among Chinese readers remains to be further examined. Greater understanding of comorbidities may have implications for understanding the causes of disabilities and could offer directions for characterization and diagnosis of children with dyslexia, SLI and ADHD and their co-morbid disabilities in different Chinese communities.

Conclusion and ways forward

Dyslexia in Chinese-speaking individuals shows a variety of different manifestations from their English speaking counterparts given that Chinese differs from English orthographies. Although weakness in phonological awareness has been characterized as the main cause of dyslexia in English orthography, deficits in rapid naming, visual-orthographic knowledge and morphological awareness have been found to be the dominant causes of cognitive deficits in Chinese dyslexia. Phonological awareness, syntactic awareness, and verbal memory are also noted as features of Chinese dyslexia. Chinese, unlike English, denotes a large family of dialects in different Chinese-speaking societies such as Hong Kong, mainland China, Taiwan, and Singapore. Chinese readers from different societies may differ in: the age at which literacy instruction begins, the literacy instruction itself, the written forms of Chinese characters, the language spoken and the foreign language learned. Thus, all these may affect the process of reading acquisition thereby yielding different cognitive profiles of dyslexia. The dual-route model has attempted to account for subtypes of Chinese dyslexia but may not be applicable. However, using the cluster-analytic approach to classify subtypes appears to be promising because it recognizes the importance of visual-orthographic knowledge, morphological awareness, syntactic awareness, rapid naming, and verbal memory in Chinese dyslexia. Overlaps between dyslexia, ADHD and SLI have also been highlighted. Weaknesses in visual-orthographic knowledge and rapid naming seem to have some degree of overlap. Findings from these investigations may further shed light on the mechanisms underlying the heterogeneous symptoms characteristic of dyslexia, ADHD and SLI.

Last but not least, several issues and questions are worth addressing from multiple perspectives in future studies. For example, research of dyslexia in Chinese societies other than Hong Kong, including mainland China, Taiwan, and Singapore, is sparse and many questions remain. Thus, the extent to which the findings obtained in Hong Kong can be generalized across different societies remains unclear. Further research is needed to investigate the various types of specific learning difficulties Hong Kong Chinese individuals face, and it might be beneficial to compare cognitive profiles among other Chinese societies to further examine the effect of diglossia. Longitudinal study designs that follow individuals with different kinds of specific learning difficulties from a developmental perspective may be very fruitful. Children can therefore be screened for early signs of SLI, dyslexia or related learning difficulties as soon as they enter formal schooling. Longitudinal research also provides further examination of the relationship between SLI, ADHD and dyslexia as one that embraces shared common and unique deficits. Brain imaging studies (e.g., Hu et al., 2010; Siok, Perfetti, Jin, & Tan, 2004) found that Chinese speakers with dyslexia showed different biological abnormalities in their brains compared to their English counterparts. Such research displays the clear dissociation between the two languages, suggesting that it is a language-specific deficit rather than a general deficit. However, similar to the studies of alphabetic speaking readers with dyslexia, a recent genetic study (Lim, Ho, Chou, & Waye, 2011) in Hong Kong identified a candidate dyslexia susceptibility gene a *DYX1C1* for Chinese speakers, suggesting this gene may exist in different populations (for further discussion of *DYX1C1*, see Newbury, this volume).

Therefore, studies of dyslexia candidate genes in different Chinese societies and non-alphabetic languages are essential to support the universality of genetic association in dyslexia. Future research should use, when possible, both brain phenotypes and genotypes and their associations and interactions that influence reading and writing in dyslexic individuals. There is a need for further studies to determine whether dyslexic individuals may be impaired in the same way on the gene–brain variables across languages, and within specific orthographies in which the spoken language differs from their written scripts. Overall, recent advances and developments shed light on dyslexia in Chinese language and provide optimistic grounds for further research and theoretical development in different cultures and languages.

Acknowledgement

This chapter was funded partly by the Hong Kong Institute of Education Research Grant (RG 3/2010–2011R) and the Hong Kong Government Research Grants Council General Education Fund (HKIED: GRF-841311) to Kevin. K. H. Chung.

References

Bental, B., & Tirosh, E. (2007). The relationship between attention, executive functions and reading domain abilities in attention deficit hyperactivity disorder and reading disorder: A comparative study. *Journal of Child Psychology and Psychiatry, 48*, 455–463.

Bishop, D. V. M., & Snowling, M. J. (2004). Developmental dyslexia and specific language impairment: Same or different? *Psychological Bulletin, 130*, 858–886.

Bowers, P. G., & Wolf, M. (1993). Theoretical links among naming speed, precise timing mechanisms and orthographic skill in dyslexia. *Reading and Writing: An Interdisciplinary Journal, 5*, 69–85.

Bryant, P. E., Maclean, L., & Bradley, L. (1990). Rhyme, language, and children's reading. *Applied Psycholinguistics, 11*, 237–252

Carlisle, J. F. (1995). Morphological awareness and early reading achievement. In L. Feldman (Ed.), *Morphological aspects of language processing* (pp. 189–209). Hillsdale, NJ: Erlbaum.

Casalis, S., & Louis-Alexandre, M.-F. (2000). Morphological analysis, phonological analysis and learning to read French: A longitudinal study. *Reading and Writing: An Interdisciplinary Journal, 12*, 303–335.

Cassar, M. T., & Treiman, R. (1997). The beginnings of orthographic knowledge: Children's knowledge of double letters in words. *Journal of Educational Psychology, 89*, 631–644.

Castles, A., & Coltheart, M. (1993). Varieties of developmental dyslexia. *Cognition, 47*, 149–180.

Catts, H. W., Adlof, S. M., Hogan, T. P., & Weismer, S. E. (2005). Are Specific Language Impairment and Dyslexia distinct disorders? *Journal of Speech, Language, and Hearing Research, 48*, 1378–1396.

Catts, H. W., & Kamhi, A. G. (2005). Defining reading disabilities. In H. W. Catts & A. G. Kamhi (Eds.), *Language and reading disabilities* (pp. 50–67). Boston, MA: Allyn & Bacon.

Chan, D. W., Ho, C. S.-H., Tsang, S.-M., Lee, S.-H., & Chung, K. K.-H. (2007). Prevalence, gender ratio and gender differences in reading-related cognitive abilities among Chinese children with dyslexia in Hong Kong. *Educational Studies, 33*, 249–265.

Chan, R. W. S., Hung, S. F., Liu, S. N., & Lee, K. K. (2008). Cognitive profiling in Chinese developmental dyslexia with attention-deficit/hyperactivity disorders. *Reading and Writing: An Interdisciplinary Journal, 21*, 661–674.

Cheng, C. M. (1982). Analysis of present-day Mandarin. *Journal of Chinese Linguistics, 10*, 281–358.

Cheung, K.-H., & Bauer, R. S. (2002). The representation of Cantonese with Chinese characters [Monograph]. *Journal of Chinese Linguistics, 18*.

Chiappe, P., Siegel, L. S., & Wade-Woolley, L. (2002). Linguistic diversity and the development of reading skills: A longitudinal study. *Scientific Studies of Reading, 6*, 369–400.

Chik, P. P.-M., Ho, C. S.-H., Yeung, P.-S., Wong, Y.-K., Chan, D. W.-O., Chung, K. K.-H., & Lo, L.-Y. (2012). Contribution of discourse and morphosyntax skills to reading comprehension in Chinese dyslexic and typically developing children. *Annals of Dyslexia, 62*, 1–18.

Chik, P. P.-M., Ho, C. S.-H., Yeung, P.-S., Luan, H., Lo, L.-Y., Chan, D. W.-O., Chung, K. K.-H., & Lau, W. S.-Y. (2011). Syntactic skills in sentence reading comprehension among Chinese elementary school children. *Reading and Writing: An Interdisciplinary Journal, 25*, 679–699.

Chow, B. W.-Y., McBride-Chang, C., & Burgess, S. (2005). Phonological processing skills and early reading abilities in Hong Kong Chinese kindergarteners learning to read English as a second language. *Journal of Educational Psychology, 97*, 81–87.

Chung, K. K.-H., & Ho, C. S.-H. (2010). Dyslexia in Chinese language: An overview of research and practice. *Australian Journal of Learning Difficulties, 15*, 213–224.

Chung, K. K.-H., Ho, C. S.-H., Chan, D. W., Tsang, S.-M., & Lee, S.-H. (2010). Cognitive profiles of Chinese adolescents with dyslexia. *Dyslexia, 16*, 2–23.

Chung, K. K.-H., McBride-Chang, C., Wong, S. W. L., Cheung, H., Penney, T. B., & Ho, C. S.-H. (2008). The role of visual and auditory temporal processing for Chinese children with developmental dyslexia. *Annals of Dyslexia, 58*, 15–35.

Corcos, E., & Willows, D. (1993). The role of visual processing in good and poor readers' utilization of orthographic information in letter strings. In S. F. Wright, & R. Groner (Eds.), *Facets of dyslexia and its remediation* (pp. 95–106). Amsterdam, The Netherlands: Elsevier Science.

DeFrancis, J. (1989). *Visible speech: The diverse oneness of writing systems*. Honolulu, HI: University of Hawaii Press.

Feldman, L. B., & Siok, W. W. T. (1997). The role of component function in visual recognition of Chinese characters. *Journal of Experimental Psychology: Learning, Memory, and Cognition, 23*, 776–781.

Grimes, B. F. (2002). *Ethnologue: Languages of the world* (14th ed.). Dallas, TX: SIL International.

Gross-Tsur, V., Manor, O., & Shalev, R. S. (1996). Development dyscalculia: Prevalence and demographic features. *Developmental Medicine and Child Neurology, 38*, 25–33.

Ho, C. S.-H., & Bryant, P. (1997). Phonological skills are important in learning to read Chinese. *Developmental Psychology, 33*, 946–951.

Ho, C. S.-H., Chan, D. W., Chung, K. K.-H., Lee, S.-H., & Tsang, S.-M. (2007). In search of subtypes of Chinese developmental dyslexia. *Journal of Experimental Child Psychology, 97*, 61–83.

Ho, C. S.-H, Chan, D., Lee, S.-H., Tsang, S.-M., & Luan, V. H. (2004). Cognitive profiling and preliminary subtyping in Chinese developmental dyslexia. *Cognition, 91*, 43–75.

Ho, C. S.-H., Chan, D., Leung, P. W.-L., Lee, S.-H., & Tsang, S.-M. (2005). Reading-related cognitive deficits in developmental dyslexia, attention-deficit/hyperactivity disorder, and developmental coordination disorder among Chinese children. *Reading Research Quarterly, 40*, 318–337.

Ho, C. S.-H., Chan, D., Tsang, S.-M., & Lee, S.-H. (2002). The cognitive profile and multiple-deficit hypothesis in Chinese developmental dyslexia. *Developmental Psychology, 38*, 543–553.

Ho, C. S.-H., Chan, D. W. O., Tsang, S.-M., Lee, S.-H., & Chung, K. K.-H. (2006). Word learning deficit among Chinese dyslexic children. *Journal of Child Language, 33*, 145–161.

Ho, C. S.-H., & Lai, D. N.-C. (1999). Naming-speed deficits and phonological memory deficits in Chinese developmental dyslexia. *Learning and Individual Differences, 11*, 173–186.

Ho, C. S.-H., Law, T. P.-S., & Ng, P. M. (2000). The phonological deficit hypothesis in Chinese developmental dyslexia. *Reading and Writing: An Interdisciplinary Journal, 13*, 57–79.

Ho, C. S.-H., & Ma, R. N.-L. (1999). Training in phonological strategies improves Chinese dyslexic children's character reading skills. *Journal of Research in Reading, 22*, 131–142.

Hu, W., Lee, H. L., Zhang, Q, Liu, T., Geng, L. B., Seghier, M. L., . . . Price, C. J. (2010). Developmental dyslexia in Chinese and English populations: Dissociating the effect of dyslexia from language differences. *Brain, 133,* 1694–1706.

Hultquist, A. M. (1997). Orthographic processing abilities of adolescents with dyslexia. *Annals of Dyslexia, 47,* 89–114.

Kamhi, A., & Catts, H. (1986). Toward an understanding of developmental language and reading disorders. *Journal of Speech and Hearing Disorders, 51,* 337–347.

Kormos, J., & Sáfár, A. (2008). Phonological short-term memory, working memory and foreign language performance in intensive language learning. *Bilingualism: Language and Cognition, 11,* 261–271.

Kuo, L.- J., & Anderson, R. C. (2006). Morphological awareness and learning to read: A cross-language perspective. *Educational Psychologist, 41,* 161–180.

Landerl, K., & Wimmer, H. (2000). Deficits in phoneme segmentation are not the core problem of dyslexia: Evidence from German and English children, *Applied Psycholinguistics, 21,* 243–262.

Leong, C. K. (1999). Phonological and morphological processing in adult students with learning/reading disabilities. *Journal of Learning Disabilities, 32,* 224–238.

Li, H., Shu, H., McBride-Chang, C., Liu, H. & Xue, J. (2009). Paired associate learning in Chinese children with dyslexia. *Journal of Experimental Child Psychology, 103,* 135–151.

Lim, C. K. P., Ho, C. S.-H., Chou, C. H. N., & Waye, M. M. Y. (2011). Association of the rs3743205 variant of DYX1C1 with dyslexia in Chinese children. *Behavioral and Brain Functions, 7,* 16. doi:10.1186/1744–9081–7–16

Luan, H. (2005). *The role of morphological awareness among Mandarin-speaking and Cantonese-speaking children.* (Unpublished doctoral dissertation). The University of Hong Kong, Hong Kong.

Lyon, G. R., Shaywitz, S. E., & Shaywitz, B. A. (2003). Defining dyslexia, comorbidity, teachers' knowledge of language and reading. *Annals of Dyslexia, 53,* 1–14.

Manis, F. R., Doi, L. M., & Bhadha, B. (2000). Naming speed, phonological awareness, and orthographic knowledge in second graders. *Journal of Learning Disabilities, 33,* 325–333.

Manis, F. R., Seidenberg, M. S., & Doi, L. M. (1999). See Dick RAN: Rapid naming and the longitudinal prediction of reading subskills in first and second graders. *Scientific Studies of Reading, 3,* 129–157.

Manis, F. R., Seidenberg, M. S., Doi, L. M., McBride-Chang, C., & Petersen, A. (1996). On the bases of two subtypes of developmental dyslexia. *Cognition, 58,* 157–195.

Mattingly, I. G. (1984). Reading, linguistic awareness, and language acquisition. In R. V. J. Downing (Ed.), *Language awareness and learning to read* (pp. 9–26). New York: Springer.

McArthur, G. M., Hogben, J. H., Edwards, V. T., Heath, S. M., & Mengler, E. D. (2000). On the 'specifics' of specific reading disability and specific language impairment. *Journal of Child Psychology and Psychiatry, 41,* 869–874.

McBride-Chang, C., & Kail, R. V. (2002). Cross-cultural similarities in the predictors of reading acquisition. *Child Development, 73,* 1392–1407.

McBride-Chang, C., Lam, F., Lam, C., Chan, B., Fong, C. Y.-C. Wong, T. T.-Y., & Wong, S. W. L. (2011). Early predictors of dyslexia in Chinese children: Familial history of dyslexia, language delay, and cognitive profiles. *Journal of Child Psychology and Psychiatry, 52,* 204–211.

McBride-Chang, C., & Manis, F. (1996). Structural invariance in the associations of naming speed, phonological awareness, and verbal reasoning in good and poor readers: A test of the double deficit hypothesis. *Reading and Writing: An Interdisciplinary Journal, 8*, 323–339.

McBride-Chang, C., Tong, X., Shu, H., Wong, A. M.-Y., Leung, K.-W., & Tardif, T. (2008). Syllable, phoneme, and tone: Psycholinguistic units in early Chinese and English word recognition. *Scientific Studies of Reading, 12*, 171–194.

McBride-Chang, C., Wagner, R.K., Muse, A., Chow, B.W.-Y., & Shu, H. (2005). The role of morphological awareness in children's vocabulary acquisition in English. *Applied Psycholinguistics, 26*, 415–435.

Morris, R. D., Stuebing, K. K., Fletcher, J. M., Shaywitz, S. E., Lyon, G. R., Shankweiler, D. P., . . . Shaywitz, B. A. (1998). Subtypes of reading disability: Variability around a phonological core. *Journal of Educational Psychology, 90*, 347–373.

Muter, V., Hulme, C., Snowling, M. J., & Stevenson, J. (2004). Phonemes, rimes and language skills as foundations of early reading development: Evidence from a longitudinal study. *Developmental Psychology, 40*, 663–681.

Nation, K., & Snowling, M. J. (2000). Factors influencing syntactic awareness in normal readers and poor comprehenders. *Applied Psycholinguistics, 21*, 229–241.

Packard, J. L. (2000). *The morphology of Chinese: A linguistic and cognitive approach.* Cambridge, UK: Cambridge University Press.

Parrila, R., Kirby, J. R., & McQuarrie, L. (2004). Articulation rate, naming speed, verbal short-term memory, and phonological awareness: Longitudinal predictors of early reading development? *Scientific Studies of Reading, 8*, 3–26.

Pennington, B. F., Groisser, D., & Welsh, M. C. (1993). Contrasting cognitive deficits in attention deficit hyperactivity disorder versus reading disability. *Developmental Psychology, 29*, 511–523.

Plaza, M., & Cohen, H. (2003). The interaction between phonological processing, syntactic sensitivity and naming speed in the reading and spelling performance of first-grade children. *Brain and Cognition, 53*, 287–292.

Purvis, K., & Tannock, R. (2000). Phonological processing, not inhibitory control, differentiates ADHD and reading disability. *Journal of the American Academy of Child and Adolescent Psychiatry, 39*, 485–494.

Rohsenow, J. S. (2004). Fifty years of script and written language reform in the P. R.C.: The genesis of the language law of 2001. In M. Zhou & H. Sun (Eds.), *Language policy in the People's Republic of China: Theory and practice since 1949* (pp. 21–43). Dordrecht, The Netherlands: Kluwer Academic Publisher.

Rose, J. (2009). *Identifying and teaching children and young people with dyslexia and literacy difficulties.* Retrieved March 1, 2010, from http://publications.dcsf.gov.uk/eOrderingDownload/00659-2009DOM-EN.pdf

Salter, R., & Smythe, I. (1997). *The international book of dyslexia.* London, UK: World Dyslexia Network Foundation and the European Dyslexia Association.

Savage, R. S., & Frederickson, N. (2006). Beyond phonology: What else is needed to describe the problems of below-average readers and spellers? *Journal of Learning Disabilities, 39*, 399–413.

Seigneuric, A., & Ehrlich, M. (2005). Contribution of working memory capacity to children's reading comprehension: A longitudinal investigation. *Reading and Writing: An Interdisciplinary Journal, 18*, 617–656.

Sergeant, J. A., Geurts, H., & Oosterlaan, J. (2002). How specific is a deficit of executive functioning for attention-deficit/hyperactivity disorder? *Behavioural Brain Research, 130*, 3–28.

Share, D. L. (2008). On the anglocentricities of current reading research and practice:

The perils of overreliance on an "outlier" orthography. *Psychological Bulletin, 134,* 584–615.

Shaywitz, S. E., Escobar, M. D., Shaywitz, B. A., Fletcher, J. M., & Makuch, R. (1992). Distribution and temporal stability of dyslexia in an epidemiological sample of 414 children followed longitudinally. *New England Journal of Medicine, 326,* 145–150.

Shu, H., & Anderson, R. C. (1997). Role of radical awareness in the character and word acquisition of Chinese children. *Reading Research Quarterly, 32,* 78–89.

Shu, H., Anderson, R. C., & Wu, N. (2000). Phonetic awareness: Knowledge of orthographic-phonology relationships in the character acquisition of Chinese children. *Journal of Educational Psychology, 92,* 56–62.

Shu, H., Chen, X., Anderson, R. C., Wu, N., & Xuan, Y. (2003). Properties of school Chinese: Implications for learning to read. *Child Development, 74,* 27–47.

Shu, H., McBride-Chang, C., Wu, S., & Liu, H. (2006). Understanding Chinese developmental dyslexia: Morphological awareness as a core cognitive construct. *Journal of Educational Psychology, 98,* 122–133.

Shu, H., Meng, X., & Lai, A. C. (2003). Lexical representation and processing in Chinese-speaking poor readers. In C. McBride-Chang & H.-C. Chen (Eds.), *Reading development in Chinese children* (pp. 199–213). Westport, CT: Praeger Press.

Shu, H., Peng, H., & McBride-Chang, C. (2008). Phonological awareness in young Chinese children. *Developmental Science, 11,* 171–181.

Siok, W. T., Perfetti, C. A., Jin, Z., & Tan, L. H. (2004). Biological abnormality of impaired reading is constrained by culture. *Nature, 431,* 71–76.

Snowling, M. J. (2000). *Dyslexia* (2nd ed.). Oxford, UK: Blackwell.

Snowling, M. J., Bishop, D. V. M., & Stothard, S. E. (2000). Is preschool language impairment a risk factor for dyslexia in adolescence? *Journal of Child Psychology and Psychiatry, 41,* 587–600.

So, D., & Siegel, L. S. (1997). Learning to read Chinese: Semantic, syntactic, phonological and working memory skills in normally achieving and poor Chinese readers. *Reading and Writing: An Interdisciplinary Journal, 9,* 1–21.

Spafford, C., & Grosser, G. (2005). *Dyslexia and reading difficulties: Research and resource guide for working with all struggling readers* (2nd ed.). Boston, MA: Pearson.

Stanovich, K. E., Siegel, L. S., & Gottardo, A. (1997). Converging evidence for phonological and surface subtypes of reading disability. *Journal of Educational Psychology, 89,* 114–127.

Taylor, I., & Taylor, M. M. (1995). *Writing and literacy in Chinese, Korean and Japanese.* Philadelphia, PA: John Benjamins.

Torgesen, J. K., & Mathes, P. G. (2000). *A basic guide to understanding, assessing, and teaching phonological awareness.* Austin, TX: Pro-ed Press.

Tunmer, W., & Bowey, J. A. (1984). Metalinguistic awareness and reading acquisition. In W. E. Tunmer, J. A. Bowey, C. Pratt, & M. L. Herriman (Eds.), *Metalinguistic awareness in children: Theory, research, and implications.* (pp. 144–168). New York: Springer-Verlag.

Wagner, R. K., & Torgesen, J. K. (1987). The nature of phonological processing and its causal role in the acquisition of reading skills, *Psychological Bulletin, 101,* 192–212.

Wagner, R. K., Torgesen, J. K., & Rashotte, C. A. (1994). The development of reading-related phonological processing abilities: New evidence of bi-directional causality from a latent variable longitudinal study. *Developmental Psychology, 30,* 73–87.

Willcutt, E. G., DeFries, J. C., Pennington, B. F., Olson, R. K., Smith, S. D., & Cardon, L. R. (2003). Comorbidity of reading difficulties and ADHD. In R. Plomin, J. C. DeFries,

P. McGuffin, & I. Craig (Eds.), *Behavioral genetics in a postgenomic era* (pp. 227–246). Washington, DC: American Psychological Association.

Willcutt, E. G., Doyle, A. E., Nigg, J. T., Faraone, S. V., & Pennington, B. F. (2005). Validity of the executive function theory of ADHD: A meta-analytic review. *Biological Psychiatry, 57*, 1336–1346.

Wimmer, H., Mayringer, H., & Landerl, K. (2000). The double-deficit hypothesis and difficulties in learning to read a regular orthography. *Journal of Educational Psychology, 92*, 668–680.

Wolf, M. (1999). What time may tell: Towards a new conceptualization of developmental dyslexia. *Annals of Dyslexia, 49*, 3–28.

Wolf, M., & Bowers, P. (1999). The "Double-Deficit Hypothesis" for the developmental dyslexias. *Journal of Educational Psychology, 91*, 1–24.

Wolf, M., & Katzir-Cohen, T. (2001). Reading fluency and its intervention. *Scientific Studies of Reading, 5*, 211–239.

Wolf, M., O'Rourke, A. G., Gidney, C., Lovett, M., Cirino, P., & Morris, R. (2002). The second deficit: An investigation of the independence of phonological and naming-speed deficits in developmental dyslexia. *Reading Writing: An Interdisciplinary Journal, 151*, 43–72.

Wong, S. W. L., & Ho, C. S.-H. (2010). The nature of the automatization deficit in Chinese children with dyslexia. *Child Neuropsychology, 16*, 405–415.

Wong, A. M. Y., Kidd, J., Ho, C. S.-H., & Au, T. K.-F. (2010). Characterizing the overlap between SLI and dyslexia in Chinese: The role of phonology and beyond. *Scientific Studies of Reading, 14*, 30–57.

Xiao, X. Y., & Ho, C. S.-H. (2011). *The role of syntactic and semantic skills for reading comprehension in Chinese elementary school children*. Manuscript submitted for publication.

Yin, W. G., & Weekes, B. S. (2003). Dyslexia in Chinese. *Annals of Dyslexia, 53*, 255–275.

Zhang, C.-F., Zhang, J.-H., Chang, S.-M., & Zhou, J. (1998). A study of cognitive profiles of Chinese learners' reading disability. *Acta Psychologica Sinica, 30*, 50–56.

Zhou, X., Zhuang, J., & Yu, M. (2002). Phonological activation of disyllabic compound words in the speech production of Chinese. *Acta Psychologica Sinica, 34*, 242–247.

Ziegler, J. C., & Goswami, U. C. (2005). Reading acquisition, developmental dyslexia and skilled reading across languages: A psycholinguistic grain size theory. *Psychological Bulletin, 131*, 3–29.

Part II

Reflections on the study of developmental disorders

7   The modern beginnings of research into developmental language disorders

Paula Hellal and Marjorie P. Lorch

Introduction

The second half of the 19th century saw growing scientific interest in the study of the child. Articles, and later books, appeared throughout Europe and the United States that focused on the infant's first three years of life. By the 1880s, the Darwinian approach to natural sciences was extended to humans and the baby came to be seen as "a biological specimen". With the founding of paediatric hospitals and the introduction of compulsory schooling for the under 12s, it became possible to investigate the developing child's mind on a scale never seen before. Concomitant with the growing interest in normal development was an increased interest in the aetiology, prognosis and treatment of developmental disorders, with the hope that increased understanding of the latter could inform the former. At the end of the century, the American philosopher Henry Davies made the following claim: "the child-mind . . . is no longer a terra incognita where pedagogues grope in the dark. We now understand the force of such words as heredity and environment as applied to children" (Davies, 1900, p. 196).

This chapter considers the neurological, psychological and therapeutic advances made during this period. The focus of the chapter is on developmental language disorders but consideration is given to the comorbidity of symptoms and the emerging diagnostic techniques applied to the speech/language difficulties accompanying motor/sensory impairments in conditions such as cerebral palsy and chorea. As well as looking at research into language delay and its perceived links to "idiocy" or general cognitive delay, we consider the early history of what is now termed Specific Language Impairment, as well as both "word blindness" and "word deafness" and the role of medicine and education in the treatment of "deaf-mutes". The latter half of the 19th century saw emerging diagnostic and treatment regimes and a growing understanding of child psychology. We discuss the ways in which these 19th-century pioneers developed techniques for making their assessments and diagnoses. We conclude by looking at the relevance of these early investigations for modern research into language acquisition and language difficulties in the child.

Background

At the beginning of the 19th century the Romantic ideal held that children came into the world "innocent" (Hendrick, 1994). By the end of that century this view had been superseded by a scientific, rational understanding of childhood. A variety of social, cultural and political factors fostered this change across Europe and North America. For example, the introduction in 1870 of compulsory elementary schooling in England and the establishment of specialist paediatric hospitals in a number of towns across the country from the mid-century onwards led to children being examined, assessed, tested and discussed on an unprecedented scale. At the same time, changes in scientific paradigm arising out of the work on evolution by Charles Darwin (1809–1882) and others led to a new research initiative focused on observing human development. Children became as legitimate a subject of scientific investigation as molluscs or lichen. By the turn of the 20th century professionals from numerous fields were engaged in investigating child development.

Language *per se* had been a topic for consideration by philosophers, classical scholars and medical professionals throughout the 19th century. One of the motivations for investigating child language acquisition was that it was believed an understanding of the developmental process in an individual might throw light on the development of language in Mankind. Charles Darwin argued for continuity between the communicative abilities in animals and those more highly developed skills seen in man (Darwin, 1871). There was also growing acceptance of the notions put forward by Herbert Spencer (1820–1903) and Ernst Haeckel (1834–1919) that ontology recapitulates phylogeny. Edinburgh physician John Wyllie (1844–1916) put the case in the strongest terms:

> Any account of the development of speech would be most incomplete if it were content merely to treat of the subject in its relations to the individual child and made no attempt to indicate the views . . . regarding the human race.
>
> (Wyllie, 1892, p. 897)

In the medical world, interest in language, its acquisition and disorders, was instigated to a large degree by the series of papers published in the early 1860s by the French surgeon and anthropologist Paul Broca (1824–1880). Broca suggested a link between impaired language function and a lesion found at autopsy in the frontal lobe (Broca, 1861 [1960]). This new syndrome of aphasia, as it came to be termed, led to great interest in determining whether a consistent relationship could be demonstrated between language disorders and localised lesions of the cerebral cortex. Aphasia was soon identified to co-occur with hemiplegia and other symptoms in cases of apoplexy and other cardiovascular diseases in both adults and children (e.g., Jackson, 1864). However reports of such case series did not take age at onset of illness to be a significant factor for either the clinical presentation or prognosis until the latter part of the century (Hellal & Lorch, 2010). Impaired speech in children who had begun to acquire language normally was also noted as a part of syndromes in conditions such as chorea and epilepsy. In the early 1870s it was suggested that the choreic child's inability to speak was not necessarily entirely due to loss of muscular control but that the physical disorder in some way "interfered" with the mental powers (West, 1871).

In this context, investigating what constituted "normal" development of language function began to interest the medical profession for the light it was hoped it could throw on these conditions. Physicians typically described the acquisition of language function in the child with reference to distinct though connected language centres in the brain; terms derived from clinical observations of aphasia and familiar to all who were interested in the localisation debate.

Methodological issues

In order to understand its social and medical meaning, a diagnosis must be placed within a contemporary classification system (Risse & Warner, 1992). In any consideration of the history of medical, psychological, or neurological research it is important to bear in mind that classifications and labels are defined and redefined over time. The fact that a particular term has been in use for a long period does not necessarily mean that its usage has remained constant throughout that time. The conditions we discuss in this paper are given their contemporaneous labels and placed in inverted commas. The evidence for the following discussion comes primarily from primary sources with some reference made to unpublished archived cases. Published cases were typically written up to illustrate the unusual, describe treatment that was successful, or describe a patient's unexpected response to standard treatment. Many of the cases were intended to establish the existence of a particular disorder and appeal to contemporary theoretical issues. For example, John Langdon Down (1828–1896), who described the eponymous Down syndrome, writes: "The medical literature of examples of defective commissures of the brain comprises so few cases, and of these the life history is so imperfect, that I need no apology in placing the records of another before the members of this Society" (Down, 1887, p. 85).

Children as scientific objects

The interest in children and childhood in the 19th century resulted in the passing of many reforming laws relating to limiting work, improving living conditions and increasing opportunities for education. In 1833 the Factories Inquiries Commission was responsible for the first extensive survey carried out to investigate child health in England. The commission was concerned solely with uncovering any physical harm suffered by the child as a result of his or her labour. The child's mental health and development were not touched upon. Only in the latter decades of the century was real concern raised about the child's mental state, but by then the children were not the factory or agricultural workers but mentally overtaxed school children cramming for their exams.

The 1870 Education Act brought about increasing access to primary education, including pupils from the most deprived areas of the cities. This brought into public view the appalling scale of poverty, sickness and mental and physical handicaps within those communities and led to a call for welfare provision. There followed a prolonged debate about the health of the nation's schoolchildren. In 1884 Francis Galton (1822–1911) opened a laboratory at University College, London, where parents could have their child's mental powers tested. Galton's interest in heredity and his realisation that the statistical analysis of data was only reliable when dealing with large sample sizes resulted in his pioneering work in anthropometry: the measurement of human characteristics. His laboratory was included in the International Health Exhibition held in London in 1885. The anthropometric measurements included scientific mental tests devised by Galton in an attempt to measure intelligence and led to the establishment of psychometrics as a field of study. Sophie Bryan (1850–1922), mathematics teacher (and later Head) at the North London Collegiate School, was inspired by Galton's work to carry out mental tests on her school children. In 1886, her presentation to the Anthropological Institute entitled "experiments in testing the character of school children" was described by Galton in his role as Institute President as "a first scientific attempt to test certain elementary characteristics in the disposition of school children" (F. Galton, 1886). Two years later, in 1888 the British Medical Association, together with the Charity Organisation Society and the British Association for the Advancement of Science, set up a committee to investigate the development of school children. The committee was set up on the instigation of Francis Warner (1847–1926), physician to the London Hospital, who was interested in studying any correlations found between physical and mental disability in childhood. Over a period of six years Warner and his colleagues examined a total of 100,000 school children. The report included recommendations as to the type of education and training most suited for handicapped children (D. S. Galton, 1895). A year later, influenced in part by the work of the influential American psychologist Stanley Hall (1844–1924), the Childhood Society was founded in England.

Despite questioning the fundamental nature of the child, the age at which adulthood began and childhood ended remained undecided throughout the century. In 1833 a Royal Commission declared that childhood ceased at 13 years of age. Britain's first paediatric hospital Great Ormond Street, London admitted children up to the age of 12. By the turn of the century the predominant school leaving age was 14. The determination of who was considered a child seemed tied to the concept of social class; for example, the older offspring of a wealthy family, still receiving education, might be considered a minor for a far longer period of time. As Walvin points out "contemporary definitions of childhood have varied greatly between social classes and, of course, across time" (Walvin, 1982, p. 12).

The early developmental psychologists

While there had been philosophical discussions on the topic throughout the previous century and in the early 1800s, by the latter half of the 19th century child development and particularly child language development had become a subject of empirical research. One key contribution which instigated interest in the topic was philosopher Hippolyte Taine's (1828–1893) diary study of his daughter's first three years of development published in French in 1876 and translated into English the following year (Taine, 1877). Upon reading this, Charles Darwin was prompted to publish selections from a diary he had kept decades earlier detailing his own children's milestones (Darwin, 1877). As a scientist of international distinction, Darwin's paper attracted widespread attention and other researchers were inspired to investigate an area that had previously been seen as belonging firmly to the domestic realm (Champneys, 1881; Pollock, 1878). Researchers working on child development in other countries and in other languages reviewed and translated each others' work (e.g., Sully, 1882). In this way, a network of colleagues and collaborators began to grow.

In these works the process of language acquisition was seen as reflecting the developing child's mind, and the role of instinct and imitation in learning new behaviours was investigated. The role of imitation in child language acquisition became an issue for evolutionary scientists from Darwin (1877) onwards in their attempt to differentiate innate versus acquired behaviours in human development (Lorch & Hellal, 2010). Vocalisation, like motor movement, Taine considered a spontaneous reflex action proposing that the repetition of these reflex actions lead by "gradual selection" to "intentional" action when the child was able to say the word (Taine, 1877, p. 252). Although he stressed the importance of imitation, Taine believed his daughter acquired her expressive behaviours by herself: "In short, example and education were only of use in calling attention to the sounds that she had already found out for herself, in calling forth their repetition and perfection, in directing her preference to them and in making them emerge and survive amid the crowd of similar sounds. But all initiative belongs to her" (Taine, 1877, p. 253).

Taine argued that as well as helping the child acquire speech sounds, the language environment played a supporting role in helping to fix the meaning of the words used. He observed that his daughter ceased to use a term when she noticed it was not produced in the speech environment. Until she noticed, "the meaning that she gives it [a word] is not what we give it, but it is only the better fitted for showing the original work of infantile intelligence" (Taine, 1877, p. 254). This overextension Taine called the "essence of language" which distinguishes human speech from animal association of sound where there was no extension in meaning. Above all, Taine stressed the originality of child language acquisition: "If language were wanting, the child would recover it little by little or would discover an equivalent . . . the child is an original genius adapting itself to a form constructed bit by bit by a succession of original geniuses" (Taine, 1877, p. 258).

Whereas Taine had focused entirely on language acquisition Darwin widened the observation to include the infant's various reflex actions and emotions such as sneezing and hiccoughing, and a range of emotional and 'moral' behaviours such as frowning and deceit. Observing his son's reflex movement, he reflected that children do not learn to blow their noses or clear their throat till they are several years old but that these same actions are performed instinctively at an early age.

Darwin comments on how such 'perfection' of movement in the infant contrasted with the 'extreme imperfection' of the voluntary ones displayed in older children due to the later development of 'the Will'. He took this as a demonstration of the important distinction between instinctual and learned behaviour, but also as an exemplar of 'gradualism' in development, in which behaviours do not appear full blown but emerge from rudimentary patterns to increasing competence.

Darwin's work inspired a whole generation of researchers to investigate child development. One of his disciples, James Sully (1842–1923), who was professor of philosophy and psychology at the University of London, began a large-scale study of children with data collected through a national public appeal to parents and teachers (Sully, 1893). This work led to the publication of what may be the first textbook in developmental psychology (Sully, 1895).

The medical perspective on developmental psychology

The mid-19th-century British physician, called upon to treat a sick child, typically relied on either books aimed primarily at guiding mothers in the care of their infants or simply on their own personal experience. The study of childhood disease was not seen as a field of specific clinical endeavour. Medical opinion had proved stubbornly opposed to specialisation *per se* (Bynum, 1994) and particularly opposed to the specialisation of child medicine. In Britain, it was widely felt that the sick child would fail to thrive if deprived of its mother, while allowing mothers to remain with their children in the hospital would permit infection to spread rapidly from person to person. As medical historians point out, 19th-century physicians tended to be conservative, keeping to tried and trusted traditional methods long after alternatives had been promoted in the medical literature (Lomax, 1996). The first paediatric hospital in Britain, Great Ormond Street in London, was not founded until 1852. Charles West (1816–1898), the hospital's founder, insisted that the developing nervous system was fragile and potentially easily disturbed and the child should not be treated as if he were a miniature adult. By the turn of the century more than twenty-five paediatric hospitals had been established in towns and cities across Great Britain and numerous medical texts had been published on childhood disease. However, paediatrics as a discipline was not to be examined in the medical schools in the UK until the early 20th century.

By the latter decades of the 19th century, physicians interested in both children and adults had motives for considering how children acquired language. It was hoped an understanding of the process would illuminate abnormal development and assist in the devising of remedial therapy for aphasia. With respect to acquired language impairments, there was a generally held view that those who suffered language loss seemed to reacquire speech in much the same manner as a child learning to talk. For developmental difficulties, increasing parental concern was an additional factor. During this time it appears that children were being brought to clinicians because they were 'late in talking' (West, 1871). These two themes will be discussed in more detail below.

Medical understanding of child language acquisition

Charles West identified three factors vital to language learning in the child: repetition, simplification and instruction (West, 1848). Other physicians followed with descriptions of their own. As well as the individual case studies, medical textbooks began to describe both developmental and acquired language disorders in childhood such as language delay, stuttering and aphasia. Literature on the subject of stammering became particularly prolific with numerous theories and therapies proposed. An objective investigation into the phenomena of language acquisition, loss and reacquisition became part of the wider scientific advance of that period. The authors of paediatric textbooks stressed the necessity of accurate, detailed observation and testing (Ashby & Wight, 1892; Keating, 1889).

This increased interest within the medical profession in normal and deviant child language acquisition made it possible for physicians to begin to compare their patient's language development with the perceived standard. A typical case description from this period is illuminating: a 7-year-old boy was admitted to a London paediatric hospital with "dementia after epilepsy". His speech was described as being "not as good as it was. (He) talks like a child learning to talk" (Dickinson, 1876). By the end of the century doctors began to compare the language skills of their patients with developmental disorders with age-matched peers. Dr. Lees of Great Ormond Street Hospital described a 15-month-old hemiplegic patient as: "makes some attempt to talk quite up to average in this respect for age" (Lees, 1898).

In writing on aphasia, the Scottish physician Byrom Bramwell (1847–1931) presented a physiologically based model of the stages of acquisition within a framework of distinct though connected language centres using terminology from studies of aphasia and associated conditions (Bramwell, 1897). His work provides a detailed account of understanding of language acquisition from a *fin-de-siècle* medical perspective before the early 20th-century move away from localisation to a more holistic view of the human brain and behaviour relations. Bramwell began his work on language disorders by describing first the order of acquisition: the initial stage being comprehension with the child learning to associate sounds with particular objects. Like other physicians and early psychologists, Bramwell thought that the infant was taught this recognition directly by the mother uttering a word while pointing to the relevant object. Repetition would fix the association in the child's auditory speech centre. Only after this would the motor centre begin to develop. The development of the motor speech centre was, in his view, directly under the guidance of the auditory speech centre and, to a lesser degree, the visual centre: "This process of co-ordination (arrangement of the cell groups and the order of their discharge) is directed, checked, corrected and governed chiefly under the guidance of the auditory centre" (Bramwell, 1897, p. 526).

Bramwell described an associationist model of learning: "the performance of these muscular movements is attended with the production of a new set of in going impressions, the memories of which are stored up in the cerebral cortex" (Bramwell, 1897, p. 538). Comprehension was noted to precede production, repetition of sounds and words was initially without meaning, and only when the connections had been consolidated could these centres be stimulated indirectly as the result of memory allowing the child to talk spontaneously.

Bramwell stated that: "In this process not only are the auditory and motor vocal speech mechanisms trained and perfected but the mental faculties and the intelligence are at the same time educated and developed. The two processes of necessity go hand in hand" (Bramwell, 1897, p. 464). This linking of the acquisition of language with the development of the mind in an individual echoes Darwin's theory of the co-evolution of language and mind in the human species. To what extent language could be said to be dependent on mind and vice versa was a topic of serious debate throughout the 19th century. Some, like Atkinson (1870), held that language was dependent on the mind: "We see in the child the mind first coming into play and then speech following. Without the first existence of mind speech is impossible; speech cannot come before the mind exists to appreciate different sounds and surrounding objects, so that in those cases where there is a decided deficiency of brain or helpless idiocy speech is absent" (Atkinson, 1870, p. 44). Another view was put forward by Thomas Smith Clouston (1840–1915) who had a long career working with mentally handicapped patients. Clouston pointed out that many 'congenital imbeciles' "can speak quite well, and yet are entirely weak in mental power" (Clouston, 1891, p. 690). He agreed only partially with those who thought, like Atkinson, that there could be no intelligent speech when the mind was impaired. "This co-equal retardation and non-development of two functions dependent on and directly related to each other, like speech and mentalization does not always occur" (Clouston, 1891, p. 690). He described language as a "lesser function" which could develop normally in a mind that showed a more general impairment in development.

However many cases of "equal co-retardation and non-development" were seen, not least in cases of infantile cerebral paralysis; this developmental disorder was first described as Little's disease with a focus on the motor aspects of the disability (Little, 1843). Interest in this group of children grew in the latter decades of the century due in part to specialist hospitals and other caring institutions, which were created to respond to these children's particular needs. This led to a number of studies carried out with large case series of infantile cerebral paralysis in the UK, USA and Germany (Bastian, 1875; Freud, 1897; Osler, 1889; Sachs & Peterson, 1890). Consideration of the aetiology led clinicians to draw distinctions among pre-, peri- and post-natally acquired nervous system injuries and between infantile cerebral paralysis which was due to central nervous system damage and paralyses caused by spinal lesions. The study of these cases contributed to 19th-century understanding of brain laterality and the role of right hemisphere involvement in the recovery of language function. The correlation of age at symptom onset with patterns of language acquisition, impairment and recovery was also investigated.

For many of these children, language difficulties were seen to co-occur with other mental impairments in development. In the case series of Sachs and Peterson (1890), various degrees of mental impairment were found, from 'weak-mindedness' to 'complete idiocy', with good mental development in only a few cases. In a major review of the aetiology, pathophysiology, risk factors, and treatment of infantile cerebral paralysis, Sigmund Freud (1856–1939) drew a clear distinction between acquired aphasia as a disturbance in someone who had already acquired speech and developmental language delay in the child (Longo & Ashwal, 1993).

William Osler (1849–1919), author of *The Principles and Practice of Medicine*, the standard text on clinical medicine for four decades, popularised the term 'Cerebral Palsy' in his monograph devoted to the condition (Osler, 1889). Osler provided data on 120 children with cerebral palsy; 13 children also had aphasic symptoms. This early longitudinal study by Osler was theoretically significant: many physicians had previously assumed that infants with brain damage would recover and develop normally for the simple reason that they did not follow up on them. Osler observed his patients' patterns of recovery and development over the course of many months and found symptoms emerging some time after the initial brain trauma. Osler (1889) observed that, as a rule, the younger the subject the greater the liability to serious and permanent damage: "usually the power of speech begins to return in a short time but recovery may be deferred for a year . . . and in (one case) the child had not spoken 6 months after the lesion. In several instances recovery was incomplete" (Osler, 1889, p. 33).

Developmental language delay

Until the 1890s, clinical interest had been restricted to children suffering from acquired language disorders due to acute illness or organic lesion (Hellal & Lorch, 2005). Children presenting with developmental language difficulties would have been less likely to come to medical attention and more likely to be referred to either an institute for the deaf or one of the asylums. Alternatively, they would receive instruction from elocution specialists. Education for the deaf had been developing since the 18th century. In Britain a school for the deaf and dumb opened in London in 1792. America soon followed with the first institution for deaf mutes established in Hartford in 1817. Pioneering work taking place on the Continent was translated into English such as Charles Michel de l'Épée's (1712–1789) 'True method of educating the deaf and dumb, confirmed by long experience' (de l'Épée, 1860). By the middle of the 19th century, teachers of the deaf were often the source of support and rudimentary therapy for such children. However by the end of the century a shift had taken place whereby difficulties in language acquisition began to be viewed as a medical rather than an educational problem.

Charles West, the leading British paediatrician interested in neurological disorders, was ahead of his time in stressing that severe communicative difficulties and consequent inability to socialise was likely to adversely affect both the mental and emotional development of the child: "The complete inability to keep up intercourse with other children, or the great difficulty in the attempt, had cast a shadow over the mind; and the little ones were dull, suspicious, unchildlike" (West, 1884, p. 289). The child's behaviour, affected by his or her inability to communicate, might be "wayward, disobedient, and passionate".

West was also one of the first to differentiate between language delay and language disorder. Evidence as to what constituted language delay came from the growing paediatric clinics in hospitals (such as West's Great Ormond Street) and the burgeoning diary studies by psychologists. Attempts were made to establish the age at which children typically acquired language and just when a parent ought to start feeling concerned. West considered all children (excepting cases of 'severe congenital idiocy') would eventually acquire language; anxiety being groundless even in the case of speech-delayed 2-year-olds. As long as the child could hear, was observed to use modulated tones when vocalising and demonstrated "any intelligence at all" West believed that speech would invariably develop.

These three yardsticks – deafness, vocalisations, and mental capacity – were far from easy to assess in the 19th century. With limited audiological tools it was very difficult to determine the existence of congenital deafness in early childhood. The fact that deafness could be partial complicated assessment and might result in the child being erroneously labelled as intellectually deficient. In other cases, problems with articulation, perhaps partly dependent on malformation of the mouth, resulted in similarly inappropriate classification. Determining the speechless child's mental capacities was a particularly complicated exercise given that the assessment of mental competence was to a large degree determined by a patient's ability to respond appropriately to questioning. The Philadelphia paediatrician Thomas Morgan Rotch (1849–1914) advised physicians to make careful note of the child's previous history as a diagnostic aid (Rotch, 1896; Wyllie, 1892). However, obtaining an accurate past medical history was itself far from straightforward as typically, the all-important early history of a condition, vital for accurate diagnosis, was acquired second hand: the informant in most cases being the child's mother.

Based on his experience of observing a large number of children (a methodology that permitted a growing understanding of childhood disease and development), West noted that the age at which children start to talk varied greatly. He did not consider that delayed speech necessarily implied a deficiency of intelligence. In certain cases he held the opposite might be true. Bernard Sachs (1858–1944), the American neurologist and psychiatrist whose treatise on the nervous diseases of children is considered the first American textbook on paediatric neurology, agreed with West that the slow acquisition of speech did not necessarily imply mental impairment, nor early utterances genius: "I have known children to be tardy in the acquisition of speech and yet in later years to show not the slightest sign of defective mental or speech development" (Sachs, 1895, p. 472). Sachs raised the possibility that late acquisition of speech might be "a family peculiarity". He considered 12 to 18 months old the age of normal language acquisition, but advised parents not to worry until their child reached the age of 2½ or 3 years old and was still not talking (Sachs, 1895).

Despite the more reassuring view of Henry Ashby (1846–1908) and George Arthur Wright (b. 1851) who suggested a longer timeframe for normal language acquisition: "if . . . the child of five or six years of age does not talk at all, there is probably some mental defect" (Ashby & Wight, 1892, p. 476), very few cases appear in the literature that would appear to show language delay (after the age of 2) without associated cognitive or physical impairment. In one such case, a boy had remained without speech until the age of 5 when he was said to have uttered "what a pity" following an accident to his toy (Wyllie, 1892). The child could not be induced to repeat these words (or any others) for a fortnight after which his acquisition of expressive language progressed rapidly and he "speedily became talkative". When re-seen at the age of 11 years his speech was described as normal and showed no sign of any language defect.

Samuel Wilks (1824–1911) presented a few cases of his own (Wilks, 1883). One of his patients was an 8-year-old boy with "perfect hearing" who was found to be "in every way . . . as intelligent as other children" and a 6-year-old boy who was "intelligent looking" and whose receptive language skills were normal. He "understood everything that was said, and did all that was told him". Wilks points out that while the child "could make noises (he made) no intelligent sound" (Wilks, 1883, p. 95). Wilks made no comment as to the possibility of motor or neurological difficulties affecting the children in these cases. Instead he suggested that "in all these cases speech will eventually come", though he professed himself somewhat surprised by the length of the delay.

Sachs (1895) was more cautious. He comments: "Inasmuch as speech is the function of special areas of the brain, it would be natural to expect that cases would occur in which speech alone was defective without the impairment of any other cerebral function, but I have not seen a single such instance although I have carefully watched for it for years" (Sachs, 1895, p. 472). As an example, Sachs described his case of a 6-year-old boy "said to come of a family that acquired speech late in life." The child, unable to utter a single word distinctly but appearing "tolerably bright" and who "evidently understood language well enough" was "on closer examination" discovered to "exhibit other than mere speech defects: ". . . he was not able to use the scissors properly, nor able to handle knife or fork (and) . . . he was entirely ignorant of the difference between colours" (Sachs, 1895, p. 472). Sachs cautioned against making a diagnosis of an exclusive speech defect before a "very careful examination" had been made.

Developmental language disorders

The debate on delayed language focused on whether children who failed to acquire speech at the normal time (whether that was considered 2 years or even 5–6 years old) were likely to be cognitively impaired or have some physical deformity that prevented the production of speech. In the last decade of the 19th century, a series of papers were published detailing the cases of children whose speech, when they did start to talk, appeared abnormal.

Walter Bough Hadden (1856–1893), a young physician at Great Ormond Street Hospital, brought his first such case to the attention of the medical community in 1891. This paper marks a turning point in the way that language development became medicalised. Hadden reported on an otherwise healthy child who was treated for a lengthy period as a hospital inpatient for his lack of progress in language acquisition. Hadden describes the boy as not speaking at all "until he was between three and four years old, when he began to make sounds":

He could not pronounce his own name properly, and even the simplest words, such as "cat", could not be rendered so as to be recognized by others. When he talked or read it was evident that he was dividing off into syllables, although the sounds were unintelligible gibberish.

(Hadden, 1891, p. 96)

Clinical case reports began to appear that described other children with difficulties in language production who had come to medical attention. These children were hospitalised and received treatment with their progress monitored over long periods. Attempts were made to conventionalise assessments and speech transcription methods.

Although linguistic science in the 19th century was in its infancy, progress was being made with books on phonetics and grammar appearing in the latter decades. However, throughout this period, physicians had to rely on their own, and their colleagues', clinical judgement and experience when presented with cases of impaired language function: speech therapy becoming a profession in its own right only in the mid-20th century. Nineteenth-century physicians' descriptions of linguistic impairments were, therefore, idiosyncratic with very little, if any, phonetic or grammatical analysis. Investigative procedures were used in the 19th century (Jacyna, 2000) but these were not standardised and there was little or no long-term follow up of patients. Hadden and his London colleagues were among the first to adopt a (for the time) consistent and rigorous assessment of language skills.

William Hale White (1857–1949) and Cuthbert Hilton Golding-Bird (1848–1939) used the new technology of the recently invented phonograph to make recordings of their patients' pre- and post-treatment speech samples (Hale White & Golding-Bird, 1891). The publication of these papers sparked medical interest in developmental language disorders. Many clinicians found that they too had seen children with similar difficulties, reflecting the general experience that once a new phenomenon is formally identified it is subsequently found to be surprisingly common. The same can be seen following the "discovery" of dyslexia and autism in the 20th century.

This growing interest in developmental language disorders led to attempts to devise treatment regimes, some involving intensive one to one remediation with specialist staff over long periods (Hadden, 1891). However this was likely to benefit only those children who came to the attention of specialist clinicians at the large teaching hospitals as was the case with adults who had acquired aphasia.

For much of the century (and well into the next), in cases where the child failed to develop language in the manner of his/her peers, loss or impairment of cognitive ability was generally believed a defining factor. In 1853 William Wilde, an Irish surgeon, carried out the first wide ranging investigation into deaf-dumbness in the British Isles. Among his many cases he found a small minority that were dumb but not deaf: "Instances of simple and uncomplicated idiopathic dumbness, independent of deafness, although rare, really do exist" (Wilde, 1853, p. 465). Many of these children would be placed in institutes for the deaf or imbeciles and would not receive a proper education. In 1867, Wilbur labelled patients presenting with disordered speech "idiotic aphasics" (Wilbur, 1867). He included in this class children who could repeat words after the observer but could not originate them. By the turn of the century, the term used for such children was 'congenital aphasia' (Gee, 1902).

Considering their plight in the early 20th century, Morison argued that they were more likely to be misunderstood than if they had been deaf and dumb "for though hearing they will be found not to comprehend" (Morison, 1930, p. 34). Fleming was concerned that the language difficulties experienced by these children meant "they may become imbeciles from deprivation" (Fleming, 1930). In spite of the fact that many patients with developmental language difficulties were described as intelligent, the idea persisted that cases of mutism or severely impaired language without deafness were due to imbecility. Indeed, so entrenched was the prevailing view well into the 20th century that some institutions for the education of mutes would not admit or even examine children who could hear and were mute or had very little speech, as it was thought that their condition was hopeless and they were unsuitable for any type of education (Worster-Drought & Allen, 1930).

Hadden was in a minority, believing therapy both possible and necessary. This Great Ormond Street physician seems to have made a special study of speech and language function in children. He found that in cases where the speech defect was minor, the condition commonly disappeared without special treatment and pointing out that the development of speech, like walking, needed special muscular coordination and was therefore "liable to variations in its rate of progress". However, in cases of extreme defects of articulation, such as those described in his 1891 paper, remediation should be attempted. Hadden and his fellow London physicians adapted treatment for their language impaired children shown to have positive effects in some deaf mute cases.

Hadden's patient spent seven weeks in hospital. The boy had learned some elementary sounds but his speech was so defective as to appear the utterances of an unknown language. He was placed in isolation with a "special nurse", given a kitten and a rabbit, regular exercise, and allowed to look at pictures but "reading to himself and conversation in his own language were forbidden". Hadden goes on to describe the rehabilitation process:

> The method adopted was really identical with that used for teaching deaf-mutes to speak. He was made to watch and then imitate the action of the lips, tongue, or teeth required for the production of the various elementary sounds; but it was often necessary actually to adjust the parts by the fingers or by forceps. After a time he succeeded in saying most of the alphabet straight through. He did not learn to roll the r or to say the soft z sound; I was apt to be n, though he could say it in one or two conjunctions; s was generally sh; th was produced readily. He had great difficulty in joining consonants and vowels to make even such simple words as 'boy', or 'cat'. At the end of seven weeks he could produce separately all the elementary sounds, except z and r, and the vowel sounds in bird and pearl, but the vowel sounds in hat, pear, and fair were still doubtful.

> (Hadden, 1891, p. 98)

The role of imitation in child language acquisition had by that time been dis-cussed in numerous publications by the early psychologists as well as Hadden's colleagues in the medical profession. Hadden's approach was to use imitation as a possible therapy in cases where the acquisition and development of lan-guage function was impaired. He also engaged parents to support their child's remediation, sending the mother of one to St. Thomas's hospital to "watch the method adopted". It is only in recent years that parent involvement in therapy has been reintroduced with, for example, the use of Parent Child Interaction Ther-apy for stuttering (Rustin & Cook, 1995) and SLI (Allen & Marshall, 2011), and the Hanen Program for autism (Sussman, 1999). Isolation was also deemed an important remedial tool by Hadden: "the results of education were far more speedy, more effective, and more permanent than they would have been had the patients not been isolated" (Hadden, 1891, p. 105). Unusually Hadden was able to follow up his patient's progress. He saw him several times after he left hospital though it isn't clear as to how long a period of time that covered. When the boy left hospital Hadden observed that the boy talked fairly quickly and quite well enough to be intelligible. When Hadden last saw him some indeterminate time later he was of the opinion that the boy speech was relatively unchanged but that he spoke "more naturally".

There was to be considerable debate over the proposed nomenclature of the condition described by Hadden and his colleagues. While "idioglossia" (the term proposed by Hale White & Golding-Bird, 1891) with its emphasis on an original language invented by the child proved, almost immediately, contentious, others suggested these children might be speaking some early form of language harking back to the speech of their ancestors. While an explanatory account was lacking, a description of the language production proved equally difficult. For example, Hun described an English speaking child with a developmental language impairment and described his productions as resembling French though the child had not been exposed to this language (Hun, 1868).

The alternative focus for those studying children with such developmental lan-guage difficulties was on aetiology. Hadden believed their "defect of articulation" was due to impairment of the motor speech centre and put forward suggestions based on the localisation debate. The central nature of the disorder was supported by the evidence that there was no mechanical impairment of the mouth, nor disease of the auditory apparatus, nor deafness, nor mental impairment. Hadden blamed a defect of part of the brain which co-ordinates the elementary sounds into more complex forms. Others blamed a faulty perception of speech with the child merely repeating the sounds as he or she heard them. In the early 20th century a number of researchers suggested difficulties in auditory perception was the result of impaired development of the auditory speech centre (Guthrie, 1907; Worster-Drought & Allen, 1930) and linked "idioglossia" to "word deafness", a term used to describe impairment in oral language understanding. Although many viewed idioglossia to be the speech complication of congenital word-deafness, Worster-Drought and Allen felt that there was a significant auditory defect which needed to be recog-nised. To those physicians, the term idioglossia was used to refer to the speech sounds made by the language impaired children, while the underlying condition of "word deafness" was the result of difficulties in auditory perception.

Worster and Allen reviewed the various papers published from the mid-19th century onwards, commenting on the plethora of terms used to identify developmental language difficulty:

> The history of the subject of congenital word-deafness and its complications is a reflection of the different phases through which the subject has passed since aphasia was first recognised as a clinical abnormality early in the nineteenth century. Hence it follows that references to the subject are to be found under the headings of idiocy in children, speech defects (and especially idioglossia), congenital aphasia, sensory aphasia, congenital word-deafness, the association of congenital word-deafness and congenital aphasia with speech defects, behaviour defects, studies in psychology and educational problems.
>
> (Worster-Drought & Allen, 1930, p. 196)

The field of developmental language impairment has a history of multiplicity of labels used to describe the same condition. Terminological considerations are to be expected in any new field of enquiry as the professionals involved work to limit and define the conditions described. Changes in meanings of these labels have occurred over time. For example, idioglossia is still in use but today tends to refer to the "special language" sometimes developed by twins. Today it is probably the case that many of the children seen by these late 19th-/early 20th-century physicians would be labelled "Specific Language Impaired"; their assessment and treatment the responsibility not of medical practitioners but speech and language therapists and teaching professionals. It is not, though, possible to know for certain. Although phonographic recordings were made of some of the children these have been lost. The 19th-century physicians, pioneers in the assessment and remediation of speech difficulties in children, nevertheless focused all their attention on phonetic analysis of speech. Clinical examination of grammatical aspects of language was very rudimentary even in adult aphasia until later in the 20th century. Testing auditory comprehension and syntactic and lexical aspects of language production did not become standard until after the First World War.

Word blindness

Another developmental condition that has attracted considerable research in recent decades (and not a little controversy) also has its roots in the 19th century and work undertaken by aphasiologists. Dyslexia is now almost entirely the preserve of educationalists and educational psychologists. This was not, however, the case until the 1960s. Prior to the 1960s, when a sea change in attitude occurred, dyslexic children were far more likely to be seen (if at all) by medical specialists. (In a similar vein, Attention Deficit Hyperactivity Disorder [ADHD] was first recognised by the medical profession before coming to the attention of educationalists.) Further back still, at the beginning of the century, the main investigators were ophthalmologists as those presenting with reading difficulties were described as having some form of impairment of the visual system. The early history of developmental reading difficulties, like that of developmental language disorders, was an area with no shortage of labels.

As was the case with developmental language disorders, clinical investigations of children with difficulty learning to read were motivated by descriptions of acquired reading disorders in adults with acquired neurological lesions towards the end of the 19th century. The terms proposed to describe this condition were "word blindness" or "alexia" and associated with lesions in the angular gyrus (Dejerine, 1892). Interestingly, although there is much less emphasis on either acquired or developmental disorders of writing today, in the 19th century investigation of difficulties producing written language (agraphia, associated with lesions of the left second frontal convolution) followed on almost immediately from the identification of aphasia (Lorch & Barrière, 2003).

In 1896 W. Pringle Morgan published the case of an intelligent 14-year-old boy with severe developmental reading and writing difficulties. The boy could not blend letter sounds and failed to understand spelling patterns. Morgan considered him "word blind" and suggested, by analogy to the pattern found in acute acquired disorders of reading, that the boy's left angular gyrus, purported to be "visual word centre", had failed to develop normally (Morgan, 1896). James Hinshelwood (1859–1919) a Scottish eye surgeon followed with a series of papers on developmental dyslexia in which he proposed that dyslexic children were using the homologous area of their right hemisphere to learn to read with expected slow progress (Hinshelwood, 1900). (This was the reasoning behind later suggestions to teach these children to write with their left hand.) Hinshelwood suggested the observed reading difficulties were due to a malfunction of eyesight as a result of a brain defect. While Nettleship observed a gender imbalance in developmental dyslexia, with the condition affecting more boys than girls (Nettleship, 1901), Fisher suggested the condition might be hereditary (Fisher, 1905).

Possible therapies were proposed: Hinshelwood recommended strengthening sight–sound association through the use of touch by having block letters that the child could feel as well as see; Fisher recommended the "look/say" method. Many others both in the UK and abroad followed the work of these early pioneers: "No less than 28 papers on the topic were published in the first decade of the twentieth century" (Benton, 2000, p. 327).

Conclusion

Unlike other areas of psychology the work in child development has its intellectual and methodological roots in the observational work of evolutionary biology rather than the experimental techniques of psychophysics. Our interest in child language acquisition can trace direct roots to those early diary studies at the end of the 19th century, with larger-scale group studies beginning to appear by the 1890s. At the same time, in the medical domain, children ceased to be treated as though they were "miniature adults". 'Age at symptom onset' became an important variable for the understanding of both congenital and acquired disorders. In addition, children with developmental difficulties in acquiring language began to be viewed as deserving clinical investigation rather than educational remediation. By the turn of the 20th century the investigation of child development and its difficulties had become a legitimate study for the new specialists in paediatric medicine, neurology, psychiatry as well as educationalists and those interested in social welfare.

By reflecting on developmental disorders with an added historical perspective it becomes clear that current theories and practices are neither inevitable nor impervious to change. Understanding the history of research in this area can offer new angles from which to evaluate current formulations of particular disorders and their treatment and throws light on the origin of contemporary questions and debates. Scientific interest in a particular phenomenon centres initially in narrowing down just what the condition actually is. What to call the phenomenon, how to accurately investigate it, what should be included or excluded in the definition are all concerns. (These concerns are presently reflected in the changes to diagnostic criteria in the *DSM-5*, which are discussed by Williams & Lind, and Byrne, Olson, & Samuelsson, in this volume.) Looking closely at this period of early modern research into developmental disorders we can follow the lines of thought pursued, the links made between what had appeared to be disparate fields of enquiry, the efficacy of various treatments and novel forms of assessment. The involvement of numerous professionals and fields of enquiry brought different skills and perceptions to the early study of language acquisition and disorder in the child.

During this early period of modern research, the volume of literature produced was small enough to permit the examination of numerous perspectives, i.e., medical, educational, and psychological. More than a century later keeping abreast of all the published material on developmental disorders in children is an impossible task. Most cases published today make reference to others published only a few years earlier. If present day authors do look further back into the literature, they typically only refer to isolated historical cases now viewed as seminal. It is important to recognise that these historical cases, which are cited for priority, were not produced in a vacuum. Most typically these observations occurred within an active research culture where large numbers of others were writing on the same topic.

Knowledge of the history of research into a particular condition illuminates how we have come to our present day conceptualisation and offers us a rich source of observation and debate arising out of different contexts that necessarily shaped their nature. Consideration of how changes in cultural values, social institutions, political attitudes, and empirical strategies impact on the formulation of child development and disorder can throw into relief our own theoretical assumptions and research agendas.

References

Allen, J., & Marshall, C. R. (2011). Parent–child interaction therapy in school-aged children with SLI. *International Journal of Language and Communication Disorders, 46*, 397–410.

Ashby, H., & Wight, G. (1892). *The diseases of children.* London, UK: Longmans.

Atkinson, F. P. (1870). A few ideas on aphasia. *Lancet, 1*, 44.

Bastian, H. C. (1875). *On paralysis from brain damage in its common forms.* London, UK: Macmillan.

Benton, A. L. (2000). *Exploring the history of neuropsychology: Selected papers.* Oxford, UK: Oxford University Press.

Bramwell, B. (1897). Lectures on aphasia. *Edinburgh Medical Journal, 11*, 1–13, 117–128, 232–245, 356–370, 454–465, 527–551.

Broca, P. (1861 [1960]). Remarks on the seat of the faculty of articulate language, followed by an observation of aphemia. In G. von Bonin (Ed.), *Some papers on the cerebral cortex* (pp. 49–72). Springfield, IL: Thomas.

Bynum, W. F. (1994). *Science and the practice of medicine in the nineteenth century.* Cambridge, UK: Cambridge University Press.

Champneys, F. H. (1881). Notes on an infant. *Mind, 6*, 104–107.

Clouston, T. (1891). The neurosis of development. *Edinburgh Medical Journal, 1*, 594–602, 689–706, 785–801, 930–938, 977–986, 1101–1119.

Darwin, C. (1871). *The descent of man.* London, UK: John Murray.

Darwin, C. (1877). Biographical sketch of an infant. *Mind, 2*, 285–294.

Davies, H. (1900). The new psychology and the moral training of children. *International Journal of Ethics, 10*, 493–503.

de l'Épée, C. M. (1860). True method of educating the deaf and dumb, confirmed by long experience. [English Translation]. *American Annals of the Deaf, 12*(1, 2), 1–58; 61–131.

Dejerine, J. (1892). Contribution a l'étude antinomique et clinique des différentes variétés de cécité-verbale. *Mémoires de la Société de Biologique, 4*, 61–90.

Dickinson, W. H. (1876). *F. Goodwin, 'dementia after epilepsy'.* Casenotes of Dr. W. H. Dickinson. Patient records, Great Ormond Street Hospital, London, UK.

Down, L. J. (1887). *On some of the mental affections of childhood and youth: being the Lettsomian lectures delivered before the Medical Society of London in 1887, together with other papers.* London, UK: J & A Churchill.

Fisher, J. H. (1905). Case of congenital word-blindness (inability to learn to read). *Ophthalmic Review, 24*, 315–318.

Fleming, G. W. (1930). Congenital auditory imperception (congenital word-deafness) and its relation to idioglossia and other speech defects. *Journal of Mental Science, 76*, 572.

Freud, S. (1897). *Die infantile Cerebrallähmung* [Infantile cerebral paralysis]. (L. A. Russin, Trans. & Translation ed.). Miami, FL: University of Miami Press.

Galton, D. S. (1895). *Report on the scientific study of the mental and physical conditions of childhood, with particular reference to children of defective constitution: And with recommendations as to education and training.* London, UK: British Medical Association.

Galton, F. (1886). Opening remarks by the President and discussion on 'Experiments in testing the character of school children,' Sophie Bryant. *Journal of the Anthropological Institute, 15*, 336–338, 350 156.

Gee, S. (1902). *Medical lectures and clinical aphorisms.* London, UK: Hodder and Stoughton.

Guthrie, L. G. (1907). *Functional nervous disorders in childhood.* London, UK: Henry Frowde.

Hadden, W. B. (1891). On certain defects of articulation in children, with cases illustrating the results of education on the oral system. *Journal of Mental Science*, 96–105.

Hale White, W., & Golding-Bird, C. H. (1891). Two cases of idioglossia with phonographic demonstration of the peculiarity of speech. *Transactions of the Medical and Chirurgical Society, 74*, 181–189.

Hellal, P., & Lorch, M. P. (2005). Charles West: A 19th century perspective on acquired childhood aphasia. *Journal of Neurolinguistics, 18*, 345–360.

Hellal, P., & Lorch, M. P. (2010). The emergence of the age variable in nineteenth century neurology: Considerations of recovery patterns in acquired childhood aphasia. In S. Finger, F. Boller, & K. L. Tyler (Eds.), *Handbook of clinical neurology* (Vol. 95, 3rd series, pp. 845–852). Edinburgh, UK: Elsevier.

Hendrick, H. (1994). *Child welfare: England, 1872–1989.* London, UK: Routledge.

Hinshelwood, J. (1900). *Letter-, word- and mind-blindness.* London, UK: H. K. Lewis.

Hun, E. R. (1868). Singular development of language in a child. *Quarterly Journal of Psychological Medicine, 2*, 525–528.

Jackson, J. H. (1864). On loss of speech: its association with valvular disease of the heart, and with hemiplegia on the right side.—Defects of smell.—Defects of speech in chorea.—Arterial regions in epilepsy. *London Hospital Reports, 1*, 388–471.

Jacyna, L. S. (2000). *Lost words: Narratives of language and the brain 1825–1926.* Princeton, NJ: Princeton University Press.

Keating, J. (Ed.). (1889). *Cyclopedia of the diseases of children.* Philadelphia: J.B. Lippincott and Co.

Lees, D. B. (1898). *A. Hook, 'Hemiplegia'.* Case notes of Dr. D. B. Lees. Patient records. Great Ormond Street Hospital, London, UK.

Little, W. J. (1843). Hospital for the cure of deformities: Course of lectures on the deformities of the human frame. *The Lancet, 41*(1053), 141–144.

Lomax, E. (1996). Small and special: The development of hospitals for children in Victorian Britain. *Medical History, Supplement No. 16.*

Longo, L. D., & Ashwal, S. (1993). William Osler, Sigmund Freud and the evolution of ideas concerning cerebral palsy. *Journal of the History of the Neurosciences, 2*, 255–282.

Lorch, M. P., & Barrière, I. (2003). The history of written language disorders: Reexamining Pitres' case (1884) of pure agraphia. *Brain and Language, 85*, 271–279.

Lorch, M. P., & Hellal, P. (2010). Darwin's 'Natural Science of Babies' *Journal of the History of the Neurosciences, 19*, 140–157.

Morgan, W. P. (1896). A case of congenital word-blindness. *British Medical Journal, 2*, 1378.

Morison, A. G. (1930). Congenital word deafness, with some observations on the accompanying idioglossia. *Journal of Neurology and Psychopathology, 11*, 28–35.

Nettleship, E. (1901). Cases of congenital word-blindness (inability to learn to read). *Ophthalmic Review, 20*, 61–67.

Osler, W. (1889). *The cerebral palsies of children. A clinical study from the Infirmary for Nervous Diseases.* (Reprint ed. Vol. 1). Philadelphia: Mac Keith Press.

Pollock, F. (1878). An infant's progress in language. *Mind, 3*, 392–401.

Risse, G., & Warner, J. (1992). Reconstructing clinical activities: Patient records in medical history. *Social History of Medicine 5,* 183–205

Rotch, T. (1896). *Pediatrics. The hygienic and medical treatment of children.* Philadelphia, PA: Young J. Pentland.

Rustin, L., & Cook, F. (1995). Parental involvement in the treatment of stuttering. *Language Speech and Hearing Services in Schools, 26*, 127–137.

Sachs, B. (1895). *A treatise on the nervous diseases of children for physicians and students.* London, UK: Bailliere, Tindall & Cox.

Sachs, B., & Peterson, F. (1890). A study of cerebral palsies of early life, based upon an analysis of one hundred and forty cases. *Journal of Nervous and Mental Diseases, 5*, 295–332.

Sully, J. (1882). Review: Die Seele des Kindes. by W. Preyer. *Mind, 7*, 416–423.

Sully, J. (1893). Appeal to parents. *Mind, n.s. 2*, 420–421.

Sully, J. (1895). *Studies of childhood*. London, UK: Longmans, Green, and Co.

Sussman, F. (1999). *More Than Words: Helping parents promote communication and social skills in children with autism spectrum disorder.* Toronto, Canada: The Hanen Centre.

Taine, H. (1877). M. Taine On the acquisition of language by children. *Mind, 2*, 252–259.

Walvin, J. (1982). *A child's world. A social history of English childhood 1800–1914.* Harmondsworth, UK: Penguin Books.

West, C. (1848). *Lectures on the diseases of infancy and childhood.* London, UK: Longman, Green, Brown and Longman.

West, C. (1871). *On some disorders of the nervous system in childhood.* London, UK: Longmans, Green and Co.

West, C. (1884). *Lectures on the diseases of infancy and childhood.* London, UK: Longman, Brown, Green and Longmans.

Wilbur, H. B. (1867). Aphasia. *American Journal of Insanity, 24*, 1–28.

Wilde, W. (1853). *Practical observations on aural surgery and the nature and treatment of diseases of the ear.* London, UK: John Churchill.

Wilks, S. (1883). *Lectures on diseases of the nervous system* (2nd ed.). London, UK: J. & A. Churchill.

Worster-Drought, C., & Allen, I. M. (1930). Congenital auditory imperception (congenital word-deafness): and its relation to idioglossia and other speech defects. *Journal of Neurology and Psychopathology, 10*, 193–236.

Wyllie, J. (1892). The disorders of speech. *Edinburgh Medical Journal, 1 & 2*, 289–314, 401–421, 501–523, 585–604, 681–693, 777–793, 897–907, 977–992.

8 What can neurodevelopmental disorders teach us about typical development?

Roberto Filippi and Annette Karmiloff-Smith

Introduction

This chapter focuses on research investigating developmental trajectories in typically developing (TD) infants and children and in those with neurodevelopmental disorders. In particular, we concentrate on studies of attention, language development, numeracy, and face processing in Down syndrome (DS), Williams syndrome (WS), autism spectrum disorder (ASD), specific language impairment (SLI), and Fragile X syndrome (FXS). We start by introducing *Neuroconstructivism* and highlighting the dynamics of gene expression and brain development through interactions with the environment. We then discuss current research on families at genetic risk for a given disorder, and how this research goes beyond the investigation of a specific cognitive ability (e.g., language development in SLI) to explore how specificity might emerge from interrelations between different abilities over developmental time, i.e., how deficits in basic-level processes, e.g., rapid timing or global processing, can in turn affect the development of higher-level cognitive-linguistic abilities to greater or lesser degrees. We also stress the importance of cross-syndrome comparisons to pinpoint what is syndrome-specific and what is syndrome-general. Finally, we argue that developmental disorders are key to understanding typical development and that the Neuroconstructivist approach provides a strong framework within which to disentangle complex cognitive processes across developmental time. We conclude that the convergence of different neuroimaging techniques that identify both the temporal and spatial signatures of brain networks may shed new light on the relationship between the brain and cognitive development, provided changing structural and functional neural modifications are traced over developmental time.

Is development domain-specific or domain-general?

A long-standing debate in the fields of philosophy, linguistics, cognitive psychology and neuroscience concerns the start state of the human brain. Is what we observe in the adult brain the result of a set of innate pre-specifications? Or is it the product of a dynamic process involving multi-directional interactions among genes, brain, cognition, behaviour and environment? The answer is not an easy one. Developmental data suggest that infants and children are capable of amazing abilities, even when their knowledge of the world is quite meagre (e.g., Baillargeon, Spelke, & Wasserman, 1985; Hyde & Spelke, 2011; Schlottman & Ray, 2010). Moreover, clinical data from neuropsychological patients indicate that selective damage in the brain of previously normal adults can lead to specific impairments (e.g., aphasia, prosopagnosia, agrammatism, agnosia, acalculia). Put together, this evidence may seem strikingly in favour of a domain-specific, nativist view: we are born pre-wired, our brain is like a Swiss army knife, an *"ensemble"* of finely-tuned, special-purpose, innate modules or tools, handed down by evolution, that operate independently of one another (Barkow, Cosmides, & Tooby, 1992; Duchaine, Cosmides, & Tooby, 2001). The argument goes that if one of them is damaged later in life, the specific function linked with it switches off, so that a selective deficit co-occurs with the preservation of all other functions. When such reasoning is applied to developmental disorders (for instance, WS), the claim is that WS "can be explained in terms of selective deficits to an otherwise normal modular system" (Clahsen & Temple, 2003, p.26). The problem with the domain-specific account is that it totally negates the constructive role of development (see Karmiloff-Smith, 1998, 2012, for discussion).

A very different view comes from those who espouse a domain-general approach. For example, the Swiss epistemologist and child psychologist, Jean Piaget (1952), argued that the brain applies three domain-general processes – assimilation, accommodation, and equilibration – to all domains of cognition. According to Piaget, assimilation is the process by which humans perceive new information and try to fit it into their existing mental representations. Accommodation, by contrast, is the process by which internal mental structures are slightly changed as a function of the new input. These domain-general processes interact such that another domain-general process – equilibration – operates to constantly re-establish stability across the entire system. For Piaget, then, the human brain is predisposed by evolution to seek equilibrium between internally-driven and externally-driven domain-general processes. Many other psychologists have explained human development in terms of domain-general processes (e.g., Chiappe & MacDonald, 2005; Penner & Klahr, 1996; Spearman, 1927). However, the domain-general approach has difficulty in accounting for uneven cognitive profiles in which some domains are defective and others not, which is why many researchers in the field of developmental disorders have opted for a domain-specific approach (e.g., Temple, 2006). But are the domain-specific and domain-general approaches the only way to understand human development? Below we offer a third alternative from Neuroconstructivism, the *domain-relevant* approach.

The domain-relevant approach

Neuroconstructivism (Elman et al., 1996; Karmiloff-Smith, 1992, 1998; Mareschal, Johnson et al., 2007; Mareschal, Sirois, Westermann, & Johnson, 2007) neither advocates innate domain-specific modules nor a general process affecting all domains in the same way. It agrees that biological constraints are likely to be more specific than those advocated by domain-general theories, but considers the constraints to be *domain-relevant* rather than domain-specific. In other words, it argues for a number of basic-level biases in the brain (different types or density of neurons, different biochemical neurotransmitters, different timing, etc.) but suggests that the differences are merely somewhat more relevant to certain types of input processing than others, and only *become* domain-specific over developmental time. It is worth recalling that the infant brain starts out highly interconnected and only with time do some circuits become strengthened and others weakened and pruned (Huttenlocher & de Courten, 1987). Under the Neuroconstructivist view, multiple bilateral regions of the infant brain initially compete to process inputs, and only with time does a specific neural circuit win out because its properties are more *relevant* to the processing of those particular inputs. Several studies on language and face processing, for instance, have shown how early in development the infant brain processes these inputs bilaterally, but with development one hemisphere (regions in the left hemisphere for language, and in the right hemisphere for faces) gradually wins out and predominates the processing of particular inputs, as it does in the adult brain (de Haan, Humphreys, & Johnson, 2002; Mills et al., 2000; Neville, Mills, & Bellugi, 1994). So the infant brain doesn't start out like the adult brain; it progressively *develops* into an adult brain, and this involves many structural, functional and biochemical changes as development proceeds. Thus, Neuroconstructivism considers domain specificity to be the *outcome* of development rather than the start state.

It is also worth recalling that the environment affects both gene expression (Szyf, McGowan, & Meaney, 2008) and cognitive outcomes, because certain regions of the human neonate brain are particularly immature compared to other species. Paradoxically, it is this lack of specialisation in early years that allow humans to *become* simultaneously both highly specialized and cognitively flexible (Karmiloff-Smith, 1992).

Evidence for the domain-relevant view

Two examples serve to illustrate how domain-specificity can progressively *emerge* from domain-relevance. The first comes from studies of the now well-known KE family (e.g., Fisher, Vargha-Khadem, Watkins, Monaco, & Pembrey, 1998), some members of which present with speech and language impairments across several generations due to a mutation of the *FOXP2* gene on chromosome 7 (Lai, Fisher, Hurst, Vargha-Khadem, & Monaco, 2001). It was initially argued that FOXP 2 must be specific to the development of a neural network specialized in language processing (e.g., Liégeois, Baldeweg, Connelly, Gadian, Mishkin, & Vargha-Khadem, 2003). In particular, the affected KE family members present with developmental verbal dyspraxia, a difficulty in making and co-ordinating the precise movements required for the production of clear speech, in the absence of damaged nerves/muscles or any other disordered traits. Initially, some authors saw the *FOXP2* gene as a likely candidate for explaining human language evolution (e.g., Gopnik & Crago, 1991), but subsequent molecular sequencing of the gene and its downstream targets tempered such claims. Interestingly, *Foxp2* is a highly conserved gene evolutionarily and is found in multiple species such as chimpanzees (Ernard et al., 2002), birds (Bolhuis, Zijlstra, den Boer-Visser, & van der Zee, 2000), mice (Lai, Gerrelli, Monaco, Fisher, & Copp, 2003), and snakes (Martinez, 2002). Studies of *Foxp2* expression in different species now show: (1) that where it is expressed in the brain changes over time (Lai et al., 2003); (2) that its expression is greatest during learning and is thus involved in plasticity (Bolhuis et al., 2000); and (3) that its most general contribution involves the rapid planning, coordination and timing of sequential movements. This is obviously critical for planning rapidly changing sequential mouth movements for speech, and would thus subsequently impact on language. Thus, the *FOXP2* mutation in humans is unlikely to be *domain-specific* to language, but definitely *domain-relevant* to speech and language over developmental time. Moreover, it is a transcription factor that impacts on other downstream genes during development (Spiteri et al., 2007; Vernes et al., 2007) and some of these genes have been found to be mutated in several disorders including *inter alia* autism, ADHD, SLI, and stuttering (see discussion by Newbury, this volume, of the *FOXP2* gene pathways). Finally, the unlikelihood that *FOXP2* is "a gene for language" comes from evidence that the affected KE family members also show deficits in the perception and production of rhythms and mouth shapes of a non-linguistic nature (Alcock, Passingham, Watkins, & Vargha-Khadem, 2000).

A second example of domain-relevance comes from a computational model of the dorsal and ventral streams, or the *where* and *what* pathways (O'Reilly & McClelland, 1992). In this model, two streams vary only by a tiny difference in the speed of change of activation levels. Both streams initially process the same inputs. However, with time and continued processing, the tiny difference in activation levels gives rise to a gradual specialization of each pathway: the slower pathway specializes in processing the features of inputs, while the faster pathway starts to process the location of the inputs in the modelling environment – mirroring the emergence of the *what* and *where* pathways in the brain, rather than their pre-specification. Without the *domain-relevant* difference in activation levels, the *where* and *what* pathways would not have emerged and both streams would have continued to process inputs in a similar fashion. So, a tiny initial domain-relevant difference in activation levels can result over time in a large domain-specific difference in outcome. While this model may not capture how this functional difference emerges in real brains, it is in our view an interesting Neuroconstructivist demonstration of how neural differentiation could emerge rather than be pre-specified.

To understand brain development, differences in brain function between children and adults must be taken into account. For example, if we consider what is known about adult aphasia, then delays in vocabulary in children ought to be most pronounced when there is damage to posterior sites in the left hemisphere. Yet in actual fact, comprehension deficits turn out to be more common in children with right-hemisphere damage (Bates & Roe, 2001; Stiles & Thal, 1993; Stiles et al., 2003; Thal et al., 1991). In other words, regions responsible for language *learning* in young children are not necessarily the same regions as those responsible for language *use* in the adult. It is also critical to recall that in the developing brain, other brain regions can compensate for damage (Lettori et al., 2008; Liégeois et al., 2004). For instance, the brains of the congenitally deaf also highlight the plasticity of the developing brain. A lack of auditory input to the deaf brain results in the emergence of visual processing in auditory areas, and vice versa for the congenitally blind; they process some auditory inputs in visual cortex (Neville & Bavelier, 2002). In other words, brains are structurally and functionally dynamic, and it is critical to differentiate between the develop*ed* brain and the develop*ing* brain (Karmiloff-Smith, 2010).

Dissociation versus association

In atypical development, is it the case that a deficit in one domain has no effect on other domains? In other words, should we think of the atypical brain as a normal brain with parts intact and parts impaired, as some researchers claim (Clahsen & Temple, 2003; Leslie, 1992)? And even when scores fall "in the normal range" in a particular domain, does this necessarily imply the same cognitive and neural processes as those used by typically developing (TD) individuals? Take, for example, studies of face processing in WS. Early research yielded scores within the normal range on two standardized tests, the Benton Test of Face Recognition (Bellugi, Wang, & Jernigan, 1994) and the Rivermead Test of Face Memory (Udwin & Yule, 1991). This led a number of researchers to conclude initially that individuals with WS had "intact" face processing abilities (Bellugi et al., 1994). Indeed, these scores "in the normal range" would seem to imply that individuals with WS have comparable performance to TD individuals. However, a closer investigation using more subtle behavioural tasks, together with electrophysiological measures, pointed to more featural processing in WS compared to more configural processing in TD controls (e.g., Annaz, Karmiloff-Smith, & Thomas, 2008; Karmiloff-Smith et al., 2004), as well as different neural processing in low-level visual perception (Grice et al., 2003). The authors concluded that such atypical visual processing in WS may affect the development of higher-level visual processing like face recognition. A recent fMRI study also highlighted the differences between individuals with WS and TD controls. It turned out that the Fusiform Face Area (FFA) in WS adults was significantly larger than that of controls, despite the fact that both groups had comparable performance on the Benton face recognition test (Golarai et al., 2010). Of course, it remains unclear whether the FFA started out larger in WS or whether it *became* larger as a function of the WS fascination with processing faces. In summary, behavioural scores in the normal range in children or adults do not necessarily indicate normal neural or cognitive processes.

These examples indicate that the search for dissociations, which characterizes much of the work in adult neuropsychology, is inappropriate for the study of neurodevelopmental disorders (Karmiloff-Smith, 1998; Karmiloff-Smith, Scerif, & Ansari, 2003). In fact, rather than neat modular dissociations, developmental disorders often reveal subtle associations across different domains which are more difficult to identify in the typical case.

The case of specific language impairment (SLI)

SLI has been a central arena for debates about domain-specificity and domain-generality. For instance, according to Fonteneau and van der Lely (2008), grammar-specific impairments exist in SLI. In an event-related potential study of temporal processing in the brains of individuals with so-called Grammatical-SLI (G-SLI), participants were presented with sentences containing either syntactic or semantic violations. The results indicated that syntactic violations failed to elicit the normal Early Left-Anterior Negative electrophysiological response (ELAN), which is held to be specific to grammatical processing. Yet, the syntactic violations did elicit a normal P600, which is associated with the re-analysis of syntactic structure or syntactic integration. Furthermore, the semantic violations did elicit a normal N400 response. This encouraged Fonteneau and van der Lely to claim that "grammatical neural circuitry underlying language is a *developmentally unique system* in the functional architecture of the brain, and this complex higher cognitive system can be selectively impaired" (2008, p. 1, italics added).

At first blush, these findings would seem to constitute an example of domain-specificity of grammatical processing within language. However, several caveats must be raised, which make it highly questionable that their albeit interesting data can be interpreted in terms of a grammar-specific deficit at the cognitive or neural levels. Pivotal to Fonteneau and van der Lely's argument against the neuroconstructivist approach are two claims: (1) that G-SLI is a purely grammatical deficit, and (2) that in their adolescents they detected no lower-level impairments in auditory processing (their measure was 'processing speed') and found all other functions to be 'normal'. But neither of these claims hold. First, the adolescents with this ostensibly domain-specific grammatical deficit had a receptive vocabulary of children half their chronological age, so their deficit did not comprise only grammar. Second, normal processing speed by the time an individual reaches adolescence does not constitute evidence of a lack of low-level perceptual problems at an earlier phase of development when such timing may have been critical, something that individuals could have overcome by adolescence (Karmiloff-Smith, 1998). This stresses how important ontogenetic timing is when trying to explain neurodevelopmental disorders. Finally, it should be recalled that the authors targeted a single age group – *adolescents* with SLI; this was therefore not a developmental study but a static snapshot of development. The authors make no attempt to address SLI developmentally.

The fact that the receptive vocabulary (measured using the British Picture Vocabulary Scale) of the SLI adolescents in this study was so delayed is clearly already indicative of atypical functioning. But the electrophysiological data also reflect atypicalities in syntactic and semantic processing at the neural level. The syntactic violations elicited an N400 electrophysiological response in the SLI participants, evidence that the neural circuitry that supported their semantic processing may have been compensating for their problems with the processing of information. Also, whereas the P600 was equally distributed on anterior sites across all the groups, in the G-SLI group it was maximally distributed on (and reached greater amplitude at) anterior sites *on the right*. This seems to indicate subtle quantitative and qualitative differences between the SLI group and the healthy controls at numerous levels of linguistic processing. To resolve these essentially *developmental* questions, it is critical to investigate such processes in the same individuals across time. Indeed, whereas the N400 response to semantic violations was distributed bilaterally in the posterior areas in the G-SLI and CA-matched participants, it was maximally negative in the right hemisphere of the younger language-matched children. This suggests that the neural substrates that give rise to the N400 are in fact dynamic, not static, i.e., they change over developmental time.

An alternative interpretation of the SLI data is that one (or more) lower-level deficits in early infancy had affected development at a critical time when they were more domain-relevant to speech and language than to other domains that they may have also affected but more subtly. Language emerges from a number of lower-level abilities, such as *inter alia* the ability to share attention, to understand communicative intentions, to segment and detect statistical regularities in the speech stream, to make phonetic and phonemic discriminations, and to increase speed of speech processing (Choudhury & Benasich, 2011; Fernald, Pinto, Swingley, Weinberg, & McRoberts, 1998; Jusczyk, Pisoni, Reed, Fernald, & Myers, 1983). A lower-level deficit in any one of these processes could disrupt development to such an extent that the emergence of higher-level processes like language comprehension and production become seriously compromised. Indeed, some studies have shown that very young children at familial risk for SLI do have problems with detecting patterns in the speech stream, specifically with the processing of rapid sequences of auditory-verbal information, necessary for processing the flow of connected speech (Choudhury & Benasich, 2011; Tallal, 2000). Furthermore, morphological markers are frequently of low salience in the speech stream and often a problem for individuals with SLI (Leonard, McGregor, & Allen, 1992). Finally, children with SLI, like other children with neurodevelopmental disorders, often also have poor auditory working memory (Bishop, North, & Donlan, 1996; Conti-Ramsden, 2003; Gathercole & Baddeley, 1990).

Other studies of SLI have repeatedly challenged the notion of a pure domain-specific deficit. For example, in a meta-analysis of research on SLI by Botting (2005), it was found that although individuals with a diagnosis of SLI scored "in the normal range" on non-verbal tests, their non-verbal scores were significantly lower than those of their siblings, pointing to subtle impairments outside language. So the very notion of SLI (*Specific* Language Impairment) should perhaps be simply replaced by LI (Language Impairment).

The importance of cross-syndrome comparisons of developmental trajectories

The discussion of SLI/LI illustrates how important it is to reflect on possible cross-domain interactions and above all on a non-static cognitive profile that frequently changes as development proceeds. A series of cross-syndrome comparisons of language acquisition and number- and face- processing within the Neuroconstructivist approach has shown that areas of strength at one point in time during development are not necessarily as strong at later or earlier points in time. For example, Paterson and colleagues (Paterson, Brown, Gsödl, Johnson, & Karmiloff-Smith, 1999) compared vocabulary performance in WS and DS. It turned out that vocabulary acquisition was equally delayed in early childhood in both syndromes. For example, typically developing children become skilled word learners by the age of 1½. Children with WS or DS acquire very little language until they reach 3 to 5 years of age (Nazzi & Bertoncini, 2003). However, the developmental trajectory subsequent to the initial delay differs across the syndromes. By adolescence and adulthood, the language of individuals with WS had developed far more than that of their DS peers. Similar differences were found in the developmental trajectory of number perception between infancy and adulthood (Paterson et al., 1999; Paterson, Girelli, Butterworth, & Karmiloff-Smith, 2006). In this case, a series of tasks measuring sensitivity to changes in numerosity showed that infants and toddlers with WS were more sensitive to differences in small numbers than their DS peers; yet by adulthood, individuals with DS significantly outperformed their WS counterparts in a battery of number tasks (Paterson et al., 2006). In other words, the adult end state cannot be used to infer the infant start state, once again highlighting the need for a Neuroconstructivist developmental perspective.

Another striking example of differences in cross-syndrome trajectories is provided by Scerif and colleagues (Scerif, Cornish, Wilding, Driver, & Karmiloff-Smith, 2004). The researchers compared visual selective attention performance in toddlers with Fragile X (FXS) compared to toddlers with WS. The participants were engaged in a computerized visual search game and instructed to "find all the monsters which were hidden under the big circles" appearing on a touch-screen. Other smaller circles were presented simultaneously on the screen and used as "distracters". However, only the big circles were programmed to reveal the monster. Both groups' performance was comparable to that of TD controls in terms of search path and reaction time, but their patterns of errors differed: toddlers with WS were more affected by a specific combination of trials that increased the cognitive demand of the task (i.e., larger display size and target-distracter similarity). By contrast, toddlers with FXS made perseveration errors, revisiting circles that they had already checked. This highlights the danger of considering only behavioural scores like search path or reaction time. While the two syndromes seemed to have the same levels of performance, the error analysis showed that they were actually processing the stimuli differently.

Obviously, the ideal way to carry out cross-syndrome, cross-domain research would be to build a developmental trajectory based on longitudinal measures in the same children (see Byrne, Olson, & Samuelsson, this volume). However, due to time, financial and logistic constraints, it may not always be possible to conduct such studies. Cross-sectional developmental trajectories are, we believe, a viable alternative, and this approach has been successfully used in a number of recent studies (e.g., Annaz, Karmiloff-Smith, Johnson, & Thomas, 2009; Karmiloff-Smith et al., 2004; Thomas et al., 2001). The aim is to build a task-specific function linking performance with chronological age on a specific experimental task (e.g., a standardised measure for language acquisition), and then use regression analyses to assess whether this function differs between the typically developing group and the disorder group (Thomas et al., 2009). An advantage of this approach is the possibility of testing large samples of TD individuals across a wide range of ages, as well as measuring their performance on a broad array of tasks specifically designed for developmental purposes. Once "normal" task-specific trajectories are built, the atypical population can be plotted on them in order to establish at which point their performance is delayed or deviant.

The cross-sectional trajectory approach makes it possible to address the question of whether the target behaviour develops typically or atypically in different neurodevelopmental disorders (Annaz et al., 2008). Following this logic, Annaz and colleagues (2009) investigated the development of featural and configural processing of faces by children with WS, DS and autism spectrum disorder (ASD) from 5 to 13 years of age. They used a modified version of the "part-whole" task (Tanaka & Farah, 1993). Cross-sectional developmental trajectories were built by linking the task performance either to chronological or to mental age measured with standardized tests for visuospatial construction, vocabulary acquisition, and face recognition. They observed atypical but different trajectories in all four groups, indicating that face recognition developed in multiple pathways and with different outcomes. In particular, they found that low-functioning children with ASD, a group that is rarely studied, outperformed the other groups on inverted featural face trials when they were very young. However, this ability decreased at about 9 years of age, whereas their accuracy on upright featural trials increased over the whole developmental period. These results clearly show that without an in-depth cross-syndrome, developmental approach, these important differences might not have come to light.

The effect of the environment in atypical development

The Neuroconstructivist point of view posits that genes, brain, cognition, behaviour and environment play a dynamic, multidirectional role in shaping developmental disorders. In particular, one key question is whether the atypically developing child receives the same level of input, quantitatively and qualitatively, from the environment as, for example, his/her TD siblings or other TD children. Let's take a simple example to clarify this. A TD child is left free to crawl and explore places and objects. The parents allow the child to take some risks. In terms of language development in the TD child, lexical or grammatical errors in the form of over-generalizations are often left uncorrected because the parents are not worried that their TD child will learn eventually the correct forms. Does the atypically developing child receive the same degrees of freedom? This is unlikely. Most parents of children with neurodevelopmental disorders are quite naturally over-protective; they fear possible dangers and tend to correct the child's language mistakes immediately in the probable fear that their child may not catch up later. Of course, they do this unconsciously with the best of intentions, for the sake of their child. However, in doing so, they change the "normal" environment and may be depriving the atypically developing child of key inputs and outputs, thereby making his/

her environment subtly different from that of TD children, even within the same family. For example, Cardoso-Martins and collaborators have studied the differences in reaction to lexical errors in parents of TD children compared to those of children with DS and found striking differences (Cardoso-Martins & Mervis, 1990; Cardoso-Martins, Mervis, & Mervis, 1985). The parents of DS children tended to correct all errors immediately. However, allowing children to refer temporarily to all four-legged animals as "cats" may well help them to form a category like "animal". By contrast, the atypically developing child whose lexical outputs are immediately corrected may learn exemplars, e.g., tokens instead of types, and thus miss out on the richness that overgeneralization makes possible. In other words, researchers need to explore more deeply how having a developmental disability subtly changes the environment in which the atypical infant/child develops.

Can bilingualism tell us anything about crucial cognitive processes in typical and atypical development?

Roughly half of the world's population (about 3 billion people) regularly speaks more than one language (Grosjean, 2010). As far as Europe is concerned, the European Commission recently published a report (2006) in which a large sample of European citizens was asked how many languages they spoke other than their mother tongue. Fifty-six percent of the people in 25 countries replied that they could have a conversation in a second language, and 28 percent spoke a third. The United Kingdom is one of the most "monolingual" countries in Europe; nonetheless, even in the UK, 38 percent of those polled replied they could speak a second language.

The first half of the 20th century was characterized by the general opinion that bilingualism or multilingualism was detrimental to cognitive functioning and so care givers avoided letting children with developmental disorders learn a second language. Indeed, the first empirical evidence to emerge on the topic influenced decades of research very negatively. Thus, in a series of studies, Saer and colleagues (1922, 1923) found that bilingual children in Wales scored significantly lower than monolinguals on a range of tests, including those of general intelligence (IQ), to the extent that bilingualism was considered to be a handicap for several decades (see Hakuta & Diaz, 1985, for a review). The turning point came in 1962 when Peal and Lambert published research that completely reshaped our views of second language acquisition. The study, conducted in Canada, involved 364 French/English bilinguals as well as English or French monolingual 10-year-old children, who were strictly matched on age, gender, SES, language, and intelligence. Results revealed that when these variables were properly controlled, bilinguals outperformed their monolingual peers on a variety of tests measuring intelligence, in particular those involving symbolic manipulation. Peal and Lambert (1962) called this ability *cognitive flexibility* and were the first to propose that the bilinguals' early skill of managing two languages may have enhanced the development of general cognition in TD children.

Anecdotes aside, there is a surprising dearth of work examining the effect of being exposed to multiple languages on those who have neurodevelopmental disorders. One of the main parental concerns relates to the possible additional burden on atypically developing children deriving from the exposure to more than one language. In theory, this could represent an extra problem, especially in those already presenting with a language delay. However, hypothesis-driven empirical research can sometimes challenge received assumptions. Indeed, a series of studies conducted in Sweden (Salameh, Håkansson, & Nettelbladt, 2004) and in Canada (Paradis, Crago, Genesee, & Rice, 2003) addressed this issue head on. For instance, the study of Paradis et al. (2003) examined 7-year-old children with SLI who were exposed to two languages (French and English) since birth. They were assessed for aspects of grammar (object pronouns, verb forms) that are particularly difficult for children with language impairments. The findings were clear: children with language deficits raised in a bilingual environment had similar language development to those raised in a monolingual setting. In other words, the simultaneous acquisition of two languages did not make their language impairment significantly worse. Their difficulties turned out to be entirely comparable to those of monolingual children with SLI who spoke either one of the two languages. Thus, learning a second language does not seem to place an extra burden on children with SLI (Genesee, Paradis, & Crago, 2004). However, despite this generally reassuring picture, at least for children with SLI, a recent survey by Kay-Raining Bird, Lamond, and Holden (2012) highlighted both parental and professional concerns about children with ASD brought up in a bilingual environment. However, as the authors themselves stressed, the pros and cons of bilingualism in neurodevelopmental disorders is a neglected area of research, which clearly deserves more targeted measures in the future.

Compelling new evidence on TD individuals indicates that bilinguals outperform monolinguals on a range of executive function tasks of a non-linguistic nature throughout their lifespan (e.g., Bialystok, 2009; Bialystok, Craik, Klein, & Viswanathan, 2004; Carlson & Meltzoff, 2008; Costa, Hernandez, & Sebastián-Gallés, 2008), even when there is a very close match between the bilinguals and monolinguals in terms of cultural and developmental history (e.g.,Yang, Yang, & Lust, 2011). The advantage may be attributable to the additional control demands placed on bilinguals relative to monolingual speakers and, intriguingly, may even delay the onset of dementia and Alzheimer's disease (Craik, Bialystok, & Freedman, 2010). Our recent work extended previous studies by revealing a bilingual advantage over monolinguals in auditory attentional processing of sentence comprehension in the presence of language interference (Filippi, Leech, Thomas, Green, & Dick, 2012). Particularly interesting is the fact that this advantage is observed even in cases where a second language has been learned later in life.

Studying bilinguals is no easy task, and many variables must be considered *a priori*, such as age of acquisition, level of proficiency, and socio-economic status. Such studies of conditions underlying the simultaneous acquisition of more than one language are obviously even more difficult when participants stem from atypically developing populations. However, given the evidence that has hitherto accrued, it is clear that research on bilingualism may help understand crucial processes underlying the development of language and cognition and could be extended to individuals with neurodevelopmental disorders. Is the advantage observed for typically developing children in terms of executive function also beneficial for bilinguals with neurodevelopmental disorders? If it is true that bilingualism enhances executive function in childhood and adulthood and curtails cognitive decline in older adulthood, it might actually help children with neurodevelopmental disorders (e.g., ADHD) to improve their executive functioning (i.e., improve their attentional abilities). Indeed, one study showed this to be the case for children diagnosed with ADHD, whose level of second language proficiency turned out to be correlated with reduced ADHD symptoms (Toppelberg, Medrano, Morgens, & Nieto-Castañon, 2002). This important research could be extended to other neurodevelopmental disorders, comparing performance in executive function tasks (e.g., the Simon Task; Lu & Proctor, 1995) of atypically developing children growing in monolingual versus multilingual environments.

Concluding thoughts

It may seem a truism to state that development always needs to be studied within a developmental perspective! Yet some researchers study infants, children and young adults in a non-developmental way, focusing on a single age group in a single domain. Neuroconstructivism, by contrast, stresses the need to study *change over developmental time* and to focus on the interaction of different domains across time (Karmiloff-Smith, 1998, 2009, 2010). In this chapter, we have highlighted the importance of studying developmental disorders across time and domains, and how this sensitizes the researcher to subtle distinctions that can subsequently be sought also in typical development at the neural, cognitive, behavioural and environmental levels. When development goes awry, differences are sometimes exaggerated and become more obvious to the researcher than in the typical case. In sum, subtle changes over developmental time really matter.

A simple metaphor helps us to see what the future might hold. In former times, taking photographs was a rather complicated matter. The photographer used very heavy cameras and had to replace the film every time he/she took a new picture. Today, not only can we take high-quality photos, but we can do so with extremely rapid clicks, highlighting all the changes in a scene within fractions of a second. Likewise in experimental psychology. We have today the tools to study developmental change with the same levels of precision; we can focus on changes across developmental time in atypical and typical development *inter alia* by using neuroimaging techniques. But with every advance, there are also potential pitfalls. Scanning brains with magnetic imaging techniques or recording temporal brain activity with electrophysiological methods can increment our knowledge of both typical and atypical development only if the experiments are hypothesis-driven. Simply looking to see where a brain "lights up" at a given age tells us little. A focus on change in neural circuitry over developmental time, as well as on change at the levels of gene expression, cognition, behaviour and the environment, however complex such interactions may be, is the only way that the study of neurodevelopmental disorders can teach us something about typical development.

References

Alcock, K. J., Passingham, R. E., Watkins, K., & Vargha-Khadem, F. (2000). Pitch and timing abilities in inherited speech and language impairment. *Brain and Language, 75*, 34–46.

Annaz, D., Karmiloff-Smith, A., Johnson, M. H., & Thomas, M. S. C. (2009). A cross-syndrome study of the development of holistic face recognition in children with autism, Down syndrome and Williams syndrome. *Journal of Experimental Child Psychology*, *102*, 456–486.

Annaz, D., Karmiloff-Smith, A., & Thomas, M. S. C. (2008). The importance of tracing developmental trajectories for clinical child neuropsychology. In J. Reed & J. Warner Rogers (Eds.), *Child neuropsychology: Concepts, theory and practice*. Oxford, UK: Blackwell.

Baillargeon, J., Spelke, E. S., & Wasserman, S. (1985). Object permanence in five-month-old infants. *Cognition, 20*, 191–208.

Barkow, J. H., Cosmides, L., & Tooby, J. (Eds.). (1992). *The adapted mind: Evolutionary psychology and the generation of culture*. NewYork, NY: Oxford University Press.

Bates, E., & Roe, K. (2001). Language development in children with unilateral brain injury. In C. A. Nelson & M. Luciana (Eds.), *Handbook of developmental cognitive neuroscience* (pp. 281–307). Cambridge, MA: MIT Press.

Bellugi, U., Wang, P., & Jernigan, T. L. (1994). Williams syndrome: An unusual neuropsychological profile. In S. Broman & J. Grafman (Eds.), *Atypical cognitive deficits in developmental disorders: Implications for brain function* (pp. 23–56). Hillsdale, NJ: Erlbaum.

Bialystok, E. (2009). Bilingualism: The good, the bad, and the indifferent. *Bilingualism: Language and Cognition, 12*, 3–11.

Bialystok, E., Craik, F. I. M., Klein, R., & Viswanathan, M. (2004). Bilingualism, aging, and cognitive control: Evidence from the Simon task. *Psychology and Aging, 19*, 290–303.

Bishop, D. V. M., North, T., & Donlan, C. (1996). Nonword repetition as a behavioural marker for inherited language impairment: Evidence from a twin study. *Journal of Child Psychology and Psychiatry, 37*, 391–403.

Bolhuis, J. J., Zijlstra, G. G. O., den Boer-Visser, A. M., & van der Zee, E. A. (2000). Localized neuronal activation in the zebra finch brain is related to the strength of song learning. *Proceedings of the National Academy of Sciences, 97*, 2282–2285.

Botting, N. (2005). Non-verbal cognitive development and language impairment. *Journal of Child Psychology and Psychiatry, 46*, 317–326.

Cardoso-Martins, C., & Mervis, C. B. (1990). Mothers' use of substantive deixis and nouns with their children with Down syndrome: Some discrepant findings. *American Journal on Mental Retardation, 94*, 633–637.

Cardoso-Martins, C., Mervis, C. B., & Mervis, C. A. (1985). Early vocabulary acquisition by children with Down syndrome. *American Journal of Mental Deficiency, 90*, 177–184.

Carlson, S. M., & Meltzoff, A. N. (2008). Bilingual experience and executive functioning in young children. *Developmental Science, 11*, 282–298.

Chiappe, D., & MacDonald, K. (2005). The evolution of domain-general mechanisms in intelligence and learning. *The Journal of General Psychology, 132*, 5–40.

Choudhury, N., & Benasich, A. A. (2011). Maturation of auditory evoked potentials from 6 to 48 months: Prediction to 3 and 4 year language and cognitive abilities. *Clinical Neurophysiology, 122*, 320–338.

Clahsen, H., & Temple, C. (2003). Words and rules in children with Williams syndrome. In Y. Levy & J. Schaeffer (Eds.), *Towards a definition of Specific Language Impairment in children* (pp. 323–359). Dordrecht, The Netherlands: Kluwer.

Conti-Ramsden, G. (2003). Processing and linguistic markers in young children with specific language impairment (SLI). *Journal of Speech, Language, and Hearing Research, 46*, 1029–1037.

Costa, A., Hernandez, M., & Sebastián-Gallés, N. (2008). Bilingualism aids conflict resolution: Evidence from the ANT task. *Cognition, 106*, 59–86.

Craik, F. I. M., Bialystok, E., & Freedman, M. (2010). Delaying the onset of Alzheimer's disease: Bilingualism as a form of cognitive reserve. *Neurology, 75*, 1726–1729.

de Haan, M., Humphreys, K., & Johnson, M. H. (2002). Developing a brain specialized for face perception: A converging methods approach. *Developmental Psychobiology, 40*, 200–212.

Duchaine, B., Cosmides, L., & Tooby, J. (2001). Evolutionary psychology and the brain. *Current Opinion in Neurobiology, 11*, 225–230.

Elman, J. L., Bates, E., Johnson, M. H., Karmiloff-Smith, A., Parisi, D., & Plunkett, K. (1996). *Rethinking innateness: A connectionist perspective on development.* Cambridge, MA: MIT Press.

Ernard, W., Przeworksi, M., Fisher, S. E., Lai, C. S., Wiebe, V., Kitano, T., Monaco, A.P., & Paabo, S. (2002). Molecular evolution of FOXP2, a gene involved in speech and language. *Nature, 418*, 869–872.

European Commission. (2006). *Europeans and their languages* [Special Survey No. 243]. Eurobarometer.

Fernald, A., Pinto, J. P., Swingley, D., Weinberg, A., & McRoberts, G. W. (1998). Rapid gains in speed of verbal processing by infants in the 2nd year. *Psychological Science, 9*, 228–231.

Filippi, R., Leech, R., Thomas, M. S. C., Green, D. W., & Dick, F. (2012). A bilingual advantage in controlling language interference during sentence comprehension. *Bilingualism: Language & Cognition.* Advance online publication.

Fisher, S. E., Vargha-Khadem, F., Watkins, K. E., Monaco, A. P., & Pembrey, M. E. (1998). Localisation of a gene implicated in a severe speech and language disorder. *Nature Genetics, 18*, 168–170.

Fonteneau, E., & van der Lely, H. K. J. (2008). Electrical brain responses in language-impaired children reveal grammar-specific deficits. *Public Library of Science ONE 3(3)*, e1832.do.

Gathercole, S. E., & Baddeley, A. D. (1990). Phonological memory deficits in language disordered children: Is there a causal connection. *Journal of Memory and Language, 29*, 336–360.

Genesee, F., Paradis, J., & Crago, M. B. (2004). *Dual language development and disorders: A handbook on bilingualism and second language learning.* Baltimore, MD: Brookes Publishing Company.

Golarai, G., Hong, S., Haas, B., Galaburda, A., Mills, D.L., Bellugi, U., . . . Reiss, A. (2010). The fusiform face area is enlarged in Williams Syndrome. *Journal of Neuroscience, 30*, 6700–6712.

Gopnik, M., & Crago, M. (1991). Familial aggregation of a developmental language disorder. *Cognition, 39*, 1–50.

Grice, S. J., de Haan, M., Halit, H., Johnson, M. H., Csibra, G., Grant, J., & Karmiloff-Smith, A. (2003). ERP abnormalities of visual perception in Williams syndrome. *Neuro Report, 14,*1773–1777.

Grosjean, F. (2010). *Bilingual: Life and reality.* Cambridge, MA: Harvard University Press.

Hakuta, K., & Diaz, R. M. (1985). The relationship between degree of bilingualism and cognitive ability: A critical discussion and some new longitudinal data. In K. E. Nelson (Ed.), *Children's language* (Vol. 5, pp. 319–344). Hillsdale, NJ: Lawrence Erlbaum Associates.

Huttenlocher, P. R., & de Courten, C. (1987). The development of synapses in striate cortex of man. *Human Neurobiology, 6*, 1–9.

Hyde, D.C., & Spelke, E. S. (2011). Neural signatures of number processing in human infants: Evidence for two core systems underlying numerical cognition. *Developmental Science, 14*, 360–371.

Jusczyk, P. W., Pisoni, D. B., Reed, M. A., Fernald, A., & Myers, M. (1983). Infants' discrimination of the duration of a rapid spectrum change in nonspeech signals. *Science, 222*, 175–177.

Karmiloff-Smith, A. (1992). *Beyond modularity: A developmental approach to cognitive science.* Cambridge, MA: MIT Press.

Karmiloff-Smith, A. (1998). Development itself is the key to understanding developmental disorders. *Trends in Cognitive Sciences, 2*, 389–398.

Karmiloff-Smith, A. (2009). Nativism versus neuroconstructivism: Rethinking the study of developmental disorders. *Developmental Psychology, 45*, 56–63.

Karmiloff-Smith, A. (2010). Neuroimaging of the developing brain: Taking "developing" seriously. *Human Brain Mapping, 31*, 934–941.

Karmiloff-Smith, A. (2012). Static snapshots versus dynamic approaches to genes, brain, cognition and behaviour in neurodevelopmental disabilities. *International Review of Research in Developmental Disabilities, 40*, 1–15.

Karmiloff-Smith, A., Scerif, G., & Ansari, D. (2003). Double dissociations in developmental disorders? Theoretically misconceived, empirically dubious. *Cortex, 39*, 161–163.

Karmiloff-Smith, A., Thomas, M. S. C., Annaz, D., Humphreys, K., Ewing, S., Brace, . . . Campbell, R. (2004). Exploring the Williams Syndrome face processing debate: The importance of building developmental trajectories. *Journal of Child Psychology and Psychiatry, 45,*1258 –1274.

Kay-Raining Bird, E., Lamond E., & Holden, J. (2012). Survey of bilingualism in autism spectrum disorders. *International Journal of Language & Communication Disorders, 47*, 52–64.

Lai, C. S. L., Fisher, S. E., Hurst, J. A., Vargha-Khadem, F., & Monaco, A. P. (2001). A novel forkhead-domain gene is mutated in a severe speech and language disorder. *Nature, 413*, 465–466.

Lai, C. S. L., Gerrelli, D., Monaco, A. P., Fisher, S. E., & Copp, A. J. (2003). FOXP2 expression during brain development coincides with adult sites of pathology in a severe speech and language disorder. *Brain, 126*, 2455–2462.

Leonard, L. B., McGregor, K. K., & Allen, G. D. (1992). Grammatical morphology and speech perception in children with specific language impairment. *Journal of Speech and Hearing Research, 35*, 1076–1085.

Leslie, A. M. (1992). Pretence, autism, and the theory-of-mind-module. *Current Directions in Psychological Science, 1*, 18–21.

Lettori, D., Battaglia, D., Sacco, A., Veredice, C., Chieffo, D., Massimi, L., . . . Guzzetta, F. (2008). Early hemispherectomy in catastrophic epilepsy: A neuro-cognitive and epileptic long-term follow-up. *European Journal of Epilepsy, 17*, 49–63.

Liégeois, F., Baldeweg, T., Connelly, A., Gadian, D. G., Mishkin, M., & Vargha-Khadem, F. (2003). Language fMRI abnormalities associated with FOXP2 gene mutation. *Nature Neuroscience, 6*, 1230–1237.

Liégeois, F., Connelly, A., Cross, J. H., Boyd, S. G., Gadian, D. G., Vargha-Khadem, F., & Baldeweg, T. (2004). Language reorganization in children with early-onset lesions of the left hemisphere: an fMRI study. *Brain, 127*, 1229–1236.

Lu, C. H., & Proctor, R. W. (1995). The influence of irrelevant location information on performance: A review of the Simon and spatial Stroop effects. *Psychonomic Bulletin and Review, 2*, 174–207.

Mareschal, D., Johnson, M. H., Sirois, S., Spratling, M. W., Thomas, M. S. C., & Westermann, G. (2007). *Neuroconstructivism: Vol. I. How the brain constructs cognition.* Oxford, UK: Oxford University Press.

Mareschal, D., Sirois, S., Westermann, G., & Johnson, M. (Eds.). (2007). *Neuroconstructivism: Vol. II. Perspectives and prospects.* Oxford, UK: Oxford University Press.

Martinez, E. (2002, August 15). The language gene, finally? Maybe not. (Op Ed). Retrieved from http://www.kuro5hin.org/story/2002/8/15/2731/86197.

Mills, D. L., Alvarez, T. D., St. George, M., Appelbaum, L. G., Bellugi, U., & Neville, H. (2000). Electrophysiological studies of face processing in Williams syndrome. *Journal of Cognitive Neuroscience, 12*, 47–64.

Neville, H., & Bavelier, D. (2002). Human brain plasticity: Evidence from sensory deprivation and altered language experience. *Progress in Brain Research, 138,* 177–188.

Neville, H. J., Mills, D. L., & Bellugi, U. (1994). Effects of altered auditory sensitivity and age of language acquisition on the development of language-relevant neural systems: Preliminary studies of Williams syndrome. In S. Broman & J. Grafman (Eds.), *Atypical cognitive deficits in developmental disorders: Implications for brain function* (pp. 67–83). Hillsdale, NJ: Erlbaum.

O'Reilly, R. C., & McClelland, J. L. (1992). *The self-organization of spatially invariant representations* (Tech. Rep. No. PDP.CNS.92.5). Pittsburgh, PA: Carnegie Mellon University.

Paradis, J., Crago, M., Genesee, F., & Rice, M. (2003). Bilingual children with specific language impairment: How do they compare with their monolingual peers? *Journal of Speech, Language, and Hearing Research, 46*, 1–15.

Paterson, S. J., Brown, J. H., Gsödl, M. K., Johnson, M. H., & Karmiloff-Smith, A. (1999). Cognitive modularity and genetic disorders. *Science, 286*, 2355–2358.

Paterson, S.J., Girelli, L., Butterworth, B., & Karmiloff-Smith, A. (2006). Are numerical impairments syndrome specific? Evidence from Williams syndrome and Down's Syndrome. *Journal of Child Psychology and Psychiatry, 47*, 190–204.

Peal, E., & Lambert, M. (1962). The relation of bilingualism to intelligence. *Psychological Monographs, 76*, 1–23.

Penner, E. P., & Klahr, D. (1996). The interaction of domain-specific knowledge and domain-general discovery strategies: A study with sinking objects. *Child Development, 67*, 2709–2727.

Piaget, J. (1952). *The origins of intelligence in children.* New York, NY: W. W. Norton & Co.

Saer, D. J. (1922). An inquiry into the effect of bilingualism upon the intelligence of young children. *Journal of Experimental Pedagogy, 6*, 232–240, 266–274.

Saer, D. J. (1923). The effect of bilingualism on intelligence. *British Journal of Psychology, 14*, 25–38.

Salameh, E. K., Håkansson, G., & Nettelbladt, U. (2004). Developmental perspectives on bilingual Swedish-Arabic children with and without language impairment: A longitudinal study. *International Journal of Language and Communication Disorders, 39*, 65–91.

Scerif, G., Cornish, K., Wilding, J., Driver, J., & Karmiloff-Smith, A. (2004). Visual selective attention in typically developing toddlers and toddlers with fragile X and Williams syndrome. *Developmental Science, 7,* 116–130.

Schlottman, A., & Ray, E. (2010). Goal attribution to schematic animals: Do 6-month-olds perceive biological motion as animate? *Developmental Science, 13,* 1–10.

Spearman, C. (1927). *The abilities of man.* New York, NY: Macmillan.

Spiteri, E., Konopka, G., Coppola, G., Bomar, J., Oldham, M., Ou, J., . . . Geschwind, D. H. (2007). Identification of the transcriptional targets of FOXP2, a gene linked to speech and language, in developing human brain. *American Journal of Human Genetics, 81,* 1144–1157.

Stiles, J., Moses, P., Roe, K., Akshoomoff, N. A., Trauner, D., Hesselink, J., . . . Buxton, R.B. (2003). Alternative brain organization after prenatal cerebral injury: Convergent fMRI and cognitive data. *Journal of the International Neuropsychological Society, 9,* 604–622.

Stiles, J., & Thal, D. (1993). Linguistic and spatial cognitive development following early focal brain injury: Patterns of deficit and recovery. In M. H. Johnson (Ed.), *Brain development and cognition: A reader* (pp. 643–664). Malden, MA: Blackwell Publishing.

Szyf, M., McGowan, P., & Meaney, M. J. (2008). The social environment and the epigenome. *Environmental and Molecular Mutagenesis, 49,* 46–60.

Tallal, P. (2000). The science of literacy: From the laboratory to the classroom. *Proceedings of the National Academy of Sciences, 97,* 2402–2404.

Tanaka, J. W., & Farah, M. J. (1993). Parts and wholes in face recognition. *Quarterly Journal of Experimental Psychology, 46A,* 225–245.

Temple, C. M. (2006). Developmental and acquired dyslexias. *Cortex, 42,* 898–910.

Thal, D. J., Marchman, V., Stiles, J., Aram, D., Trauner, D., Nass, R., & Bates, E. (1991). Early lexical development in children with focal brain injury. *Brain and Language, 40,* 491–527.

Thomas, M. S. C., Annaz, D., Ansari, D., Scrif, G., Jarrold, C., & Karmiloff-Smith, A. (2009). Using developmental trajectories to understand developmental disorders. *Journal of Speech, Language, and Hearing Research, 52,* 336–358.

Thomas, M. S. C., Grant, J., Barham, Z., Gsödl, M., Laing, E., Lakusta, L., . . . Karmiloff-Smith, A. (2001). Past tense formation in Williams syndrome. *Language and Cognitive Processes, 16,* 143–176.

Toppelberg, C. O., Medrano, L., Morgens, L. P., & Nieto-Castañon, A. (2002). Bilingual children referred for psychiatric services: Associations of language disorders, language skills, and psychopathology. *Journal of the American Academy of Child and Adolescent Psychiatry, 41,* 712–722.

Udwin, O., & Yule, W. (1991). A cognitive and behavioural phenotype in Williams syndrome. *Journal of Clinical Experimental Neuropsychology, 13,* 232–244.

Vernes, S. C., Spiteri, E., Nicod, J., Groszer, M., Taylor, J. M., Davies, K. E., . . . Fisher, S. E. (2007). High-throughput analysis of promoter occupancy reveals direct neural targets of FOXP2, a gene mutated in speech and language disorders. *American Journal of Human Genetics, 81,* 1232–1250.

Yang, S., Yang, H., & Lust, B. (2011). Early childhood bilingualism leads to advances in executive attention: Dissociating culture and language. *Bilingualism: Language and Cognition, 14,* 412–422.

Glossary and abbreviations

Angelman syndrome   A chromosomal disorder that affects about 1 in 25,000 live births. Diagnosis is usually made between 3 and 7 years of age, and characteristics include developmental delay, lack of speech, seizures, walking and balance disorders, hand flapping movements and frequent laughter and smiling. The majority of cases are caused by a small deletion of part of the maternally-inherited copy of chromosome 15. Interestingly, this is a similar genetic fault to that found in another chromosomal condition, Prader-Willi syndrome, but in that syndrome the affected copy of chromosome 15 is inherited from the father.

Asperger's disorder (also known as **Asperger's syndrome**)   A disorder on the autism spectrum, characterised by qualitative impairment in social interaction, by stereotyped and restricted patterns of behaviour, activities and interests, but by no clinically significant delay in cognitive development or general delay in language.

Attention deficit and hyperactivity disorder (frequently abbreviated to **ADHD**)   The most commonly studied and diagnosed psychiatric disorder in children, primarily characterised by inattention, hyperactivity, and impulsivity. Common symptoms include a short attention span, restlessness, being easily distracted and constant fidgeting.

Autistic disorder (also known as **autism**)   A disorder characterised by a triad of symptoms: impairments in social interaction, impairments in communication, and restricted interests and repetitive behaviour. These signs all begin before three years of age.

Autism spectrum disorder (frequently abbreviated to **ASD**)   Autism spectrum disorders or pervasive developmental disorders (PDD) are a spectrum of psychological conditions that are characterised by abnormalities of social interaction, verbal and nonverbal communication, and by restricted and repetitive interests and behaviour. Currently five disorders fall on the autism spectrum: (1) Autistic disorder, (2) Asperger's disorder, (3) Rett's disorder, (4) Childhood disintegrative disorder, and (5) Pervasive developmental disorder–not otherwise specified, each of which has its own entry in this glossary.

Central auditory processing disorder (frequently abbreviated to **CAPD**, or just **APD**)   An umbrella term for a variety of disorders that affect the way the brain processes auditory information. Individuals with CAPD usually have normal peripheral hearing ability, but have problems processing the information they hear, which leads to difficulties in recognising and interpreting speech sounds. Consequently they may have trouble paying attention to and remembering information presented orally, have problems carrying out multistep directions and need more time to process verbal information.

Cerebral palsy   A group of non-progressive motor conditions, caused by damage to the motor control centres of the developing brain during pregnancy or childbirth, and with an incidence of around 1 per 400 births. Resulting limits in movement and posture cause activity limitation and are often accompanied by disturbances of sensation, depth perception and other sight-based perceptual problems, impaired communication ability, and sometimes cognitive impairments.

Childhood disintegrative disorder   A rare condition on the autism spectrum that is characterised by late onset (>3 years of age) of developmental delays in language, social function and motor skills. Its cause is as yet unknown. The characteristics that distinguish it from Autistic disorder are the age of onset and evidence of normal development prior to the presence of symptomatology.

Chorea   An abnormal involuntary movement disorder, characterised by brief, quasi-purposeful, irregular contractions that are not repetitive or rhythmic, but appear to flow from one muscle to the next. Chorea is a primary feature of Huntington's disease, a progressive neurological disorder.

Developmental coordination disorder (also known as **Dyspraxia**)   A motor learning difficulty that can affect the coordination and performance of purposeful movements and gestures.

DiGeorge syndrome   See Velocardiofacial syndrome.

Down syndrome (frequently abbreviated to **DS**)   A chromosomal condition characterised by the presence of an extra copy of genetic material on chromosome 21, either in whole (trisomy 21) or part (such as due to translocations). Its incidence is estimated at 1 per 733 births. It is associated with some impairment of cognitive ability and physical growth, and a particular set of facial characteristics.

Dyscalculia   A specific learning disability involving difficulties in simple mathematics, including understanding numbers, learning how to manipulate numbers, and learning mathematical facts.

Dyslexia   A specific learning disability that impairs fluency and/or accuracy in reading and spelling.

Dyspraxia   See Developmental coordination disorder.

Fragile X syndrome (frequently abbreviated to **FXS**)   A genetic syndrome that is the most common inherited cause of intellectual disability and the most common single-gene cause of autism. It results in a spectrum of characteristic physical and intellectual limitations and emotional and behavioural features which range from mild to severe. The syndrome is associated with the expansion of a single CGG sequence on the X chromosome, and results in a failure to express the protein coded by the *FMR1* gene, which is required for normal neural development.

Gilles de la Tourette syndrome (also known as **Tourette syndrome**)   A neuropsychiatric disorder with onset in childhood, characterised by multiple physical tics and at least one vocal tic; these tics characteristically wax and wane. Tourette's syndrome is defined as part of a spectrum of tic disorders, which includes transient and chronic tics.

Intellectual disability   A broad concept encompassing various intellectual deficits, including mental retardation, deficits too mild to properly qualify as mental retardation, various specific conditions such as dyslexia, and problems acquired later in life through acquired brain injuries or neurodegenerative diseases such as dementia. The term is increasingly being used as a synonym for mental retardation.

Neurofibromatosis type 1   A tumour disorder that is caused by the malfunction of a gene on chromosome 17 that is responsible for controlling cell division. The incidence is about 1 in 3,500 live births, and the most common complications are a learning disability (in approximately 80 percent of cases), speech and language delays (in approximately 70 percent of cases), and ADHD (in approximately 40 percent of cases).

Pervasive developmental disorder–not otherwise specified (frequently abbreviated to **PDD-NOS**)   PDD-NOS is one of the five autism spectrum disorders, and is often referred to as "atypical autism" because it is a diagnosis given to individuals who do not fully meet the criteria for the other disorders on the autism spectrum.

Phenylketonuria   A metabolic genetic disorder characterised by a mutation in the gene for the liver enzyme phenylalanine hydroxylase. If left untreated, the condition can cause problems with brain development, leading to progressive mental retardation, brain damage and seizures.

Prader-Willi syndrome   A rare genetic disorder in which up to seven genes on chromosome 15 are deleted or unexpressed on the paternal chromosome. The incidence is between 1 per 10,000 and 1 per 25,000 births. Affected individuals are at risk of learning and attention difficulties.

Rett's disorder (also known as **Rett's syndrome**)   A disorder on the autism spectrum caused by mutations in the gene *MECP2* located on the X chromosome. It occurs worldwide in 1 of every 10,000 to 23,000 female births (male foetuses with the disorder rarely survive to term). The onset and course are distinctive. The child develops normally during the first five months of life, but after the fifth month head growth slows down and she loses purposeful hand movements. After 30 months, she frequently develops repetitive hand-washing or hand-wringing gestures. Rett's disorder is also associated with severe or profound intellectual disability and communication impairment.

Selective mutism   An anxiety disorder in which an individual who is normally capable of speech is unable to speak in certain situations or to particular people.

Specific language impairment (frequently abbreviated to **SLI**)   SLI is diagnosed when a child's language does not develop normally and the difficulties cannot be accounted for by generally slow development, physical abnormality of the speech apparatus, autistic disorder, acquired brain damage or hearing loss.

Speech sound disorder   Disorders of speech in which some speech sounds are either not produced, not produced correctly, or are not used correctly. Within this group, articulation disorders are caused by a difficulty learning to physically produce the intended sounds, whereas phonological disorders are caused by a difficulty learning the sound system of the language, thereby failing to recognise which sounds are involved in contrasting meaning.

Stuttering   A speech disorder in which the flow of speech is disrupted by involuntary repetitions and prolongations of sounds, syllables, words or phrases, and involuntary silent pauses or blocks in which the stutterer is unable to produce sounds.

Tourette syndrome   See Gilles de la Tourette syndrome.

Tuberous sclerosis   A rare genetic disease caused by a mutation of genes that act as tumour growth suppressors. Non-malignant tumours grow in the brain and on other vital organs such as the kidneys, heart, skin and lungs. Symptoms may include seizures, developmental delay, behavioural problems, skin abnormalities, and lung and kidney disease. Between 25 percent and 61 percent of affected individuals meet the diagnostic criteria for autism. Other conditions, such as ADHD, can also occur.

Turner syndrome   A chromosomal abnormality occurring in 1 in every 2,000 to 5,000 of phenotypic females, in which one of the X chromosomes is absent in part or in its entirety. In some cases, the chromosome is missing in some cells but not others ("Turner mosaicism"). A specific pattern of cognitive deficits is often observed, with particular difficulties in visuospatial, mathematical, and memory areas.

Velocardiofacial syndrome (also known as **DiGeorge syndrome**)   A syndrome caused by the deletion of a small piece of chromosome 22, at a location designated q11.2 (hence a third name, **22q11 deletion syndrome**). The prevalence is estimated at 1 per 2,000 to 4,000 live births. The features of this syndrome vary widely, and may include congenital heart disease, defects in the palate, intellectual disabilities, mild differences in facial features, and recurrent infections. Autoimmune disorders and psychiatric illnesses are common late-occurring features.

Verbal dyspraxia   A difficulty in making and co-ordinating the precise movements required for the production of clear speech, but with no evidence of damage to nerves or muscles. Affected individuals have difficulty producing individual speech sounds and sequencing sounds together in words, and as a result their speech is often unintelligible even to family members.

Williams syndrome (frequently abbreviated to **WS**)   A rare genetic disorder, caused by a deletion of about 26 genes from the long arm of chromosome 7, and with an estimated prevalence of 1 per 7,500 to 1 per 20,000 births. It is characterised by hypercalcaemia of infants, heart defects, characteristic facial features, a sociable personality, and a relatively high verbal aptitude, but mild to moderate intellectual disability.

Index

DATE DUE	RETURNED
OCT 2 8 2015	OCT 2 0 2015
OCT 0 3 2016	
OCT 0 3 2016	OCT 0 4 2016